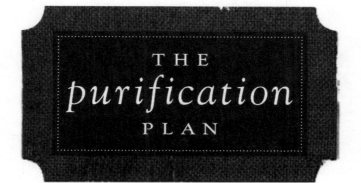

THE
purification
PLAN

RODALE

LIVE YOUR WHOLE LIFE™

Every day our brands connect with and inspire millions of people to live a life of the mind, body, spirit — a whole life.

pure vitality

pure resilience

pure health

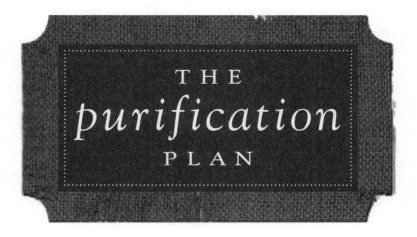

THE
purification
PLAN

FEATURING AN EXCLUSIVE 7-DAY DETOX PROGRAM

BY PETER BENNETT, N.D.,

CO-AUTHOR OF *7-Day Detox Miracle*

RODALE

© 2005 by Rodale Inc.
Photographs © 2005 by Rodale Inc.

First published 2005
First published in paperback 2006

Printed in the United States of America
Rodale Inc. makes every effort to use acid-free ∞, recycled paper ♺.

The recipes Barley with Ginger and Broccoli, page 54, and Fenugreek Kichari, page 55, are courtesy of the Himalayan International Institute of Yoga Science and Philosophy of the U.S.A.

Book design by Christina Gaugler
Photographs by Mitch Mandel

ISBN-13 978–1–59486–130–7 hardcover
ISBN-10 1–59486–130–7 hardcover
ISBN-13 978–1–59486–131–4 paperback
ISBN-10 1–59486–131–5 paperback

Distributed to the trade by Holtzbrinck Publishers

4 6 8 10 9 7 5   hardcover
2 4 6 8 10 9 7 5 3 1 paperback

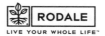

We inspire and enable people to improve their lives and the world around them

For more of our products visit **rodalestore.com** or call 800-848-4735

CONTENTS

The Role of Purification in a Healthy Lifestyle

As a naturopathic physician, I've been treating patients with detoxification strategies for 20 years. I use purification and detoxification methods because they bring results. Commonly I will see immediate results in healthy people who just want more energy, want to lose some weight, or want to renew their minds and spirits.

Some are like Nellie, a 39-year-old accountant at a bank, who came to see me because she was slowly starting to gain weight, despite having a regular exercise plan. She also noticed that she was losing her focus at work and was needing more sleep, even though her daily routine had not changed. Yet in 1 week, with the help of a simple fast with a modified diet and hydrotherapy, she enjoyed immediate results. She lost 7 pounds and was once again feeling refreshed after her normal 7 hours of sleep. Most important, her mind was more clear and focused at work.

I have also seen severely ill patients achieve dramatic results with an incurable diagnosis from their conventional physician. Using purification strategies, they were able to reverse the course of chronic degenerative disease and beat the odds of their prognosis. I have seen gastrointestinal, rheumatological, immune, and neurological diseases respond to the strategies described in this book. One patient, Alan, came in with chronic fatigue ever since being diagnosed with mononucleosis in his early twenties. Fifteen years later he still struggled with low energy. After using a simple 1-week detox program, he found dramatic improvements in his energy level. Following the detoxification, he adopted a new healing diet and has remained in good health ever since.

Suffice it to say, I am firmly convinced that detoxification and purification are important strategies we should all use to boost our health and promote healing. Purification and medical detoxification are so effective because they stimulate the body's own healing mechanisms and enhance the body's ability to filter and clean the blood. By resting the immune and detoxification organs of the digestive tract and promoting elimination, we can recharge our body's ability to heal itself.

To accomplish this, doctors who use detoxification medicine focus on healing the liver. Many chronic health problems arise from "sluggish" liver function. A sluggish liver causes toxins to accumulate in the bloodstream. If the hormone estrogen, for example, is not dismantled during detoxification, the buildup can reach potentially harmful levels and trigger premenstrual tension. As we age, our body's natural detoxification processes slow. What's more, use of certain medications; exposure to cadmium,

lead, and mercury; and consumption of large amounts of sugar and hydrogenated fats all hinder detoxification pathways. These kinds of often unavoidable external factors make it even more important that we assist our bodies in removing poisons through regular and well-targeted purification strategies like those described in this book.

Of course, my generation of naturopathic doctors did not discover all of this knowledge or invent all of these techniques. Shamans, yogis, medicine men, and healers have used various methods of purification to benefit themselves and their communities since the beginning of time. There is a rich heritage in the history of medicine for the use of detoxification medicine. Going back to Hippocrates, fasting, diet therapy, and hydrotherapy have been used with great effect to successfully treat a wide range of health disorders. More recently, over the last 100 years, holistic physicians have relied on the traditional methods of detoxification therapy to assist their patients in achieving optimum health. Even with the recent advancements in biochemistry, physiology, and pharmacology, the ancient wisdom of detoxification therapy in maintaining health and curing a wide range of disease processes remains unequaled.

Yet even now, despite valid clinical results in the United States, Canada, and across the world, detoxification techniques are little understood and still underprescribed in the medical treatment of chronic conditions like asthma, heart disease, migraines, and fatigue that defy treatment by other means.

That's why the editors of Rodale Health Books have done such a great service to readers in bringing together this vast assortment of purification and detoxification techniques in *The Purification Plan.* With the practical details provided in this book, you can gain immense benefits from adopting purification methods in your own self care. Through a detoxifying diet you can boost your immunity to disease. With the use of safe and effective herbs you can improve digestion and fight infection. Healing exercises and meditation can help to stimulate your circulatory and nervous systems to keep stress from poisoning your body. You'll also be introduced to the world of more intensive, professional detoxification methods like panchakarma and lymphatic drainage massage to help you decide whether they offer the healing you seek.

In addition to describing the immediate health benefits that these purification methods can bring you, this book offers the hope that you will be able to protect yourself and your family from the scourge of everyday toxins in your life. The threats in your life may be chemicals in your water, airborne toxins in your home or workplace, or the aftermath of a diet that is too heavy in processed foods and sugars. In any case, you will find safe, simple, yet powerful ways to reverse the damage and smart advice on reducing or preventing further exposure.

Armed with the tools provided in this book, you can now be ahead of the medical health-care delivery system. In some ways, modern medicine is like the Titanic. You'll remember that even though the crew could see the iceberg ahead, they could not turn the ship fast enough to protect its passengers. Modern medicine knows about the negative impact of pollution, toxins, dysbiosis, heavy metals, and stress hormones, but it cannot provide a drug or surgical therapy to deal with such a complex mess of problems facing society.

But now, in the pages of *The Purification Plan,* you have at your disposal some of the most effective healing methods ever developed. When you use these purification strategies in your life, every day will be a little farther down the road to happiness and healing.

Peter W. Bennett, N.D.
Coauthor, 7-Day Detox Miracle

How to Use This Book

In *The Purification Plan: Clear Your Body of the Toxins That Contribute to Weight Gain, Fatigue, and Chronic Illness,* you will find the largest and most diverse collection of detoxification tips ever collected in one volume. You are about to discover techniques that range from simple recipes and exercise advice to herbal remedies to professional treatments developed from ancient healing practices—all brought together in one place and explained for maximum safety and effectiveness.

The first section of the book (chapters 1 through 10) will help you understand why detoxification is so critical to restoring and maintaining your health and vitality. You will learn the practical strategies that you can use in your path to better health. For each of the primary means of detoxification, you will find in-depth discussions of how to employ what are familiar aspects of healthy living put to use in remarkable new ways. The result will be to purify your body and build immunity to toxins you encounter at home, at work, and in the environment. With these secrets, you can unlock the full promise of better health and healing by applying the purifying power of food, herbs, exercise, fasting and cleansing, emotional healing, home spa treatments, and professional therapies.

In the second section of the book, you'll discover the three-part strategy that makes it so easy to make detoxification a part of your healthy lifestyle. The strategy starts with a general-purpose 7-day plan that is a great place for virtually everyone to begin on the path of purification (chapter 11). You'll then find targeted plans and tips for specific conditions of particular concern for you (chapters 12 and 13). You may be surprised to find that detoxification techniques can help with conditions as serious as preventing cancer and reversing heart disease, as common as headaches and weight gain, and as annoying as bad breath and ear infections. In all, more than 50 specific health problems are addressed. The plan concludes with hints and tips for "staying clean." Consider chapter 14 as a simplified road map of safe and easy, yet powerful ways you can avoid toxic exposure and keep your newly purified body in a fully functioning state of health.

Your strategy for putting *The Purification Plan* into action can be as simple as 1-2-3.

1. Try the 7-Day Purification Plan to begin to reverse the toxic buildup in your body.

2. Choose a targeted Purification Plan for a condition that concerns you, or build on the 7-Day Plan using your preferred methods of general detoxification such as healing foods, herbs, fasting, cleansing, exercise, spa treatments, or professional techniques.

3. Reduce your exposure to more toxins by following the advice in chapter 14, "Staying Clean: 45 Steps to Toxin-Free Living."

At Rodale Health Books, it is our hope that you find this book as useful and fascinating as we have in creating it. It's been a privilege for us to work alongside some of the world's leading practitioners of detoxification in the research, writing, and editing of *The Purification Plan*. Particular thanks go to Peter Bennett, N.D., who provided guidance and the foreword to the book.

May the healing power of purification bring you the health and peace you seek.

THE ESSENTIALS OF PURIFICATION:
Your Path to Better Health

THERE ARE MANY PATHS TO HEALING. But all paths share one common goal: to restore your body's natural ability to heal itself.

In this section, you'll discover the remarkable capacity that detoxification has to provide the restorative balance that your body craves. What's more, you'll learn the secrets of the safest, most effective purification methods you can use in your own home. From familiar remedies like healing foods, herbs, and exercise to fasting and relaxing therapeutic spa treatments, you'll be able to find the paths to healing that best suit your health needs and lifestyle.

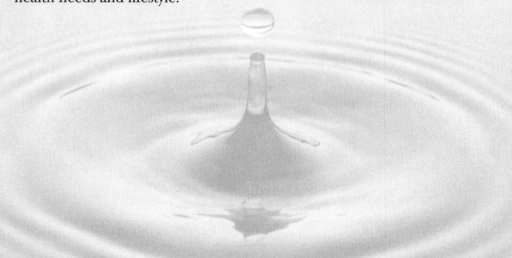

Chapter 1

Healing with Purification: When and Why Your Body Needs a Little Help

YOUR BODY CLEANS ITSELF ALL THE TIME. Constantly. Day and night, no matter what else you're doing, the biological machinery of your body goes about its household chores: sweeping, cleaning, scrubbing your cells, hauling away the trash left over from last evening's meal, venting noxious gases, sweating out toxins from every pore, collecting wastewater, and blocking the harmful actions of invading toxic microbes. Your body functions like a self-cleaning machine, and it's all the more magnificent because it all happens automatically. If you had to consciously pay attention to all the work that goes on all the time, you'd never get anything else done.

All of this amazing biomachinery was set on automatic when you were still in your mother's womb. And it's been doing its self-cleaning thing 24/7 ever since. But does that mean you can just ignore it and go about your business?

Yes and no. Your liver, for example, is going to clean your blood of toxins whether you tell it to or not. But if you eat a fatty meal, belt down a couple of martinis, and then take a hefty dose of acetaminophen to banish a headache, you overload your liver's ability to detoxify your body, and you run the risk of compromising the long-suffering organ that helps keep you from getting cancer. So it's a good idea to do what you can to avoid exposure to toxins whenever you can. It's also a good idea to increase your body's ability to detoxify itself in every way that you can. These two goals have become increasingly important in today's world, and both strategies are what this book is all about.

But we're getting ahead of ourselves. Before we delve into the details of the

The Body's Waste-Treatment Plant

ACCORDING TO ALTERNATIVE PRACTITIONERS, five specific organs play critical roles in helping to escort toxins from your body. Collectively, they're known as the organs of elimination. Here's a miniprofile of each.

The liver. The size of a football, this is your body's purification powerhouse. Your liver filters toxins from your blood, removing bacteria, viruses, and environmental pollutants such as pesticides, drugs, and household and industrial chemicals.

The lungs. Your lungs take in oxygen, which cells need to live and carry out their normal functions, and get rid of volatile gases and carbon dioxide, a waste product of your body's cells. Your lungs also produce mucus, which traps toxins and impurities so that they can be coughed out.

The kidneys. These two organs, each about the size of a fist, are located in the small of your back. Every day, they process about 200 quarts of blood to sift out about 2 quarts of waste products and extra water, which come from the normal breakdown of active tissues and from food. The waste and extra water become urine.

The skin. Sweat glands cover every inch of your skin. These glands eliminate waste—primarily urea and ammonia—in the form of perspiration.

The intestines. Your small intestine absorbs nutrients from the food you eat. The remains enter your large intestine, called the colon, which absorbs needed water and minerals and transports waste to the rectum for elimination.

proven ways to defend yourself from the modern toxic onslaught, we need to take a brief look at how the self-cleaning actions of your body's systems work. Then we'll look at the toxic challenges that your body comes up against on a daily basis.

MOTHER NATURE'S CLEANING MACHINE

Every single cell of your body comes equipped with protection against toxins, and there are trillions of cells in your body. That's *trillions*; we're talking 12 zeros here. Every single one of these cells is surrounded by a protective membrane, the main function of which is "selective permeability." This simply means that the membrane lets in only stuff that's good for the cell, while it blocks stuff that's bad for the cell from entering. And it expels waste material—any stuff left over from metabolism that the cell doesn't need. In other words, it acts as a barrier against toxins. So your body comes equipped with a powerful set of toxic shields right down at the cellular level.

On top of this, you have millions and millions of cells whose sole function in life is to guard against invaders, quickly dispatching any organism or foreign object that doesn't belong in your body.

For example, white blood cells known as macrophages work to clear your lungs of pollutants, picking up individual bits of dust and debris to carry off. Some things, like asbestos fibers, simply stymie these hard-working cells. If there's no way the macrophages can haul off a particular substance, it just accumulates and ultimately causes inflammation. If you're a smoker or you're exposed to a lot of secondhand smoke, these macrophages can get so overwhelmed with what they need to haul away that the debris just accumulates to the point where it can cause disease.

In addition to all these cells, you have entire organ systems that are devoted almost exclusively to cleansing and detoxifying your body.

APPRECIATE YOUR LIVER

Along with creating bile, which helps you digest fats, your liver serves as a blood filter. It's like the oil filter in your car. As your blood circulates around and around in your body, it goes through your liver again and again. Every minute 2 quarts of blood flow through your liver to be filtered and detoxified.

Any medications you've taken, any pesticides that rode in on your food, and any pollutants that got into your blood from the air you breathe ideally get filtered out and removed by your liver. Your liver is your main organ of detoxification.

Of course, if you're exposed to a lot of toxins, your liver can get overwhelmed and can't quite manage to dispose of everything that needs to be disposed of. When that happens, toxins get stored in your body, mostly in your fatty tissues, and—no surprise—can make you sick in any number of ways.

Your liver requires a multitude of different chemical compounds—hundreds, actually—to do its job of detoxifying your body of a mind-boggling variety of toxic substances. And all of those chemical compounds come from the foods you eat. Of course, it's not just your liver that needs nutrients in order to do its detoxification work. All of your other detox systems need nutrients, as well.

WORKING TOGETHER TO CLEAN YOUR SYSTEM

In tandem with your liver, your kidneys work constantly to filter from your blood any toxins that have gotten in through your food. The reason you urinate and defecate every day is because your body has taken in what it needs from your food and is throwing off what it doesn't need.

The entire length of your intestines also gets into the act. Your intestines have a lining that absorbs nutrients and water. That lining lets in only what's good for you and shuts out what's bad for you. At least that's what it should be doing. If this protective lining becomes inflamed or irritated, it can let toxic material through and into your bloodstream. That's what's known as a leaky gut.

You may not think of your skin as an organ of elimination, but it is. So many toxins are removed through the pores of your skin via sweat that some naturopaths even refer to skin as the third kidney.

Even your nose comes equipped with a trash-disposal system. Your nose is lined with tiny hairs that help keep dust, pollens, mold, and pollutants from getting into your lungs. And any particles that do get through stick to the mucous membranes at the back of your nose and throat. These mucous membranes are lined with cells that contain tiny hairlike structures, called cilia, that beat in unison and push the particles down your throat to be destroyed by stomach acid.

This is only a very brief introduction to your body's detoxifying system. Suffice it to say that you are a living, breathing, detoxifying machine. But these days that magnificent machine is under assault as never before.

The Hormone "Impostors"

WHAT DO BABY DOLLS, FOOD-STORAGE CONTAINERS, and cling wrap have in common? And what do they have to do with low sperm counts and breast cancer?

They're all sources of environmental estrogens (also known as xenoestrogens). These chemicals, which occur naturally in plants and are found in toys and other plastic goods, household products, pesticides, and industrial chemicals, act like the female sex hormone estrogen. They mimic, alter, or stop estrogen's natural effects within the body.

In women, environmental estrogens mimic natural estrogen. High estrogen levels have been linked to cancers fueled by estrogen, such as some forms of breast cancer.

Some scientists believe that environmental estrogens may explain why young girls are reaching puberty at younger and younger ages. The compound bisphenol-A, used to make reusable plastic bottles, dental sealants, and other plastic goods, is released in food and water.

While there's no research on how bisphenol-A affects humans, researchers at the University of Missouri in Columbia have exposed pregnant lab animals to the same levels of bisphenol-A that humans are exposed to. They found that the chemical caused the offspring of the mice to grow faster after birth and to enter puberty earlier than usual.

Environmental estrogens are thought to affect men, too. Some scientists believe that they may be behind the rapidly falling sperm counts in the United States, the rising rates of genital defects in male infants, and the rise in testicular cancer among young American men.

FACING THE TOXIC ONSLAUGHT

Toxins are in the air you breathe, the water you drink, the food you eat, your household cleaners and body-care products, your child's plastic toys, and the freshly dry-cleaned clothing in your closet. And they're in you. Your body generates them as it carries out its normal functions—breathing, eating, even going for your daily walk.

"Everyone has chemical residues stored in their bodies," says Chris Spooner, N.D., postdoctoral fellow at the Environmental Medicine Center of Excellence at Southwest College of Naturopathic Medicine and Health Sciences in Tempe, Arizona. "Scientists have found them in blood, urine, body fat, organs, hair and nails, even breast milk."

Your body also struggles under the burden of "emotional toxins" such as stress, anger, and depression, says Peter Bennett, N.D., a naturopathic physician in Vancouver and coauthor of *7-Day Detox Miracle.* "Toxins affect the ways in which we think and feel, and thoughts and feelings affect the ways in which we process environmental toxins."

There is compelling evidence that chronic stress contributes to a host of maladies and slows the activity of detoxification enzymes in the liver, the body's prime purification organ. If the body can't rid itself of toxins, they back up in the blood, cells, and tissues, causing a kind of low-grade poisoning. The weaker the body's ability to cleanse itself, the more vulnerable to illness it is. "Our clinic sees many people who have been fairly healthy," says Dr. Spooner. "Something happens—they become overstressed, start eating badly, or are prescribed a medication that affects the way their bodies clear toxins. All of a sudden, their bodies are pushed over the edge, and they get sick."

The good news is, there's much you can do to build up your body's ability to eliminate the internal and external poisons that threaten it. The key? Taking charge of your health. "You have to educate yourself about environmental toxins and how they can affect your health," says Dr. Spooner. "Yes, there are toxins out there, and yes, they are causing health problems, but you're not helpless. You can protect yourself against them."

YOUR BODY'S BURDEN

In 2003, researchers at the federal Centers for Disease Control (CDC) drew samples of blood and urine from 2,500 men, women, and children to find out which man-made chemicals were finding

Kids Most at Risk

THERE'S GROWING EVIDENCE THAT CHILDREN ARE MOST susceptible to environmental toxins. Their vulnerability may even begin before birth.

Pregnant women use their stores of body fat to nourish the fetus, says Chris Spooner, N.D., postdoctoral fellow at the Environmental Medicine Center of Excellence at Southwest College of Naturopathic Medicine and Health Sciences in Tempe, Arizona. But because many toxins, including dioxins and PCBs, are stored in body fat, mothers can unknowingly pass them along to their unborn children. After birth, babies may continue to be exposed because the toxins are found in breast milk, as well.

Pound for pound, children eat, drink, and breathe more than adults, which means that they absorb proportionally larger doses of toxins, says Dr. Spooner. Children also have faster metabolisms, which speeds up their absorption of these chemicals. For example, children absorb about 50 percent of the lead they swallow, while adults absorb about 10 percent. Plus, they play on the floor, where the highest concentrations of pollutants settle.

"There are a lot of pesticide and solvent residues in that 1 or 2 feet above the ground," says Dr. Spooner. "Some pesticides and solvents have been shown to be toxic to the nervous system, and the nervous systems of babies and children are not fully developed. These neurotoxins may be linked to conditions like attention deficit hyperactivity disorder (ADHD) and autism."

The jury is still out on that, but the research is intriguing—and disturbing, says Dr. Spooner. For example, researchers at the State University of New York at Oswego showed that babies who had significant amounts of PCBs in their umbilical cords performed more poorly than babies who didn't in tests designed to assess overall intelligence, recognition of faces, and the ability to shut out distractions. Another study conducted in 2000 by the National Academy of Sciences suggested that a combination of neurotoxins and genes may account for nearly 25 percent of developmental problems in children.

No One Is Immune

SCIENCE HAS LINKED THE MAN-MADE TOXINS in the environment to a wide variety of chronic degenerative diseases like asthma, Alzheimer's disease, cancer, and coronary artery disease, to name just a few. But some studies have associated these substances with specific conditions that affect men, women, and children. The table below lists some of these conditions.

Women
Breast, ovarian, and uterine cancers
Endometriosis
Infertility/sterility
Miscarriage
Premenstrual syndrome (PMS)
Uterine fibroids

Children*
Attention Deficit Disorder
Attention Deficit Hyperactivity
    Disorder
Autism

Birth defects of the penis and testicles
    in boys
Childhood cancers, including brain
    tumors and leukemia
Early puberty in girls (increases risk of
    breast cancer in adulthood)

Men
Decreased fertility/sterility
Diminished sperm count
Testicular cancer

*Many forms of childhood cancer have been linked to exposure to toxic chemicals such as pesticides in children, parents, or both.

their way into the American people. The researchers found every single one of the 116 chemicals they tested for. That's right, every one of the 116 toxic chemicals the researchers went looking for, they found in at least one person. Included in this chemical cocktail were toxic metals such as lead, aluminum, and mercury; cotinine, a by-product of secondhand smoke; and various pesticides, plastics, and disinfectants. They even found DDT, a pesticide that has not been used in this country since the early 1970s but which can persist in the environment—and in the body's fat cells—for up to 50 years.

The CDC findings—part of its ongoing assessment of Americans' exposure to environmental toxins—show that no matter how well you care for your health, you can't completely escape environmental toxins. Quite simply, you're polluted. Scientists call this personal pollution "body burden," and there's clear evidence that there are health consequences to our cradle-to-grave exposure.

That's precisely why it's so critical that you make detoxification an important part of your health care. While there's no way you can avoid all the toxins coming at you, you can take steps to avoid unnecessary exposure to a great many. There are also a number of strategies that you can incorporate into your life to help support your body's efforts to throw off any toxins that do make it into your body. Throughout this book you'll find details on how to customize a purification plan to meet your personal needs.

HAVING A "BAD AIR DAY"?

The very air we breathe is swirling with toxins. All told, more than 40 million pounds of toxic chemicals were released into the air through 1994. (And that was more than 10 years ago!) While some air toxins come from natural sources, such as forest fires, most are man-made. These include benzene, found in gasoline; perchloroethylene, used in dry cleaning; and methylene chloride, an industrial solvent.

Then there are dioxins, the by-products of burning wastes and chemical manufacturing. Considered to be some of the most toxic chemicals known to man, dioxins don't dissolve in water, but they do dissolve in fat—our fat. Once we absorb dioxins, it's hard to get them out again.

And let's not forget acid rain. When fuels such as coal and oil are burned at high temperatures, they form gases called nitrogen oxides and sulfur dioxide. These gases interact in the atmosphere and fall in the form of rain, snow, and fog. When they evaporate, they form dry gases and particles that are transported by winds and inhaled.

Thinking this isn't much of a problem these days? Not so fast. Even though we've cut way back on coal burning in this country, it's still the primary fuel used in China. And, yes, those particles and gases do blow all the way across the Pacific Ocean and show up on the West Coast.

These toxic air pollutants have been linked to cancer, reduced fertility, birth

A Witch's Brew of Threats

THE TOXINS WE MUST ALL DEAL WITH ARE CATEGORIZED by their effects on human health:

Carcinogens cause genetic alterations that lead to cancerous tumors or promote the growth of cancer cells.

Developmental toxicants harm a fetus in the womb, causing birth defects or behavioral problems.

Reproductive toxicants damage the male and female reproductive systems, which can cause infertility.

Immunotoxic chemicals interfere with or damage the body's immune system.

Endocrine disrupters affect the functioning of hormones, including the female sex hormone estrogen, raising the risk of hormone-fueled cancers such as breast cancer. The chemical DDT is thought to be an endocrine disrupter. A study by Belgian researchers found that women with breast cancer were at least five times more likely to have residue of DDT in their blood than those without.

Volatile organic compounds (VOCs)—a class of substances widely used in industry and manufacturing and found in household products such as cleansers, aerosol sprays, air fresheners, and dry-cleaned clothing—are a significant source of our body burden, says Dr. Spooner. These include solvents, which are substances used to dissolve other substances and which are found in paint, paint strippers, and gasoline. "Solvents are toxic to both the nervous system and immune systems," says Dr. Spooner. They have been linked to brain tumors and leukemia in children.

Phthalates are used to manufacture countless household items, from toys and shower curtains to nail polish and wallpaper. These chemicals have been linked to birth defects, liver and thyroid damage, a decline in the quantity and quality of sperm in men, and miscarriages in women. At least one phthalate, Di(2-ethylhexyl) phthalate (DEHP), is likely to cause cancer.

defects, and heart and lung problems. According to a 2002 Environmental Protection Agency (EPA) study, at least two-thirds of Americans live in areas where toxic chemicals in the air raise the risk of cancer. What's more, a study conducted by the Natural Resources Defense Council (NRDC) and the University of California at San Francisco (UCSF) School of Medicine suggests that diesel exhaust doesn't just aggravate asthma, it may cause it. The fine particles in diesel exhaust may cause alterations in the immune system, and these changes may cause asthma in otherwise healthy people. According to the CDC, the incidence of asthma rose by 42 percent from 1982 to 1992, and it's been on the rise ever since.

But you don't just breathe in air toxins. They can also get into water and soil, which means that you can absorb them by drinking water polluted by these chemicals; eating fish from polluted waters or meat, milk, or eggs from animals that fed on contaminated plants; or eating fruits and vegetables grown in soil in which these toxins have been deposited. Children can absorb them when they place their soil-covered hands or toys in their mouths.

The good news here—and there is some—is that it is possible to avoid some of these toxins by paying careful attention to the sources of the foods you eat and by making careful choices about the kinds of products you use in your home. And even though you've undoubtedly been exposed to many of these toxins and have some stored in your tissues, you don't need to carry them around with you forever. Throughout this book you'll find remedies using herbs, foods, and even spa treatments that will help enhance the ongoing cleansing process that lessens your body's burden.

Toxins on Tap

That water rushing out of your kitchen or bathroom tap might seem to be sparkling clear, but looks can be deceiving. According to one independent study conducted by the Ralph Nader Research Institute, the water we drink contains more than 2,000 toxic chemicals, including industrial chemicals, pesticides, and toxic metals.

For example, perchlorate, the main ingredient in rocket and missile fuel, has been found in the drinking water, groundwater, or soil in at least 43 states, according to a study of government data by the Environmental Working Group, a nonprofit organization based in Washington, D.C. Perchlorate affects the thyroid's ability to use iodide, a nutrient the body needs to manufacture thyroid hormones, and may cause thyroid cancer.

In pregnant women, perchlorate interferes with the thyroid gland's ability to produce the hormones needed for the normal development of a fetus. This interference may cause learning disabilities and developmental delays in children.

Lead is one of the most pervasive contaminants in drinking water. Typically, the lead isn't in the water itself, but in lead pipes, joints, and solder, usually found in very old homes. Babies and children who drink lead-tainted water may develop physical and developmental delays. Adults who drink it over many years can develop kidney problems or high blood pressure.

Outdated treatment plants also threaten our drinking water, according to a study by the NRDC. Treatment plants were designed to remove organic wastes such as bacteria, not man-made chemicals. So when this chemical-laced water passes through the treatment plant, the chemicals remain.

Think you're safe if you drink well water? Think again. If you live within a few miles of a farm (especially a farm with livestock), gas station, or landfill, the chances are good that your water is laced with chemical toxins or bacteria, says Bruce Fife, N.D., a nutritionist and naturopath in Colorado Springs and author of *The Detox Book.*

Sound grim? Well, you definitely don't have to subject yourself and your family to toxins in your water supply. To find out how to secure a clean water supply, see "Water Fit to Drink" on page 45.

A PLATEFUL OF POISONS

Whether you savor a bowl of luscious berries, slice into a juicy steak, or sip a glass of skim milk, the chances are good that you're also ingesting a chemical stew of pesticides (used to prevent crop damage by weeds, insects, rodents, and molds) or other potentially dangerous substances. About 20 percent of our food supply is contaminated with pesticide residue, according to a 2002 study published in the *Journal of Epidemiology and Public Health.* Even organic fruits and vegetables aren't totally safe. In 2002, analysts from Consumers Union, the publisher of *Consumer Reports,* and the Organic Materials Research Institute (OMRI), an independent research organization in Eugene, Oregon, analyzed government data and found that 23 percent of organic fruits and vegetables contained pesticide residues.

The meat and milk we eat and drink are laced with chemicals as well. Beef cattle are given hormones to fatten them up for market, while dairy cows are injected with recombinant growth hormone (rBGH) to increase the amount of milk they produce. According to some researchers, consuming the meat or milk of animals given these substances may raise the risk of breast cancer in women and colorectal and prostate cancers in men.

A junk-food diet is also toxic to the body, says Elson M. Haas, M.D., director of the Preventive Medical Center at Marin in San Rafael, California, and author of *The Detox Diet*. It's high in calories and refined carbohydrates, like white flour and white sugar, and low in vitamins, minerals, and phytonutrients—the good-for-you substances in fruits, veggies, and whole grains shown to reduce the risk of cancer and other degenerative diseases.

Processed foods such as salty snack foods and boxed baked goods contain trans fatty acids, now known to be as unhealthy for your heart as the saturated fat in bacon and butter. (A positive development: The Food and Drug Administration has ruled that, starting in January 2006, food manufacturers must reveal the amount of trans fatty acids in their products.) Chemicals added to food to preserve its freshness or add flavor can also "poison" the body, says Dr. Haas. For example, aspartame (Nutrasweet) and monosodium glutamate (MSG) can cause headaches and other symptoms in genetically susceptible people. Sodium nitrite, used in some hot dogs and lunch meats, can combine with chemicals already in the stomach to form nitrosamines, cancer-causing substances.

While you can't eliminate all the toxins from your food—the pesticide residues found in organic produce are just one example—the food choices you make every day are among your most important tools for detoxification. You'll find a wide variety of suggestions in the pages that follow. Pay special attention to chapter 3 on page 30.

HOME, TOXIC HOME

"People tend to be most concerned about outdoor air pollution, but indoor air is much more toxic than the air outside," says Dr. Spooner. In fact, concentrations of volatile organic compounds (VOCs) are two to five times higher inside our homes than they are outdoors. "And don't forget about cigarette smoke, perhaps the deadliest household toxin," says Dr. Spooner. Studies have shown that secondhand smoke invades the lungs of about 88 percent of nonsmokers in this country.

The very materials used to build your home may contain health-threatening chemicals. For example, the formaldehyde used in cabinetry, furniture, and decorative wall coverings can sting your eyes and throat, make you queasy, and make it difficult to breathe. It also causes cancer in test animals and may cause cancer in people.

Asbestos, a mineral fiber used for insulation, has been shown to cause lung cancer. While asbestos is no longer used, homes built before 1986 (the year it was banned) may have it in ductwork, pipe wraps, siding, or other materials, and removing it improperly can cause its fibers to be released into the air and inhaled.

Perchloroethylene, commonly used in dry cleaning, has been shown to cause cancer in animals. Research shows that people breathe low levels of this chemical at home, where their dry-cleaned clothing is stored.

Work is no less toxic. An investigation conducted in 2000 by the newspaper *USA Today* found that employees in more than 35 states unknowingly carried toxins from work to home in their cars and on their shoes, clothes, hair, tools, and briefcases, potentially exposing their families to mercury, radioactive material, lead, asbestos, PCBs, and pesticides.

Office workers are frequently trapped in office buildings with windows that don't open—so-called tight buildings, says Dr. Bennett—and inhale fumes emitted by plastic chairs, new carpets, and formaldehyde-permeated particleboard. People with on-the-job exposure to solvents, paints, or other chemicals can absorb them either by inhaling the fumes or through direct contact. "People usually find out about chemical sensitivity after they have already become sick," says Dr. Bennett.

Body-care products are another source of potentially toxic chemicals. Because makeup is not considered a food or drug, the Food and Drug Administration (FDA) does not regulate cosmetics for the safety of their ingredients. But some cosmetics contain nitrosamines, which have been found to cause cancer. (Nitrosamines can be difficult to find on ingredients labels; they can be found in ingredients with "tea" or "dea" in the name. The solution here is clear—simply avoid any products that contain these ingredients.)

Talc is an asbestos-like material commonly used in powders and other makeup. What's more, a study by the Fred Hutchinson Cancer Research Center in Seattle found that women with ovarian cancer are more likely to have used powder products and sprays in the genital area than women without the disease.

For a good, overall look at how to select body-care products and use them wisely, see chapter 9 on page 188. And throughout the book you'll find tips and techniques for avoiding exposure to other toxins and for flushing them out of your system after you've been exposed.

Chapter 2

Purification Partners: Safe and Effective Ways to Detox

PICTURE YOURSELF WITH MORE ENERGY AND MENTAL CLARITY, with more radiant hair and skin, and as thin as you've ever dreamed of being. See yourself sailing through cold and flu season with barely a sniffle or cough. See yourself free from chronic aches and pains. Envision reducing (or even eliminating) your medications for diabetes, allergies, or high blood pressure. Imagine yourself calmer and more content, with the ability to shrug off stress and fatigue. In short, imagine looking and feeling better than you have in years.

Detoxification can help you reap all of these benefits and more. Practiced for centuries by cultures around the world, detoxification is the process of eliminating the body's "toxic buildup," helping it to repair and renew itself.

"The body has its own natural healing system, and detoxification enhances this system," says Peter Bennett, N.D., a naturopathic physician in Vancouver and coauthor of *7-Day Detox Miracle*. "It rejuvenates the body's natural ability to cleanse itself of waste generated by cells and tissues as they do their work, as well as man-made chemicals in air, water, and food."

Detoxification is more important than ever before, adds Dr. Bennett. "In addition to the health problems we've experienced for thousands of years, we are now exposed to a huge variety of environmental poisons," he says. Detoxification can ease your body's toxic burden because it helps to eliminate the toxins already in your body and minimize the absorption of new ones.

Detoxification isn't a New Age fad. Although it has taken many forms, detoxifying the body is a serious healing concept practiced for centuries in cultures around the world. For example, Native Americans used sweat lodges to purify and renew their bodies and spirits, while Scandinavians prescribed the sauna for their ills. Practitioners of ayurveda, the ancient system of medicine in India, view many diseases as the accumulation of toxic materials in the digestive system and recommend fasting.

Today, more and more Americans are discovering detoxification's rejuvenating powers. Alternative practitioners contend that, properly used, a number of detoxification practices can strengthen the body's immune system, as well as the "purification system," made up of the liver, kidneys, and other organs. "Without its toxic burden, the body is better able to repair itself and stay at peak health," says Phoebe Yin, N.D., a naturopathic physician at the Bastyr Center for Natural Health in Seattle.

Purification should be an ongoing process. Still, it's wise to undergo a more formal cleansing at least once a year, says Dr. Bennett. You can certainly detoxify more often than that, if you wish. The exceptions: pregnant women, nursing mothers, children, and people with cancer, low body weight, psychiatric illness, or other serious diseases. Anyone in doubt should consult a qualified naturopathic physician.

There are many purification methods, all of which can be used alone or in combination. Here are the techniques most commonly used by alternative practitioners.

HEALING DIET

Eating the right kinds of foods is the cornerstone of the detoxification process, says Elson M. Haas, M.D., director of the Preventive Medical Center at Marin in San Rafael, California, and author of *The Detox Diet*. A diet of whole, organic, natural foods gives the body the nutrients it needs to nourish cells and tissues and cleanse stored poisons from the colon (large intestine) and other organs. It also gives your intestinal tract a break from the white flour, white sugar, artery-clogging fats, and chemicals in the typical American diet.

Are You Having a Healing Crisis?

YOU'VE CLEANED UP YOUR DIET, quit smoking, and started taking a brisk walk each day. You're feeling great and then, out of nowhere, you're hit with fatigue, headaches, and an all-over ill feeling. What's going on?

Chances are, you're in the midst of what alternative practitioners call a healing crisis—a temporary surge in symptoms that often occurs during the purification process. Believe it or not, a healing crisis signals that the body is on the mend.

Here's what happens: As your body begins to purify itself and get healthier, it begins to eliminate toxic residues that it has stored for a long time, sometimes for years. These residues include stool in the bowels, traces of old chemicals stored in fat tissue, remnants of prescription medications from your blood, and other wastes. This influx of toxins causes symptoms that may include constipation or diarrhea, headaches, nausea, and canker sores or fever blisters. If you've suffered from skin rashes in the past, you may erupt anew, as you release poisons through your skin. You may feel better for a day or two, suddenly feel worse again, and then feel better again. One healing crisis may not purge all of the toxins that have built up in your body over the years, but each successive crisis will become milder and of shorter duration.

To help minimize the healing crisis, get lots of rest, drink plenty of water, and reduce stress as much as possible. If the symptoms don't pass after 3 or 4 days, however, consult your doctor. It can be difficult to determine the difference between a healing crisis and an illness.

How a Healing Diet Works

A detoxifying diet helps your body release substances that it might not otherwise be able to release, thereby relieving poor digestion, headaches, fatigue, joint pain, and other symptoms. How? By eliminating foods and beverages that disturb your body's detoxification machinery, such as processed and refined foods, caffeine, alcohol, and fatty foods. What a healing diet does include is fresh fruits and vegetables and whole grains. These foods are filled with fiber, which helps your colon eliminate toxins.

Ideally, a detoxifying diet is something that you do for a lifetime. However, it is possible to follow a stricter form of eating for a short period of time—anywhere from a few days to a week or more—and experience considerable benefits. This kind of diet is typically paired with herbs and supplements known to eliminate toxins. Most alternative practitioners recommend following a strict 1- to 2-week detoxification diet twice a year—once in spring and again in fall.

Benefits

When you give your body a break from the toxins in the typical American diet, even for as little as a few days, your body comes alive, says Dr. Haas. You can shed pounds of excess water weight, boost your energy and mood, and lose that vaguely sick, bloated feeling—what nature-oriented practitioners call congestion. "Even mild changes from your current way of eating will produce some benefits, while more dramatic changes can produce a profound improvement in health," says Dr. Haas.

Drawbacks

Some people may experience headaches, fatigue, and an overall "blah" feeling for the first few days of a detox diet. This is entirely normal as the body releases toxins, says Dr. Haas. These symptoms usually fade by the third or fourth day to be replaced with energy and feelings of well-being. And folks who are not used to eating a lot of fiber may experience gas and abdominal discomfort.

A Healing Diet Works Best For

Men and women in good general health stand to benefit from this diet. Although children should generally not be put on a strict "cleansing diet," they can benefit from following its guidelines in a milder form, says Dr. Haas. That is, they should eat lots of fresh fruits and veggies and whole grains, and fewer (or no) processed junk foods.

HEALING HERBS

Herbs have a long medical tradition. For example, herbal remedies are in the Papyrus Ebers, a medical guide used by doctors in ancient Egypt. Thousands of years later, alternative practitioners now use specific herbs to support detoxification and promote healing, says Bruce

Fife, N.D., a nutritionist and naturopath in Colorado Springs and author of *The Detox Book.*

How Healing Herbs Work

There are two main classes of detoxification herbs. The first class of herbs, the "housekeeping" herbs, speeds toxins out of the body by increasing production of urine, sweat, and bile (an enzyme produced by the liver that aids digestion) or by revving up immune cells. For example, buchu encourages urine production while helping to prevent kidney stones from forming, and dandelion enhances bile production while helping to speed digestion. The second class of herbs, known as adaptogens, raises the body's resistance to toxins, as well as physical and emotional stresses. Ashwagandha, for example, increases an individual's vitality and resistance to disease. You'll learn more about these herbs in chapter 5 on page 81.

Benefits

Herbs are easy to take. They're available in almost any form, including easy-to-swallow capsules, tablets, liquid drops (tinctures), and teas made from fresh or dried herbs. What's more, most herbs are nontoxic and are not habit-forming.

Drawbacks

Herbs don't normally work quickly. They may take weeks or even months to work, so be patient. Some herbs may also cause side effects, especially when used in combination with prescription or over-the-counter drugs, or when used by people with preexisting health conditions. Generally, side effects from herbs are not as serious as those caused by prescription and over-the-counter medications.

Healing Herbs Work Best For

Healthy adult men and women. Unless you're working with a health care professional experienced in prescribing herbs, don't take herbs if you're pregnant or have kidney disease, high blood pressure, diabetes, or any other serious health condition. While certain herbs are safe for children, they should not be given herbs with a powerful laxative effect. Let a naturopathic health care professional work with "little ones"; their needs are special and require extra training.

EXERCISE

More than 2,000 years ago, the Greek philosopher Aristotle wrote, "A man falls into ill health as a result of not caring for exercise." Science has since proved him right. "Regular exercise is essential to the purification process," says Dr. Haas. While any sweat-inducing physical activity will aid the body's detoxification efforts, three in particular—yoga, tai chi, and qi gong—are particularly associated with the purification process.

How Exercise Works

Regular exercise boosts your circulation of blood and lymph, the fluid produced by your lymph glands. Improved circulation carries nutrients, oxygen, and immune cells to damaged cells or tissues and carries away cellular waste and other toxins, says Dr. Bennett. Physical activity also promotes sweating, which eliminates toxins through the skin, and increases the frequency of bowel movements.

Even moderate exercise on a regular basis helps melt excess body fat. Since fat is a primary storage site for toxins, getting rid of excess body fat is an important part of detoxification, says Dr. Bennett.

Benefits

Dr. Bennett is particularly enthusiastic about yoga. "The benefits of yoga for detoxification are unequaled," he says. "It encourages the proper circulation of blood and lymph fluid, enhances digestion, and lubricates the joints, among other benefits."

Studies show that moderate exercise boosts the body's immune system, which can help the body resist the effects of environmental toxins. For example, regular brisk walking has been shown to bolster specific aspects of the immune system, including cancer-fighting natural killer (NK) cells. In one study, researchers at Texas Christian University found that exercisers who rode a stationary bike for 1 hour twice a day—once in the morning and again in the afternoon—had significantly higher counts of important immune system cells than nonexercisers. Being active also reduces your risk of degenerative diseases, including heart disease, high blood pressure, and diabetes; improves flexibility and sleep; and relieves stress.

Drawbacks

While moderate-intensity exercise helps eliminate toxins, too much exercise can actually weaken the immune system, says Thomas J. Slaga, Ph.D., scientific director of the AMC Cancer Research Center in Denver and author of *The Detox Revolution*. "For example, athletes have been shown to become very susceptible to colds after a competition," he says. That's because during intense physical exertion, the body produces cortisol and adrenaline, stress hormones that temporarily suppress the immune system. Generally speaking, most Americans are not exactly in danger of overdoing it in the exercise department.

Exercise Works Best For

Everyone. Federal guidelines call for adults and older people to engage in moderate physical activity five or more times a week for at least 30 minutes at a time. Children need at least an hour of moderate activity most days of the week. If you are over 50 or have health issues, get your doctor's okay before you embark on an exercise program. For more information on safe and healthful exercise as part of your detoxification efforts, see chapter 6 on page 115.

FASTING

Fasting—going without solid food for a day or longer—is one of the oldest therapeutic practices in medicine. While the most stringent form of fasting allows only water, most alternative practitioners recommend juice fasts, featuring the freshly made juices of fruits and vegetables. Unlike water alone, fresh juices supply nutrients the body needs to help eliminate toxins and rejuvenate cells and tissues.

How Fasting Works

The typical juice fast consists of drinking 2 to 3 quarts of water and freshly squeezed fruit and vegetable juices over the course of a day. Fruits are considered the best purifiers and vegetables the best cellular rebuilders, says Dr. Fife.

Ideally, the fruits and vegetables you juice should be organic—grown without the use of pesticides. If organic produce isn't available, fruits and vegetables should be thoroughly washed and peeled.

During a fast, cells begin to release stored fat. When this fat is burned, the toxins within are released and eventually eliminated from the body. Experts recommend that beginners start with a 1-day fast before attempting a longer fast. Several days before a fast, experts suggest eliminating caffeine, nicotine, alcohol, and animal foods from the diet and eating only fruits and vegetables.

Benefits

A juice fast allows many of the body's systems a rest, says Dr. Haas. Cells have the opportunity to repair themselves and eliminate their waste, and the liver can

The Benefits of Emotional Detox

DETOXIFICATION DOESN'T JUST BENEFIT YOUR BODY; it can also increase your emotional well-being. Similarly, neutralizing emotional "toxins" such as anger and depression can reduce your body's vulnerability to physical ills.

Cleansing your mind and spirit of past hurts and resentments is just as important as cleansing your body of toxins, says Elson M. Haas, M.D., director of the Preventive Medical Center at Marin in San Rafael, California, and author of *The Detox Diet*. "Emotionally, detoxification helps us uncover and express feelings, especially hidden frustrations, anger, resentments, or fear, and replace them with forgiveness, love, joy, and hope," he says.

Some research links forgiveness with better health. For example, a study from Duke University Medical Center in Durham, North Carolina, demonstrates that among people who have chronic back pain, those who have forgiven others experience lower levels of pain and fewer associated psychological problems (such as anger and depression) than those who have not forgiven. In another study conducted at the University of Pittsburgh, researchers studied 680 women with chest pain and found those who harbored feelings of anger were four times more likely to have unhealthy cholesterol levels and a higher body mass index (a measure of weight and body proportion), both of which are linked to heart disease.

"On a spiritual level, many people experience new clarity and/or an enhancement of their purpose in life during cleansing processes," says Dr. Haas. "When your body has eliminated much of its toxic buildup, you feel lighter and are able to really experience the moment and be open for the future."

spend more time on the important process of detoxification. Fasting is also a good way to break bad eating habits and commit to healthy lifestyle changes, he says.

Drawbacks

Juices must be made with a machine designed specifically for juicing; tossing chunks of fruits or vegetables into a blender just won't work. If you don't already have a juicer, be prepared to do some research to find one that will meet your needs without putting too big a dent in your wallet.

During a fast, you may experience unpleasant symptoms, such as weakness, headaches, fatigue, and dizziness. However, these symptoms usually pass in 2 or 3 days, and if you do a shorter fast or a modified fast, you may not experience them at all.

Fasts that consist only of water can actually hinder the process of detoxification if done for a few days, says Dr. Bennett. That's because water-only fasts deplete the body of nutrients critical to the detoxification process, such as antioxidant vitamins and the enzyme glutathione. They're also bereft of protein, which the liver uses to do its detoxification work, and fiber, which sweeps the digestive tract clean, escorting toxins out of the body.

It is possible to benefit from longer, water-only fasts, but these must be done only under the supervision of a health care professional experienced in supervising therapeutic fasts.

Fasting Works Best For

Adult men and women in good health. Do not fast if you're pregnant or nursing, if you're underweight, or if you have recently had or will soon have surgery. People with chronic health problems such as cancer or heart disease should fast only under the supervision of a doctor experienced with using fasts as therapy. Children should not fast.

CLEANSING

Methods to cleanse the colon have been around for centuries. As far back as the ancient Egyptians, enemas and other cleansing techniques were commonly used to rid the body of toxins believed to cause ill health. In the early 20th century, cleansing was advocated by the American physician and breakfast-cereal magnate John Harvey Kellogg at his health sanatorium in Battle Creek, Michigan. According to proponents of cleansing, a poor diet, too much stress, and too little exercise lead to "autointoxication"—the poisoning of the body with its own waste. Over time, undigested food and left-behind fecal waste harden and accumulate on the walls of the bowels, hindering the bowels' attempts to eliminate it. These materials decay and become toxic, poisoning the body and leading to a host of symptoms that range from frequent headaches to overall ill health.

How Cleansing Works

There are three main ways to cleanse: natural laxatives, such as the soluble fiber psyllium or herbs; enemas; and colonics. An enema is a self-administered injection of warm, distilled water or other healing substances, such as aloe vera or coffee, into the colon by way of a tube inserted into the rectum. It cleanses the lower portion of the large intestine and uses about 2 quarts of liquid. A colonic is a more extensive cleansing technique. Performed by a trained colon therapist, a colonic uses 20 or more gallons of water to cleanse the colon's entire 5-foot length. It requires the use of a special machine that pumps the water into the bowel with a hose and then drains the waste. In either method, the water or liquid loosens waste in the colon so it can be eliminated through the rectum.

Benefits

Flushing out impacted fecal matter, toxins, mucous, and parasites, which build up in the intestines over time, eliminates the toxic buildup that causes ill health and disease, says Dr. Fife. Cleansing also allows the bowel to better absorb nutrients from food, which can help improve the symptoms of vitamin and other nutrient deficiencies. Many people with intestinal problems or chronic headaches say they experience almost immediate relief after cleansing, he says.

Drawbacks

Not all health care practitioners advocate cleansing, so the practice is somewhat controversial. Some people may find colon cleansing to be physically or mentally unpleasant. While most people are used to taking gentle, natural laxatives, enemas and colonics require time and a matter-of-fact attitude. When properly performed, enemas and colonics cause a feeling of bloating or fullness, but not pain. And, of course, proper sanitation is crucial for at-home procedures and for those done in a professional setting.

Cleansing Works Best For

People who suffer from chronic constipation, overweight, and stress will find cleansing particularly helpful, says Dr. Fife. These conditions tend to make the bowels sluggish and hinder digestion. Don't cleanse if you have a gastrointestinal condition such as Crohn's disease or diverticulitis, or a serious condition such as heart disease or high blood pressure. If you opt for a colonic, make sure it's performed by a certified member of the International Association for Colon Hydrotherapy (I-ACT). For more information on fasting and cleansing, see chapter 7 on page 143.

HYDROTHERAPY

The practice of using water to promote healing, hydrotherapy has been part of the healing tradition of almost every civilization and is a cornerstone of detoxification therapy. Even the Old Testament mentions the healing powers of mineral waters. Today, people travel to hot springs to "take the waters," believing that their healing powers can improve health or cure disease.

How Hydrotherapy Works

Hydrotherapy consists of alternating hot and cold water in various ways to improve circulation and stimulate the immune system. Methods include hot and cold baths and showers, steam and sauna therapy, and constitutional hydrotherapy, in which alternating hot and cold packs are placed on the body, front and back. Various ways of using water, baths, and other spa treatments are discussed throughout this book.

Benefits

Hydrotherapy intensifies blood circulation to the liver, kidneys, and intestines, which helps these organs excrete waste, says Dr. Bennett. In steam and sauna therapy, toxins are eliminated through the skin via sweat. "The body stores toxins in fatty tissue," he says. "Sweating therapy reduces fat stores quickly, releasing these poisons through excretion."

Drawbacks

Some forms of hydrotherapy can be time-consuming and, for some people, uncomfortable. For example, the wet-sheet method calls for lying in a tub filled with water as hot as possible, then quickly wrapping up in a cold, wet sheet. Also, excessively hot or cold water applied directly to the skin for long periods may cause discomfort or even tissue damage.

Hydrotherapy Works Best For

Healthy men and women can use most forms of hydrotherapy. However, sauna

A Fragrant Way to Cleanse the Spirit

AROMATHERAPY HAS BEEN USED to increase physical and emotional well-being at least since the time of the ancient Egyptians. While this therapy has a wide variety of uses, including relieving pain, nausea, colds, skin problems, and other conditions, its stress-relieving qualities are also used in detoxification.

Aromatherapy uses the essential oils of plants, which have been chemically extracted from aromatic flowers, herbs, and even woods. Each essential oil has its own characteristic aroma and therapeutic effects. There are oils to soothe, to invigorate, and to relieve negative emotions, such as depression, stress, and anxiety. Still other essential oils are believed to battle bacteria and fungi and reduce inflammation.

Essential oils are used in many different ways, including massage, inhalation, aromatic baths, compresses, and vaporization. Some of the oils commonly used for detoxification purposes include angelica root, fennel, grapefruit, and juniper berry.

Essential oils are very concentrated, so never apply them directly to your skin. Before you use them, you must dilute them in a pure, natural "carrier" oil, such as sweet almond oil, apricot oil, or grape seed oil.

Aromatherapy isn't for everyone, however. Avoid it if you have asthma, high blood pressure, cancer, sensitive skin, or allergies, or if you are pregnant. Also, avoid using essential oils on babies and children.

therapy is not for everyone. Avoid these techniques if you are pregnant or have a serious health problem such as diabetes, high blood pressure, heart disease, or a seizure disorder, says Dr. Bennett. And sauna therapy should not be used by children—they can become dangerously dehydrated.

Chapter 3

The Essential Foods: Choosing a Diet for Detoxification

DOES ANY OF THIS SOUND FAMILIAR? Chances are it does.

"Consume a wide variety of whole grains, fruits, and vegetables, preferably organic."

"Stay away from processed foods, fatty foods, hydrogenated oils, food additives, and sugar."

"Drink plenty of pure, clean water."

If you've been paying attention to what you need to eat in order to be healthy and vital, prevent disease, have plenty of energy, keep your weight down, and remain youthful as long as possible, then you've encountered these rules again and again.

These rules are also what it takes to not only detoxify your body, but to keep it clean inside once you've gotten the toxins out.

In fact, most every health care professional who places an emphasis on detoxifying the body as a means to a longer, healthier life emphasizes the importance of eating the right kinds of foods on a regular basis.

"I'd rather clean my house all the time than give it a really good cleaning once a year," says Suzzanne Myer, M.S., R.D., who is on the nutrition faculty at Bastyr Center for Natural Health in Seattle. By "cleaning my house all the time," she means eating on a daily basis the foods that keep her system clean.

"The bottom line is that I eat from the Earth to me, whole grains, fruits, vegetables, eggs, dairy," says Carrie Demers, M.D., director of the Himalayan Institute's Center for Health and Healing in Honesdale, Pennsylvania. In her own life, she says, she concentrates on "food that's really fresh and whole, food that's rich in life force—*prana*." ("Prana," the Sanskrit word for life force or life energy, is a concept that has become widespread as untold thousands of people worldwide turn to yoga as their exercise of choice.) If you don't do anything else, advises Dr. Demers, "add more fresh food to your diet. Those fresh foods have fiber."

"Eat close to the Earth," agrees Geoff Lecovin, D.C., N.D., L.Ac., a chiropractor, naturopath, and acupuncturist who practices in Kirkland, Washington.

Interesting how health care professionals from different fields of study and opposite ends of the country use the same kind of language when talking about how to eat right, detoxify, and keep the body clean. They even choose the same words: Eat close to the Earth.

Why is this? What is it about this kind of eating that helps the body purify itself?

Let's take a look at just one of the body's cleansing mechanisms to help get a handle on how foods that are "close to the Earth" actually make a difference. We'll look at the liver, because that's one of the body's main detoxifying organs. We can concentrate on just the liver as a way to clarify the whole picture because—again, no surprise—the same foods that support the liver also support the other organs and cleansing systems as well.

FIBER POWER

By now, you probably understand that the liver is perhaps your body's best filter of toxins. It's where everything from caffeine and alcohol to pesticide residues, heavy metals, and prescription medications gets filtered out of your body. But you may not realize that by eating a high-fiber diet, you can actually help this filter do its job better. Most of the detailed explanation that follows of what to eat to support your liver's detoxification efforts comes from Gayle Povis Alleman, R.D., a health educator specializing in obesity prevention who administers nutrition education programs for Washington State University.

As part of the digestion process, your liver manufactures bile, a substance made partly from cholesterol. (Yep, there's actually a good use for that stuff.) Bile gets squirted into your gallbladder, where it's stored until you eat something. Then it gets squirted into your small intestine to help your body digest fats. Being an efficient and economical biomachine, the liver uses the bile as a runoff place for toxins. This is just one of the places it stashes toxins. Under *ideal conditions,* the bile is destined to leave the body anyway. It does its job of helping to digest fats and then it gets swept from the body along with the waste products of digestion.

And what are those "ideal conditions"? When you eat a natural diet high in fiber, you form a good bulky stool, the soluble fiber binds up the bile, and it moves through your body swiftly. The remains of a meal eaten one day should come out the other end in 24 hours or less.

But if you don't eat a high-fiber diet— let's say you eat the stereotypical American meat-and-potatoes-white-bread diet, instead—it will take a lot longer for stool to move through your body. It can take 2 days, 3 days, or even longer. And since your liver is an efficient machine, it can reuse bile. Instead of sliding out of your body the way nature intended, the bile

gets reabsorbed, moves back to your liver, and gets used again the next time you eat a meal that contains fat.

What's wrong with this picture?

Number one, your liver uses cholesterol to make bile. So if it doesn't need to make new bile, some cholesterol that you could have gotten rid of will just stay in your blood. And number two, if your liver has stashed some toxins in that bile, you've just reabsorbed them back into your body.

Doesn't that make things like apples, bean soup, and oatmeal sound a lot more important?

Your best sources of fiber are, of course, whole grains, fruits, and vegetables. There are all kinds of ways to add considerably to the fiber you're already taking in. Here are just a few suggestions to get you started:

Double your oat power. If you enjoy oatmeal for breakfast, you can rev up its fiber power by sprinkling a tablespoon of oat bran directly onto the cooked cereal. Give it a good stir and dig in. You won't even taste the difference, but you've just added a little more scrubbing power to your body's cleansing system. Actually, you can add oat bran to any hot cereal. You can also add it to things like chili and meat loaf.

Try some apple fries. Before the family

sits down in front of the TV for the evening, peel and core a few apples. Cut them into 8 to 12 slices to resemble "steak fries" that you might get at a chain restaurant, and put them in a bowl. Don't say anything about this being a healthy snack. Add a side of chunky peanut butter for dipping, then start munching. Pretty soon you'll see other hands reaching into the bowl.

Bring it with you. Packing an orange or a peach or a little baggie of sliced carrots along with those lunchtime sandwiches is always a good idea. This will help you spread your fiber consumption out over the whole day, too, rather than eating a whole day's worth at one sitting.

Put beans in your salads. Open and rinse a can of kidney beans or chickpeas and throw a couple of handfuls into your salad. You can even do this with prepared salads that you've picked up on the way home from work. It's a good way to make a "low-cal, light bite" feel like a really substantial meal. Salads already pack a high-fiber wallop. A half-cup of canned kidney beans has 7.9 grams of fiber; a half-cup of canned chickpeas has 7 grams. That's a lot of fiber in just a little bit of food.

Pop your own. In place of potato chips (no fiber), put out bowls of air-popped popcorn. Lack of flavor is one reason so many people find air-popped popcorn unappealing. An easy fix for this is to drizzle some olive oil over the popcorn, toss it like a salad, and sprinkle it with salt. Voilà! The salt will now stick to the popcorn just the way you like it to. Just one tablespoon is enough olive oil to cover a whole big salad bowl full of popcorn, but feel free to use two if you like the taste. It's still a low-cal snack when you figure in how much appetite-satisfying popcorn (and fiber!) is in that bowl.

Bump it up slowly. If you and your family aren't used to getting a lot of extra fiber, you might want to ease into it slowly. If you jump on the fiber bandwagon too quickly, you could experience bloating, abdominal discomfort, and gas. If you gradually increase the amount of fiber you eat, your body will take it in stride.

Wash it down. If you eat a lot of fiber, you also need to drink plenty of water to keep things moving. You should drink at least eight 8-ounce glasses a day. Young children, of course, can drink less, but they still need to get three or four glasses a day. The water needs to be as toxin-free as you can make it. (See "Water Fit to Drink" on page 45 to learn how to assure that your water is pure.)

Of course, you can always take a fiber supplement, and that might be a good idea if you're also dealing with high cholesterol. But there are some really good reasons why you should plan on getting your key nutrients from food.

NUTRIENTS TO INCREASE YOUR FILTERING POWER

The liver uses some 50 to 100 separate enzymes to filter and detoxify food wastes, pesticide residues, alcohol, and other poisons that get into your blood. Think about that for a minute. That means your liver needs literally dozens of separate chemicals in order to do its job correctly and keep your body toxin-free and healthy. And all of these biochemicals—or the components to manufacture them—must come from the foods you eat. Every last one of them.

Nutrition researchers know about dozens of these biochemicals. They know where they come from, and they know which foods you need to eat in order to take in adequate amounts. But do they have a handle on every single enzyme that your liver has to have? No one thinks that they do.

Every year researchers learn more. Every year dozens of articles on new findings get published in professional nutrition journals. There's no way you could take a couple of supplements and cover all your bases. That's one of the reasons that health care professionals point to a nature-based diet, rather than supplements, as a way to be sure of meeting your needs.

Actually, professionals who work in this cleansing and detoxifying field do recommend taking a good multivitamin supplement as insurance that you're getting at least some of what you need. And if you have problems with aspects of detoxification and get tested by a health care practitioner experienced in this field, you might also find yourself taking some additional supplements prescribed to meet your individual needs. But all of the experts on nutrition for detoxifying the body insist that the most important factor is eating right on a daily basis.

FOODS THAT PROTECT YOUR BODY

So what kinds of foods does the liver need in order to protect your body from toxic buildup?

Keep in mind that medical research has yet to uncover all the details of what the liver needs, so you should make a real effort to incorporate a wide variety of foods into your diet. However, the following foods, which we call transformers and escorts, have shown themselves to be the best places to start when you are ex-

Two-Stage Cleansing Power

RESEARCHERS HAVE FOUND that the liver does its detoxification work in two main phases, says Gayle Povis Alleman, R.D., a health educator specializing in obesity prevention who administers nutrition education programs for Washington State University.

During the first stage, a set of enzymes known as cytochrome 450 transforms toxic substances into intermediate chemicals. Then the second stage of detoxification, which takes place in several separate steps, turns those intermediate chemicals into water-soluble substances that can be flushed from the body.

"Sometimes our poor liver is detoxifying things it's never seen before in our chemical world," says Alleman. "It gets through phase one, then doesn't know what to do with the substances." That can slow things down. One challenge that your body is faced with, explains Alleman, is that these intermediate chemicals are frequently even more toxic than the chemicals that you're trying to get rid of in the first place. If the second stage of your liver's detox system is not adequately supported by good nutrition, your body has to deal with serious toxic buildup.

panding your diet. (See "Two-Stage Cleansing Power" for a deeper explanation of the liver's two-phase approach to keeping your body free of toxins.)

The Transformers

Here's what you can do to help your liver with its first job: transforming toxic substances into intermediate chemicals that can later be removed from your body.

Eat more foods rich in vitamin C. These include citrus fruits, red bell peppers, papaya, cantaloupe, broccoli, and tomatoes.

Learn to love limonene. This powerful detoxifier is found in citrus fruits such as oranges, lemons, limes, and tangerines.

Go easy on grapefruit. The one citrus exception is grapefruit. While grapefruit does contain limonene, it also has a substance that actually slows down the first stage of detoxification, says Alleman. If you're taking prescription drugs, the drugs will clear from your body more slowly if you eat a lot of grapefruit. Grapefruit also hinders your body's ability to rid itself of the toxic effects of alcohol, which makes mixed drinks that include grapefruit a "double whammy." It's okay to consume grapefruit in moderation, Alleman says. But you should probably forgo it altogether if you either work in a polluted environment, take a lot of prescription medications, or consume too much alcohol.

Get more vitamin E. The best food sources are nuts, seeds, and vegetable oils. Since it's hard to get all the vitamin E you need from food, you can safely take a daily supplement of 150 IUs.

Make sure you get enough B vitamins. You can increase your B vitamin intake with brewer's yeast, lean beef, chicken, eggs, kidney beans, chickpeas, peanuts, whole wheat flour, brown rice, cheese, and other dairy products. If you're a vegetarian, it is possible to get adequate amounts of B vitamins by eating whole grains and dairy products, but do take a B_{12} supplement.

Reach for the bioflavonoids. There are hundreds of them, found in a variety of fruits, vegetables, and beans. They are also found in tea, which is a really good reason to switch from coffee to tea, at least some of the time. And if you drink either green or black tea, you get the added benefit of the antioxidant catechin, which not only protects against heart disease and cancer, but also boosts metabolism. If you prefer stimulant-free tea, keep in mind that removing caffeine also reduces the catechin content.

Embrace your brassicas. Foods from the *Brassica* family actually help support both stages of your liver's detoxification efforts. These include cabbage, broccoli, kale, and bok choy.

The Escorts

Here are some additional suggestions for eating to support the second stage of your liver's detoxification efforts. This phase takes place in several separate steps, turning those intermediate chemicals from stage one into water-soluble substances that can be escorted from your body.

Make lots of glutathione. Your body needs good protein to make this important detoxifier. Besides lean meats, you can get protein from dairy products, eggs, and beans. Whey powder is one of the best foods to boost glutathione. It also helps if you eat sulfur-containing foods, such as cabbage, garlic, onions, eggs, and red peppers.

Remember molybdenum. You're probably not used to thinking about this trace mineral, but your liver loves it. It's found in whole grains and legumes. (Beans, again!)

Learn to love curries. Turmeric, a key spice in curries, slows down the first phase of the liver's detoxification efforts, but it speeds up the second phase. That means that when you eat turmeric, you're less likely to have a problem with a buildup of the intermediate toxic chemicals. *Note:* It is possible to buy turmeric in capsules called curcumin and take this important detoxifying herb as a supplement.

GUT CHECK

Of course, your liver is not your only detoxifying organ. There's another organ, in which most of your food digestion and absorption actually takes place. No, not your stomach, which is actually a sort of storage bag where food is attacked by strong acids and broken down into tiny slippery pieces before it's passed along to the organ that does the *most* work to get nutrients into your blood. Your small intestine, otherwise known as your gut, actually digests your food.

Your small intestine, which is a thin tube about 20 feet long, is not as small as it seems. This organ is lined by a rough field of microscopic fingers called villi and microvilli. If you smoothed out all the roughness and flattened it out, it would be the size of a tennis court. All these tiny rifts and valleys are lined with capillaries, tiny blood vessels that absorb nutrients directly from your small intestine and carry them to your liver and then on to waiting hungry cells throughout your body.

The small intestine is designed to let only the good stuff into your blood and to block out the bad stuff—the toxins from bacteria, from your food, and from any pollutants that ride in on your food. But guess what? If you are allergic to a food or even sensitive to a food, your small intestine can get irritated, possibly even inflamed, and start to leak. What's it leaking? The contents of your intestine include undigested food, thriving colonies of bacteria, and waste matter. A lot of it is toxic stuff that you don't want in your bloodstream. If your intestine starts letting some of it through—this is known as a leaky gut—your immune system views the substance as alien and acts accordingly. If the substance happens to be a partially digested food, your immune system will react to that food the next time it comes along, according to Peter Bennett, N.D., a naturopathic physician in Vancouver and coauthor of *7-Day Detox Miracle.*

SCOPING OUT PROBLEM FOODS

If you've ever eaten a food that gives you that "my guts are on fire" feeling, you're sort of right. What you're feeling is not flames, but it could be inflammation.

Life would be a lot easier if every food you were sensitive to gave you a "guts on fire" reaction. Then those foods would be easy to identify and eliminate. Unfortunately, that's not the case. Instead, food sensitivities show up as other kinds of symptoms, things like joint pain, fatigue, skin disorders, sinus problems, and headaches.

It's fairly easy to find out that you're allergic to a food, says Myer. Food allergies usually cause such dramatic negative reactions that you soon figure out that you're allergic. Food sensitivities, on the other hand, are a little harder to pinpoint. In fact, people often crave the very foods that they are sensitive to, she says.

Myer specializes in what is known as the elimination diet—a special kind of diet that lasts just a few weeks and helps people figure out which foods they are sensitive to.

The most common offenders? Dairy products, wheat, chocolate, oranges, corn, and soy. All of these are perfectly healthy foods, fine for most folks, problematic only for those who are sensitive to them. However, people can also be sensitive to things that are not typical offenders.

Myer says that in her clinical work she's encountered people who are sensitive to just one vegetable or fruit, or just tropical fruits. She even found a few people who are sensitive to rice, which is supposed to be one of the least likely foods to cause bad reactions.

The elimination diet is the "gold standard" for figuring out which foods you're sensitive to so you can get them out of your diet and plug that leaky gut, says Myer.

A supervised elimination diet, says Myer, is done immediately following a brief fast. The strategy is to add foods back in one at a time while watching carefully for reactions. The reactions may be as obvious as a rash or as subtle as the sniffles. Reactions may also include headaches; runny nose; hives; gas-

Detox Makeover

Suzzanne Myer did not like what she was seeing in the mirror. After enjoying a lifetime of clear skin, she decided that the sudden appearance of adult acne simply wouldn't do.

As a registered dietician on the nutrition faculty at Bastyr Center for Natural Health in Seattle, Myer now makes her living as a kind of food detective, helping clients ferret out the foods that they have sensitivities to—sensitivities that cause a wide range of unpleasant symptoms, including acne.

In fact, it was in part her own success in clearing her complexion that caused Myer to gravitate toward this field as her specialty. Myer was familiar with the elimination diet as a tool, and she had reason to suspect dairy products as a possible culprit. As they had entered adulthood, many members of her immediate family had developed sensitivities to diary products. Her own father got pimples on his back whenever he overindulged in his favorite food—buttermilk.

Myer knew what she needed to do. After a few days' fast she began adding suspect foods back into her diet one at a time. The fact that she loved dairy products so much (craved them, in fact) was another clue. "Please, please don't let it be dairy," she thought. But it was. As soon as she added dairy products back into her diet, she developed the tell-tale sniffles—a sign that her body was reacting negatively and was, indeed, sensitive to dairy products.

Myer stopped eating dairy products almost completely, and ever since then her skin has been clear.

Almost completely?

Myers says, "I save my poker chips for what I really like, which is cheese. I don't eat a lot of cheese. And I buy really good cheese, so I really can enjoy it when I eat it."

Clear skin, a new career, and she still gets to eat an occasional morsel of really good cheese—not a bad payoff for one elimination diet.

trointestinal symptoms, like diarrhea, gas, or abdominal discomfort; or even emotional reactions, such as anxiety or depression. But reactions tell the tale. If you discover that you're sensitive to a particular food, your best bet is to either eliminate it entirely or to eat it only on rare occasions, in moderation, notes Myer.

Unfortunately, it's difficult to do an elimination diet on your own, says Myer. A health care practitioner who is experienced in supervising this procedure begins with an interview—a careful medical history that is likely to reveal suspect foods right from the start. As the individual resumes eating after a fast, foods are carefully reintroduced one at a time.

The problem with trying this on your own is that there are so many emotional issues that surround food, she says, that it's all too easy to misread or overlook reactions. It's also dangerously easy to either trigger an eating disorder or revive an old eating disorder. And it's easy to make a mistake, either refusing to believe that a favorite food is actually causing a reaction or to misinterpret results and needlessly eliminate a food that's perfectly good for you. Why deprive yourself of something if you don't really need to?

A health care practitioner such as a naturopath or a registered dietician who supervises elimination diets is rather like a detective who follows clues to solve a mystery, says Myer. The clues are the subtle and not-so-subtle reactions to problematic foods. At the end of 2 weeks or so the culprits—the offending foods—have been identified.

Eliminating foods that you are sensitive to can make a dramatic difference in your health. Plugging that leaky gut can bring improvement to such wide-ranging health problems as arthritis symptoms, migraines, chronic fatigue, many skin conditions, obesity, and numerous digestive disorders.

While you need supervision to do an elimination diet, there are a number of things you can do on your own, in addition to eating a nature-based diet from the Earth, to promote your body's ongoing detoxification efforts.

JUICE UP YOUR LIFE

One of the most efficient ways to take advantage of the multitude of nutrients in fruits and vegetables is through juicing. Juicing simply allows you to take in more nutrients, period. Your liver loves juices. Your small intestine loves juices. And so do all the other organs in your body.

If you eat a carrot, you get the nutrients of one carrot. Even the most avid health enthusiast is not going to sit and eat eight carrots at one sitting. But you can juice eight carrots with relative ease. Eight carrots yield approximately 1 cup of sweet, delectable juice that is so full of nutrients that it almost feels electric after it goes down, especially if you drink it while fasting. In fact, many experts who supervise therapeutic fasts recommend supporting your detoxifying efforts with freshly made juices whenever you fast.

"Juices are absorbed readily, easily, with very little effort," says Dr. Demers. Juices are also an easy way to get all the nutrients that you need to help your body do its cleansing and detoxifying work on a daily basis. They support a fast, and they also support your daily diet.

When you drink juices throughout the day, "your body gets the nutrients it needs to support the detox process," explains Alleman.

Although juice bars that prepare fresh juices are proliferating around the country, many cities still don't have even one. And machines that juice vegetables are not exactly cheap. Should you take the plunge?

If you're serious about detoxifying your body, and especially if you plan to fast on a regular basis, the answer is yes.

But only if you're going to really use the machine. Just as there are lots of treadmills and stationary bikes sitting unused in dusty corners, there are plenty of juicing machines hidden away in dark kitchen cabinets.

There are two keys to buying a machine that you will use on a regular basis.

Look for easy cleanup. Unless you're going to be juicing for a large family, consider buying a machine that uses a filter. (If you routinely juice for several people at a time, you'll have to change the filter so often that it's impractical.) Then, instead of having to deal with fruit and vegetable fibers that get into every nook and cranny of the machine, you simply pull out the filter and toss it into the compost. You can clean the machine parts afterward with just a quick rinse.

Try new recipes. If you juice carrots, you'll love it. But you probably won't love it every day, especially since you have to clean the machine every time you make a glass of juice. But if you buy a few books that contain juice recipes and try new ones on a regular basis, you're more likely to continue using your juicer. The "I can't believe that tasted so fabulous" recipes will keep you coming back for more.

If you use the juicer often enough in the first months after you buy it, you'll begin to see the difference in your body and feel the difference that it makes in your health. Then you'll be hooked. In any case, if you're going to fast on a regular basis, you need a juicer.

CLEAN UP YOUR FOOD ACT

We've been talking about making the kinds of food choices that will help your body's detoxification efforts. But it's also important to clean up your food act, literally.

Choose organic produce whenever possible. You can detoxify your body to the best of your ability, but if you continue to take in more poisons, you're more or less running in place. Study after study has shown that pesticide residues are found in nonorganic produce. (Some residues are even found in organic produce, but the quantities are minute in comparison.)

"I am a promoter of organic produce for lots of reasons," says Myer. While pesticide residues are not good for anybody—especially children and the elderly—some people are more sensitive than others. These are the "canaries" of our society, she explains. (In the old days, miners used to take canaries down into the mines to alert them when poison gases were present. When the canary keeled over, the miners would hightail it out of the mine.) The ever-increasing numbers of people with asthma, chronic fatigue, skin conditions, joint pain, and cancer are the canaries, letting us all know that we're being exposed to too many pollutants. Short of moving, there's not much you can do about poisons in the air; however, you can limit the poisons you consume by turning to organic produce and by limiting the amount of processed foods that you eat.

Learn the secret signs of a clean restaurant. Food poisoning comes from toxic bacteria. Just about everyone has experienced an episode of vomiting or diarrhea a day or two after eating in a restaurant. But did you know that every year a couple hundred people in the United States *die* from food poisoning?

While there's no way to ever be 100 percent certain that a restaurant's kitchen is clean, here's a tip from the long-time owner of an Italian restaurant in Spokane, Washington. Look at three things in a restaurant:

⑥ The restroom
⑥ The menus
⑥ Any glass around the entryway

If the owner of the restaurant doesn't take steps to see that these things that are seen by the public are kept clean, there's a good chance that the kitchen is filthy. Find somewhere else to eat.

Strictly avoid anything that's rancid. Ever pick up a can of nuts and notice that they taste a little odd? Ever open a bottle of cooking oil and notice a slightly "off" smell? You might be tempted to nibble the nuts or use the oil anyway. Many people do, because these things just don't smell spoiled the way a bad chicken or a bad piece of fish smells spoiled. Big mistake!

Rancid oils won't make you obviously sick the way spoiled meat can. But rancid oils produce vast numbers of free radicals—very active oxygen molecules that do serious damage in the body. Bad oils are seriously toxic, contribute to aging, and can even trigger cancerous changes in cells.

Set realistic limits. If fruits and vegetables are good for you, what about going on a diet that's exclusively fruits and vegetables? What about being a vegetarian or vegan? What about the raw foods diet that's getting so much attention of late? (Don't the celebrities on that diet just *glow*?) What about macrobiotics? And so on and so on.

Any diet that incorporates a lot of fruits and vegetables is good for you, says Myer. And it's good for you precisely because it contains lots of fruits and vegetables. Vegetarianism and veganism can be healthy diets, but adherents need to be careful of ending up with chronic protein, essential fatty acid, and mineral deficiencies.

BUY FOODS THAT WORK FOR YOU

Of course, there are any number of other things you can do to get more detoxification "oomph" from the foods you eat on a regular basis. Take a look at what's available around you in your day-to-day world of shopping and cooking and eating out. Many of the decisions that you make every day can make a significant difference in whether your body's detoxification efforts are being adequately supported. You should make it your mission to find ways to add detoxifying foods to your life.

Here are a few examples of the kinds of things you can do.

Buy real yogurt. Your body contains a lot of bacteria. Amazingly enough, there are more bacteria in your gut than there are cells in your body. (Bacteria, obviously, are much smaller than most cells.) You have a pretty important relationship with them, too. When you have the right kind of bacteria in your gut, these friendly guys help you digest your food and keep the bad bacteria from moving in.

Whenever you use antibiotics, you kill off most of the bacteria in your body—the bad ones that you're targeting and the good ones, as well. If you fast, many bacteria get flushed away. And as you age, the right kind of bacteria can move out, to be replaced by bad neighbors. To keep the right kind of bacterial colonies thriving in your gut, it's helpful to eat yogurt that contains "live cultures" on a regular basis.

Read the label to make sure it specifically says that the microorganisms are *Lactobacillus acidophilus*. These bacteria will take up residence in your gut, taking the place of the kind of bacteria that exude toxins and can make you sick.

Note: It's no longer enough to simply find "live cultures" on the label. (Keep in mind that most commercial yogurt is now thickened with dead bacteria, not the live ones that you want.) Some yogurt manufacturers have found that other kinds of bacteria work better as thickeners, while still delivering a tasty product. Unfortunately, the bacteria that they are using, while they won't hurt you, are not able to provide the health-giving functions of *Lactobacillus.*

One other little thing to look for on the label: See if you can find a product that is 100 percent yogurt. Most low-fat and nonfat yogurt today is made with gelatin. That's a meat product, not a dairy product. While there's nothing wrong with eating gelatin, you can make a gelatin dessert for a lot less money than it costs to buy real yogurt.

Fortunately, you can still find good commercial yogurt if you take the trouble to read the label. Best bet: Buy plain yogurt, not the flavored kind. Drizzle it with honey or maple syrup, add a handful of berries or chopped peaches and a sprinkle of your favorite nuts, and you'll be in breakfast heaven.

Buy real juice. Of course, it's best to make your own juice. But if you're like most folks, you sometimes need the convenience of prepared juices. Don't assume that a juice product that you buy in a natural food store is healthy. Some of the expensive juices that come in earthy, healthy-looking individual serving bottles are full of sugar and "natural flavors" that are only remotely related to fruit juice. At the same time, it's possible to buy 100 percent juice in a big, clunky, inexpensive can in the supermarket. Just make sure you read the labels.

Expand your garlic repertoire. Garlic

really does a couple of detoxification jobs for you. First, it contains nutrients that help the second phase of your liver's detoxification system. Second, it helps eliminate harmful bacteria and yeasts from your intestines.

There are numerous ways to enjoy raw garlic. Try throwing a handful of raw garlic on top of the next commercial frozen pizza that you heat up. (We're assuming here that you're not eating things like commercial frozen pizza every night!) Follow the package directions, except slide the pizza out exactly 1 minute before it's done. Sprinkle a tablespoon (or two, if you can take it) on top of the pizza. Then let it heat for 1 more minute.

A handful of raw garlic is also great on pasta drizzled with a little olive oil and sprinkled with grated Parmesan cheese.

WATER FIT TO DRINK

About 40 percent of Americans use some kind of filter or purifier to treat their drinking water. Should you? Or might you stay just as healthy—and perhaps a bit happier—if you spent that cash on, say, a seaweed wrap at your favorite day spa?

That depends on where you live.

"Water quality varies tremendously from one water supply to another," explains Erik Olson, head of the Natural Resources Defense Council's drinking-water program. If you live in Chicago, for example, you can probably save your money. According to a report released in 2003, when the NRDC tested water in 19 American cities, Chicago was the only one that got an "excellent" rating. Most were rated "good" or "mediocre."

If you live in Boston, Phoenix, or San Francisco, you may need to shell out for at-home treatment. Those cities' water systems were rated "poor" because they contained contaminants such as bacteria, potentially cancer-causing chemicals, and lead.

Looks Clean, but Is It?

To determine whether you need to treat the water you drink, first find out what, if any, unhealthy contaminants are lurking in it. To do that:

Get the report. The federal Safe Drinking Water Act requires water companies to issue annual reports on contaminant levels. Yours should come with your water bill. If it doesn't, call the water company and ask for a copy. You may also find the reports at the local library or, if your water company is large enough, at the Environmental Agency Web site. (Go to www.prevention.com/links.)

Read the whole thing. In its investigation, the NRDC found that several water companies buried bad news inside their reports. The cover page of the Washington, D.C.'s, for example, announced, "Your drinking water is safe." But the pages that followed revealed that the city's water contained worrisome levels of lead and potentially harmful chemicals.

Double-check the numbers. In addition to revealing levels of contaminants in your water, your report should specify the Environmental Protection Agency's "MCL" or "maximum [allowable] contaminant level" for each. If a contaminant level exceeds the MCL, the EPA will require your water company to fix it. But don't rest easy, figuring that your water is safe.

It Came from the Faucet

Lead, which can lower children's IQs and cause developmental delays; in adults it can boost blood pressure and cause kidney problems.

Potential carcinogens, including asbestos, radium, benzene, trichloroethylene, radon, the pesticide atrazine, and perchlorate, a chemical known for causing thyroid tumors and, in fetuses and infants, delaying development.

Microorganisms, including giardia and cryptosporidium; fecal bacteria, such as fecal coliform; and viruses. These are a particular risk for infants and anyone with a weakened immune system, including those with HIV, transplant recipients, chemotherapy patients, and the frail elderly.

By-products of chlorination, such as trihalomethanes and halocetic acids, which may cause cancer, reproductive problems, and birth defects.

Nitrate (from fertilizers and human and animal waste), which can interfere with the blood's ability to carry oxygen and is especially hazardous to infants; it also may be linked to miscarriages and birth defects.

Heavy metals, such as mercury and cadmium, which may cause kidney and neurological damage.

You should also pay attention to contaminants that come *close* to the MCL, says Olson. Since companies are required to test only periodically, a contaminant that nears the MCL during testing could exceed it at other times.

If you are pregnant or have an infant at home, look for levels of nitrate, a contaminant from fertilizer and feces, and chlorination by-products called trihalomethanes, Olson says. These may increase risks of miscarriage, birth defects, and other health problems.

Call the company. Most water companies test for more contaminants than the EPA requires. Call yours and ask if it has found high levels of any contaminants it tests for voluntarily, since these may not appear in your annual report, says Olson. Ask if they've taken steps to remove the contaminants.

Got kids? Test for lead. If your kids are 6 years old or younger, test for lead, even if your annual report shows low levels of this toxic metal in your water supply, Olson says. These days, lead contamination often originates *inside* the house, he explains.

Most cities have replaced old lead water mains with iron ones. But older buildings may be plumbed with lead pipes or copper pipes welded with leaded solder. Even new "lead-free" faucets may be made from brass that contains enough lead to cause problems, such as lower IQs, Olson says.

FIND THE RIGHT TREATMENT

If you do find something in your water, which treatment system should you use? Again, that depends—on what's in there, on whether you want to treat every drop that enters your home, and on how much you're willing to spend. There are several different types of treatment devices, from carbon filters to more complex ion exchange systems and distillers, and they range in price from $20 to $2,500. Unfortunately, there's no single system that removes all contaminants, explains Joseph Harrison, technical director of the Water Quality Association (WQA), an industry group. So you might need more than one device.

Complicating matters (just a little): Most types come in a variety of models. There are pitchers, devices that screw to faucets, and under-the-sink units that attach to the cold-water line and feed treated water to a third faucet that's installed on the sink board. There are also more pricey point-of-entry or whole-house systems (installed where the water enters your home) that treat all your

TREAT YOUR WATER RIGHT

System	What It Removes	Available As	Cost
Activated granular carbon filters	Atrazine, benzene, mercury, trichloroethylene, trihalomethanes, and radon *Note:* These filters may include other materials, in addition to carbon, that remove additional contaminants, such as lead.	Pitchers,* faucet-mounted, under-sink, and whole-house	From about $20 for faucet-mounted to $1,800 for whole-house
Solid block carbon filters	Asbestos, atrazine, benzene, lead, mercury, trichloroethylene, trihalomethanes, giardia, and cryptosporidium	Pitchers,* faucet-mounted, and under-sink	From about $30 for faucet-mounted to $400 for under-sink
Reverse osmosis system	Arsenic, asbestos, atrazine, lead, mercury, nitrate, radium, cryptosporidium, and fluoride *Note:* These systems usually include carbon filters that also remove benzene, radon, trichloroethylene, and trihalomethanes.	Faucet-mounted and under-sink	$200 to $1,000
Distillers	Arsenic, asbestos, lead, mercury, nitrate, trichloroethylene, trihalomethanes, radium, coliform bacteria, cryptosporidium, and fluoride *Note:* These usually include charcoal filters that also remove atrazine, benzene, and radon.	Faucet-mounted and under-sink	$100 to $500
Ion exchange systems (water softeners)	Calcium and magnesium (minerals that shorten the life of household plumbing and make it harder to scrape away soap residue) *Note:* Some ion exchange systems also remove iron, manganese, aluminum, lead, and radium. Anion exchange systems, a variation on ion exchange systems, may remove arsenic, nitrate, mercury, sulfate, and perchlorate, in addition to the contaminants ion exchange systems remove.	Whole-house	$800 to $2,500 *Pitchers range from about $20 to $45.

water for drinking, dishwashing, bathing, and laundering. Why choose one of these? Showers are a particular problem because you can inhale trialomethanes, which have been linked to cancer and miscarriage, says Olson.

On the opposite page there's a guide that compares several different types of water-treatment systems. When shopping, look for a model certified by an independent lab such as NSF International, the WQA, or Underwriters Laboratories, and check the manufacturer's specifications to make sure it removes the contaminants in your supply.

Chapter 4

Recipes for Purification

FRUIT, VEGETABLES, WHOLE GRAINS . . . with all of Nature's bounty from which to choose ingredients, preparing food that purifies and detoxifies your body should be an ongoing delightful adventure. If you do the main part of your shopping in the produce aisle and keep packaged foods to a minimum, you're on the right path. Here are some scrumptious recipes to get you started.

Breakfast
Apple Pancakes

These ginger-spiced pancakes are terrific, and they're ready in just 20 minutes.

⅔ cup whole wheat flour

⅔ cup unbleached flour

⅓ cup cornmeal

1 tablespoon baking powder

1 teaspoon ground ginger

½ teaspoon baking soda

2 cups fat-free plain yogurt

¾ cup fat-free egg substitute

¼ cup honey

2 tablespoons canola oil

1 apple, shredded

Coat a large, nonstick skillet with nonstick cooking spray and heat over medium heat.

In a blender or food processor, pulse the whole wheat and unbleached flours, cornmeal, baking powder, ginger, baking soda, yogurt, egg substitute, honey, and oil until just combined. By hand, stir the apple into the batter.

For each pancake, spoon 2 or 3 tablespoons of the batter into the skillet. Cook until lightly browned and cooked through, about

2 minutes on each side. Repeat with the remaining batter.

Good for:

> Digestion
>
> Improving liver function
>
> Colon health

Apples contain pectin, a kind of water-soluble fiber that sweeps the intestines clean of toxins. Whole wheat flour and cornmeal are also rich in fiber.

Makes 12 servings

Per serving: 137 calories, 5 g protein, 25 g carbohydrates, 3 g fat, 1 mg cholesterol, 223 mg sodium, 1 g fiber

Berry Morning Crush

Reduced-fat cottage cheese provides a good supply of lean protein to help the liver carry out its detoxification duties; the fruit and nuts offer health-promoting antioxidants.

> 1 cup plain yogurt
>
> 2 tablespoons honey
>
> ½ cup reduced-fat cottage cheese
>
> ½ cup blueberries and/or sliced strawberries
>
> 2 tablespoons crushed walnuts or almonds

In individual cups or a large bowl, mix the yogurt, honey, cottage cheese, berries, and nuts. Serve.

Good for:

> Heart health
>
> Digestion

Cottage cheese is high in protein, which the body needs to do its detoxification work, while walnuts are rich in omega-3 fatty acids, good fats that combat heart disease. Berries are excellent sources of fiber and disease-fighting antioxidants.

Makes 2 servings

Per serving: 259 calories, 14 g protein, 37 g carbohydrates, 7 g fat, 20 mg cholesterol, 312 mg sodium, 3 g fiber

Breakfast Rice Pudding *yummy*

Eat dessert for breakfast—we turned this homey favorite healthy with tofu and brown rice.

 9 ounces soft tofu

 ¼ cup honey

 2 teaspoons vanilla

 ½ teaspoon cinnamon

 1½ cups cooked brown rice

 ¼ cup raisins

 ¼ cup almonds

In a blender, blend the tofu until smooth. Spoon into a bowl and add the honey, vanilla, cinnamon, rice, raisins, and almonds. Mix well. Chill for several hours to blend the flavors.

Good for:

 Immune function
 Heart health
 Digestion

Tofu is a good source of zinc, necessary for good immune function, while cinnamon may help stop the growth of bacteria and fungi, including candida yeast. Brown rice is rich in fiber, which helps the body eliminate toxins, as well as manganese, selenium, and magnesium, enzymes that help in the detoxification process.

Makes 4 servings

Per serving: 272 calories, 7 g protein, 47 g carbohydrates, 7 g fat, 0 mg cholesterol, 6 mg sodium, 3 g fiber

Fruit Melba Breakfast "Sundae"

Yummy fruit and nuts spooned over smooth and creamy yogurt. This is a "sundae" you can feel good about eating!

 ½ package (5 ounces) frozen raspberries, thawed

 1 medium fruit of your choice (we suggest 1 ripe peach—unpeeled if organic, peeled if not—a banana, or an orange)

 4 ounces fat-free plain yogurt

 2 tablespoons sliced toasted almonds

Place the raspberries in a food processor. Process until the berries form a smooth puree. Pit and slice the peach or other fruit. Divide the yogurt between two goblets. Spoon the puree over the yogurt, and top with the peach or other fruit. Garnish with the almonds.

Good for:

 Heart health
 Digestion
 Bone health

Raspberries are rich in anthocyanins, plant chemicals with potent antioxidant powers, while yogurt is a good source of protein, B vitamins, and minerals, including calcium.

Makes 2 servings

Per serving: 127 calories, 5 g protein, 19 g carbohydrates, 5 g fat, 1 mg cholesterol, 34 mg sodium, 3 g fiber

Fruited Yogurt Muesli

Plain yogurt comes alive with bursts of sweet and tangy flavor in a high-fiber treat.

1⅓ cups rolled oats

2⅔ cups water

1 tablespoon fat-free plain yogurt

1 tablespoon honey

2 tangerines, peeled and sectioned

2 unpeeled apples, chopped

In a large bowl, soak the oats in the water overnight, or let stand in the water for about 1 hour right before preparing. Stir in the yogurt, honey, tangerines, and apples. Refrigerate any leftovers.

Good for:

Reducing candida yeast

Improving liver function

Colon health

Digestion

Lowering cholesterol

Yogurt contains probiotics, good bacteria that take up residence in the intestine and protect the body from the bad bacteria and yeast overgrowth. Tangerines contain lycopene, which helps the liver do its job of detoxifying the body. Apples and rolled oats contain fiber, which cleanses the digestive system, lowers cholesterol, and protects heart health.

Makes 4 servings

Per serving: 180 calories, 5 g protein, 38 g carbohydrates, 2 g fat, 0 mg cholesterol, 9 mg sodium, 6 g fiber

Mandarin-Kiwifruit Parfaits

Is it breakfast or is it dessert? It's good for you. It tastes scrumptious. Eat it anytime!

2 cups fat-free lemon yogurt

1 can (11 ounces) mandarin oranges, drained

2 kiwifruit, halved and sliced

4 gingersnap cookies

In each of 4 parfait glasses, alternately layer the yogurt with the oranges and kiwi. Cover with plastic wrap and refrigerate until ready to serve. Serve with a gingersnap.

Good for:

Improving liver function

Antiaging

Colon health

Reducing candida yeast

Kiwis and oranges are both rich in vitamin C, an antioxidant that cleanses the body of harmful free radicals and thereby has an antiaging effect. Oranges also contain limonene, a nutrient that supports the liver's work of detoxifying the body. Yogurt contains probiotics, good bacteria that prevent toxic bacteria and yeasts from growing in the intestines.

Makes 4 servings

Per serving: 150 calories, 5 g protein, 30 g carbohydrates, 1 g fat, 3 mg cholesterol, 81 mg sodium, 1 g fiber

Entrees

Barley with Ginger and Broccoli

This dish offers nutritional support to the liver without adding to its toxic burden.

6 cups water

1 cup dry barley

1 one-inch cube of fresh ginger, sliced

1 small head of broccoli, chopped into pieces

1 teaspoon thyme

1½ teaspoons oregano

1½ teaspoons basil

Black pepper and ghee to taste

Place the water, barley, and ginger together in a medium saucepan, and bring to a boil. Lower the heat, cover the pan, and let the mixture simmer for 35 minutes. Add the broccoli and continue to simmer until the barley is cooked, about 25 minutes more. Add the thyme, oregano, basil, black pepper, and ghee. Simmer a few minutes more, then serve.

Good for:

Fasting and cleansing

Constipation

Liver support

Broccoli contains sulphorophanes, biochemicals that the liver needs in order to carry out its work of detoxifying the body. Both broccoli and barley are high in fiber, which helps reduce cholesterol while sweeping toxins from the body. This cleansing dish can be used during a semi-fast.

Makes 2 servings

Per serving: 181 calories, 7 g protein, 37 g carbohydrates, 1 g fat, 0 mg cholesterol, 31 mg sodium, 10 g fiber (Analysis does not include ghee, which can be added to taste.)

Fenugreek Kichari

Kichari is a traditional Indian rice dish. Most variations are appropriate for use during semi-fasts. You're not likely to feel deprived if you include this nourishing and satisfying dish in your diet.

¼ cup fenugreek seeds

1½ cups water

1 cup basmati rice

¼ teaspoon turmeric

1 teaspoon salt

3 tablespoons ghee

1 tablespoon cumin seeds

Soak the seeds overnight in the water.

Put the rice in a pot with the seeds and water and bring to a boil. Scrape off the foam and add the turmeric and salt. Cover loosely and simmer over medium-low heat until all the water is gone, about 20 minutes.

In a skillet, heat the ghee to the smoking point and add the cumin seeds. Cover and remove from heat. Let it stand 15 to 30 seconds before adding to the rice mixture.

Good for:

Fasting and cleansing

The flavored rice in this dish is unlikely to provoke food sensitivities of any kind. It offers gentle nutritional support during a semi-fast.

Makes 4 servings

Per serving: 297 calories, 7 g protein, 43 g carbohydrates, 12 g fat, 25 mg cholesterol, 594 mg sodium, 5 g fiber

Ghee Whiz

You can buy ghee (pronounced like the *gee* in "geek") in Indian specialty shops and many natural foods stores. You can also make your own by melting a pound of butter and carefully skimming off the foam that rises to the top. The clear oil that remains behind is ghee. It will keep in the refrigerator for several weeks. It can be used for frying, as it doesn't burn the way butter does. (Note that in a detoxifying diet, fried foods should be kept to a minimum.) Traditional Indian detoxification techniques, especially those in ayurvedic medicine, rely on the scrumptious, buttery taste of ghee to flavor simple foods. It's viewed as a food particularly high in life force (*prana*).

Chicken Tamale Pie

Tired of the same old chicken breast recipes? Try this spicy alternative that is both easy to make and a real crowd-pleaser.

½ cup cornmeal

½ cup unbleached flour

1 tablespoon sugar

1½ teaspoons baking powder

¾ pound boneless, skinless chicken breast, cubed

½ cup chopped onions

2 tablespoons chili powder

1 can (14½ ounces) low-sodium tomatoes

1 cup corn

1 cup chopped green bell peppers

1 cup canned kidney beans, rinsed

1 teaspoon dried oregano

⅓ cup fat-free milk

¼ cup fat-free egg substitute

Place the cornmeal, flour, sugar, and baking powder in a resealable plastic bag. Set aside.

Coat a nonstick skillet with nonstick cooking spray; heat for 1 minute. Add the chicken, onions, and chili powder. Cook, stirring often, until the chicken is browned and cooked through. Add the tomatoes, corn, peppers, beans, and oregano, stirring to break up the tomatoes. Spoon into an 8-inch-square baking dish. At this point you can finish making the casserole or cover it with foil and refrigerate it until the next day.

To finish the casserole, cover it and bake at 400°F for 10 minutes. Pour the milk and egg substitute into the bag containing the cornmeal mix. Seal the bag and knead to mix the ingredients. Stir the casserole. Cut a corner from bag and squeeze the batter over the casserole. Bake until a toothpick inserted into the cornbread comes out clean, about 20 minutes.

Good for:

Detoxifying the colon

Prostate health

Improving liver function

Antiaging

Peppers and kidney beans are high in fiber, which helps speed waste through the colon. Green peppers and tomatoes are high in vitamin C, an antiaging antioxidant. Onions contain sulfur and chicken has protein, both of which promote liver function.

Makes 4 servings

Per serving: 384 calories, 32 g protein, 60 g carbohydrates, 3 g fat, 50 mg cholesterol, 327 mg sodium, 9 g fiber

Eggplant Casserole with Herbed Tomato Sauce

Bursting with the robust flavors of tomato, garlic, olive oil, and herbs, this tofu-based casserole only tastes decadent.

- 10 ounces firm tofu
- 1 can (15 ounces) tomato sauce
- 1 cup canned tomato puree
- 1½ tablespoons dried oregano
- 4 cloves garlic, minced
- Black pepper
- 3 medium zucchini
- 2 medium fresh tomatoes
- 1 medium eggplant
- ¼ teaspoon olive oil
- 1 medium onion, diced
- 6 slices whole grain bread

Drain the tofu on a paper towel; cut into ¼-inch slices. Preheat the oven to 350°F.

In a large mixing bowl, blend the tomato sauce, tomato puree, oregano, garlic, and black pepper; set aside.

Wash the zucchini, tomatoes, and eggplant well. Cut the zucchini lengthwise into ¼-inch slices. Cut the tomatoes crosswise into ¼-inch slices. Peel the eggplant and cut it crosswise into ¼-inch slices.

Rub the inside of a 3½-quart casserole dish with the olive oil. Spread ¼ cup of the blended sauce in the bottom of the dish. Top with a layer of eggplant, then a layer of zucchini. Distribute ½ of the onion over the zucchini, then top evenly with the tofu and bread. (The slices may overlap.) Top the bread evenly with the tomato slices and half of the remaining sauce. Add the remaining onion, the remaining eggplant, and the remaining zucchini. Spread the remaining sauce evenly over the zucchini. Cover and bake for 45 to 50 minutes, or until the vegetables are tender when pierced with a fork. Remove the lid and allow the casserole to stand at room temperature for 5 to 10 minutes before cutting. Serve hot.

Good for:

- Heart health
- Digestion
- Eye health
- Cancer protection

Eggplant contains nasunin, an antioxidant shown to protect cell membranes from damage. Tomatoes are rich in lycopene, which protects against cancers of the stomach, colon, mouth, and esophagus. Zucchini is a good source of fiber, potassium, and vitamin C, and also contains the carotinoids lutein and zeaxanthin, which protect eye health.

Makes 4 servings

Per serving: 304 calories, 17 g protein, 54 g carbohydrates, 6 g fat, 0 mg cholesterol, 1,103 mg sodium, 13 g fiber

Chicken Cassoulet

This elegant meal takes its name from a classic French recipe made with fatty duck meat and ham hocks. We slimmed it down by using chicken breasts and low-fat turkey kielbasa.

1 can (15 ounces) no-sodium small white
     beans, rinsed and drained

4 boneless, skinless chicken breast halves

¼ teaspoon pepper

1 tablespoon olive oil

6 ounces turkey kielbasa, sliced ¼-inch thick

½ can (14½ ounces) reduced-sodium chicken
     broth

1 cup chopped onions

¾ cup seasoned bread crumbs

¼ cup sun-dried tomatoes (not packed in
     oil), thinly sliced

2 tablespoons fresh basil or
     2 teaspoons dried chopped basil

Preheat the oven to 350°F. Spread half of the beans in a 2-quart casserole.

Season the chicken on both sides with the pepper. In a large skillet over medium heat, brown the chicken in the oil for 5 minutes, turning once. Transfer the chicken to the casserole. Top with the kielbasa slices, remaining beans, and broth.

In the same skillet, cook the onions for 4 minutes, stirring to loosen any browned bits from the pan. Stir in the bread crumbs, tomatoes, and basil. Cook, stirring, for 2 minutes. Spread over the beans, patting to create a thick crust. Cover and bake for 10 minutes. Remove the cover and bake for 15 minutes or until the crust is browned. Serve. Alternately, the casserole can be frozen at this point. To serve, thaw in the refrigerator first, then reheat in the oven.

Good for:

Improving liver function
Antiaging
Detoxifying the colon

Basil and sun-dried tomatoes are rich in body-protecting antioxidants. Beans are high in fiber, which helps sweep waste from the body. Chicken and turkey kielbasa are good sources of low-fat, high-quality protein to support the liver's detoxification efforts.

Makes 4 servings

Per serving: 400 calories, 43 g protein, 35 g carbohydrates, 10 g fat, 95 mg cholesterol, 6 g fiber

Mexican Red Rice and Beans ✗

Got fiber? You do when you enjoy this spicy and flavorful dish!

  1 teaspoon olive oil

  ½ cup chopped onions

  ½ clove garlic, minced

  ¾ cup plus 1 tablespoon water

  ½ cup uncooked brown or basmati rice

  1 small can (4 ounces) tomato sauce

  ½ small green bell pepper, chopped

  ¼ teaspoon chili powder

  ¼ teaspoon dried oregano leaves

  ¼ teaspoon dried cumin

  Pinch salt (optional)

  1 or 2 drops hot pepper sauce ┼

  1 can (8 ounces) reduced-sodium kidney
    beans, rinsed and drained

  2 tomatoes, chopped

In a large saucepan, combine the oil, onions, garlic, and 1 tablespoon of the water. Cook over medium heat, stirring frequently, for 6 to 7 minutes, or until the onions soften.

Add the rice, tomato sauce, green pepper, chili powder, oregano, cumin, salt (if using), hot pepper sauce, and the remaining ¾ cup of water. Stir, bring to a boil, and simmer for 20 minutes, or until the rice is tender and the liquid has been absorbed. Stir in the beans and tomatoes. Cook over low heat for 2 minutes, or until heated through. Makes 2 servings.

Good for:

  Heart health

  Digestion

  Cancer protection

Tomatoes are a good source of vitamins A and C, and they contain the antioxidant lycopene, which helps prevent cancer. Kidney beans contain phytic acid, shown to prevent colon cancer in animals.

Makes 2 servings

Per serving: 230 calories, 9 g protein, 42 g carbohydrates, 4 g fat, 0 mg cholesterol, 566 mg sodium, 10 g fiber

Orange Roughy Veracruz

Fish is always a heart-healthy choice. Fish is not only lower in fat than red meat, but it also contains a kind of fat that's good for you. With this lively, spicy dish, eating more fish is a pleasure.

   4 orange roughy or red snapper fillets (4 ounces each)

   1 tablespoon lime juice

   1 teaspoon dried oregano

   2 teaspoons olive oil

   1 onion, chopped

   1 garlic clove, minced

   1 can (15 ounces) Mexican-style diced tomatoes

   12 pimiento-stuffed olives, coarsely chopped

   2 tablespoons parsley, chopped

Preheat the oven to 350°F. Coat an 8-inch-square baking dish with nonstick cooking spray. Place the fillets in the baking dish. Sprinkle with the lime juice and oregano. Set aside.

Warm the oil in a medium skillet over medium heat. Add the onion and garlic. Cook, stirring occasionally, for 5 to 6 minutes or until soft. Add the tomatoes, olives, and parsley. Cook, stirring occasionally, for 5 minutes, or until thickened. Spoon over the fillets. Cover tightly.

Bake for 18 to 20 minutes, or until the fish flakes easily.

Good for:

   Lowering cholesterol

   Arthritis

   Improving liver function

   Weight loss

   Prostate health

Fish oils have been shown to lower cholesterol. Onions contain sulfur, which helps support the liver's detoxification efforts. Tomatoes contain lycopene, a phytochemical that helps protect the prostate gland. This entree is also low in calories.

Makes 4 servings

Per serving: 160 calories, 18 g protein, 23 g carbohydrates, 5 g fat, 23 mg cholesterol, 513 mg sodium, 2 g fiber

Shrimp with Ginger, Broccoli, and Corn

Exotic tasting yet easy-to-find flavorings make this stir-fry extra-special.

2 cups broccoli florets

1½ tablespoons reduced-sodium soy sauce

1 tablespoon rice vinegar

½ tablespoon chopped fresh ginger

½ teaspoon chile-garlic paste

1¼ teaspoons toasted sesame oil

2 scallions, thinly sliced

1 cup corn kernels

½ pound large shrimp, peeled and deveined

Place the broccoli in a steamer, and gently steam over low heat until crisp-tender, about 4 minutes. In a small bowl, whisk together the soy sauce, vinegar, ginger, and chile-garlic paste.

Just before serving, heat a large nonstick skillet over high heat. Add the oil. When it ripples, add the scallions, corn, and shrimp. Stir-fry for 2 to 3 minutes, or until the shrimp are no longer translucent. Add the broccoli and the soy mixture, and stir-fry until all the ingredients are coated with the sauce and heated through.

Good for:

Cancer protection

Heart health

Immune function

The main active components of ginger, gingerols, may inhibit the growth of cancer cells. Shrimp is an excellent source of the mineral selenium, shown to protect cells from damage, support heart health, and boost immunity.

Makes 2 servings

Per serving: 270 calories, 29 g protein, 28 g carbohydrates, 6 g fat, 172 mg cholesterol, 576 mg sodium, 5 g fiber

Very Veggie Omelet

The fresh veggies provide flavor as well as a decent dose of fiber, which helps satisfy even the heartiest of appetites.

2 eggs, well beaten

3 tablespoons chopped red bell pepper

2 tablespoons chopped green bell pepper

2 tablespoons chopped tomato, seeded

2 tablespoons chopped zucchini

2 tablespoons chopped mushrooms (optional)

Salt and ground black pepper

Coat a large skillet with olive oil cooking spray and place it over medium heat. When the skillet is warm, add the eggs, allowing them to cover the bottom of the pan. Cook for 3 minutes, or until the bottom begins to set. When nearly cooked, top half of the omelet with the red and green bell peppers, tomato, zucchini, mushrooms (if using), salt, and black pepper. Carefully fold the remaining half over the filling and cook for 2 minutes, or until cooked through.

Good for:

Improving liver function

Heart health

Cancer protection

Digestion

Eggs are rich in choline, a substance that assists with the removal of fat in the liver. The vegetables provide fiber, which reduces the risk of heart disease and cancer, and the peppers are rich sources of the disease-fighting antioxidants vitamin C and beta-carotene.

Makes 1 serving

Per serving: 164 calories, 13 g protein, 5 g carbohydrates, 10 g fat, 425 mg cholesterol, 129 mg sodium, 1 g fiber

Tuna Tater

This good-for-you combo of lean protein (tuna and Cheddar) and healthy carbs makes a delicious and satisfying meal.

1 medium baking potato

½ package (5 ounces) frozen broccoli florets, thawed

½ can (3 ounces) albacore tuna in water, drained

2 tablespoons low-fat shredded Cheddar cheese

Prick the potato with a fork, and microwave it on high for 8 minutes. In a medium microwave-safe bowl, microwave the broccoli on high for 4 minutes, then add the tuna. Cut the potato lengthwise. Top with tuna-broccoli mixture, then microwave on high for 1½ minutes. Top with the cheese.

Good for:

Heart health

Cancer prevention

Potatoes are high in vitamin C, which combines with certain toxins in the body and destroys them. Tuna is rich in omega-3 fatty acids, which benefit the heart. Broccoli contains cancer-fighting isothiocyanates.

Makes 1 serving

Per serving: 263 calories, 33 g protein, 33 g carbohydrates, 2 g fat, 28 mg cholesterol, 429 mg sodium, 7 g fiber

Shrimp Tabbouleh

The addition of seafood to this timeless Middle Eastern favorite turns it into a complete entree. Nutri-bonus: This dish provides 47 percent of the recommended Daily Value for fiber!

1 package (6 ounces) bulgur

1¼ cups boiling water

2 tablespoons olive oil

1 pound small shrimp, peeled, deveined, and cooked

1 cucumber, peeled and diced

1 cup finely chopped red onions

½ cup fresh mint, snipped

½ cup fresh parsley, snipped

Juice of 1 lemon

Place the bulgur in a large bowl and add the boiling water and oil. Cover and let stand for 30 minutes.

Stir in the shrimp, cucumber, onions, mint, parsley, and lemon juice. Serve warm, or chill for at least an hour and serve cold.

Good for:

Digestion
Colon health
Lowering cholesterol
Heart health
Improving liver function
Antiaging

Parsley and bulgur both contain fiber, which helps check excess cholesterol and keep the digestive system running smoothly. Parsley is also rich in vitamin C, an antiaging, heart-protecting nutrient. Onions contain sulfur, a chemical that the liver needs for its detoxification efforts. The liver also needs good-quality protein, which is found in shrimp.

Makes 4 servings

Per serving: 272 calories, 14 g protein, 40 g carbohydrates, 8 g fat, 67 mg cholesterol, 95 mg sodium, 10 g fiber

Salads, Soups, and Side Dishes

Barley Salad with Smoked Cheese

Smoky Gouda cheese, garlic, and olive oil, as well as a variety of veggies, turn barley into a surprisingly satisfying salad.

1 cup quick-cooking barley

⅛ cup balsamic vinegar

2 tablespoons fat-free plain yogurt

½ tablespoon olive oil

½ tablespoon minced garlic

Pinch of salt (optional)

Freshly ground black pepper

¼ cup chopped red onions

¼ cup chopped parsley

1 scallion, chopped

1 cup halved cherry tomatoes

¼ cup shredded carrots

¼ cup smoked Gouda cheese, cubed

Place the barley in a large saucepan. Add cold water to cover. Bring to a boil. Cook for 10 minutes, or until the barley is soft but not mushy. Drain, rinse to remove excess starch, drain again, and set aside to cool.

In a medium salad bowl, whisk together the vinegar, yogurt, oil, garlic, salt (if using), and pepper to taste. Stir in the onions, parsley, and scallion. Add the tomatoes, carrots, Gouda, and barley. Toss to mix well.

Good for:

Heart health

Improving liver function

Digestion

Barley is a good source of soluble fiber, which can help lower levels of total cholesterol. It also contains tocotrienol, a nutrient that helps suppress cholesterol production by the liver, and beta glucans, a specific type of soluble fiber that helps prevent dietary fats and cholesterol from being absorbed by the intestines.

Makes 2 servings

Per serving: 558 calories, 19 g protein, 96 g carbohydrates, 13 g fat, 33 mg cholesterol, 674 mg sodium, 18 g fiber

Emerald Sesame Greens

Kale, a much underappreciated vegetable, has a deep, rich taste that combines nicely with ginger and sesame. Enjoy kale as a robust alternative to the milder taste of spinach.

2 bunches kale

½ teaspoon sesame oil

½ teaspoon canola oil

1 teaspoon minced garlic

1 teaspoon minced ginger

1 tablespoon water

1 teaspoon low-sodium tamari or soy sauce

1 teaspoon sesame seeds

¼ teaspoon ground red pepper

Wash the kale but do not pat it dry. Coarsely chop it.

In a 12-inch nonstick skillet or wok, warm the sesame and canola oils over medium-high heat. Add the garlic and ginger, and sauté until the garlic is lightly browned. Add the kale with the water that clings to it and sauté it, sprinkling with water as needed until it's tender, 5 to 7 minutes.

Transfer the kale to a bowl and toss with the tamari or soy sauce, sesame seeds, and ground red pepper.

Good for:

Antiaging

Clear vision

Kale, a delicious, leafy member of the cruciferous family of vegetables, is high in beta-carotene, a nutrient that supports the liver's detoxification effort. Beta-carotene is an antioxidant that mops up free radicals—molecules that damage the body.

Makes 4 servings

Per serving: 100 calories, 6 g protein, 17 g carbohydrates, 3 g fat, 0 mg cholesterol, 113 mg sodium, 6 g fiber

Indian-Spiced Potatoes and Spinach

Potatoes as a side dish are too often ho-hum. In this dish, they positively sing with flavor. And it's always a good idea to incorporate turmeric into your diet. Not only a tasty spice, it's also a powerful detoxifying herb.

2 medium russet potatoes, peeled, scrubbed, and cut into ½-inch chunks

2 tablespoons canola oil

3 cloves garlic, minced

1 medium onion, chopped

1¾ teaspoons ground cumin

¾ teaspoon ground coriander

½ teaspoon ground turmeric

¼ teaspoon ground ginger

¼ teaspoon salt

¼ teaspoon freshly ground black pepper

½ teaspoon ground cinnamon

2 cups frozen cut leaf spinach

2 to 4 tablespoons water

½ cup (4 ounces) fat-free plain yogurt

Place a steamer basket in a large saucepan with ½ cup of water. Place the potatoes in the steamer. Bring to a boil over high heat. Reduce the heat to medium, cover, and cook for 20 minutes, or until the potatoes are very tender.

Place the potatoes in a bowl and keep warm. Drain and dry the saucepan.

Heat the oil in the same saucepan over medium heat. Add the garlic and onion and cook, stirring frequently, for 5 minutes or until soft. Add the cumin, coriander, turmeric, ginger, salt, pepper, and cinnamon and cook, stirring, for 30 seconds to cook the spices.

Add the potatoes and cook, stirring frequently, for 5 minutes or until crisp and golden.

Add the spinach and 2 tablespoons of water. Cover and cook, tossing gently. Add additional water 1 tablespoon at a time, if needed, for 5 minutes or until heated through.

Place in a serving bowl. Spoon the yogurt on top, but don't stir it in. Serve hot.

Good for:

Improving liver function
Intestinal health
Eliminating candida yeast

Turmeric helps the liver balance the different aspects of its efforts, shortening the transit time for the worst chemical by-products of detoxification. Yogurt contains probiotics, a good kind of bacteria that promote better digestion, prevent candida yeast overgrowth, and keep the intestines healthy.

Makes 4 servings

Per serving: 195 calories, 8 g protein, 24 g carbohydrates, 7 g fat, 1 mg cholesterol, 350 mg sodium, 6 g fiber

Fresh Fruit Salad with Almonds

A simple but satisfying way to get a daily dose of fiber. The lime and mint add a burst of flavor.

- 2 cups assorted chopped or sliced fresh fruit (such as berries, grapes, mango, or kiwifruit)
- Juice of ½ lime
- ½ teaspoon finely chopped fresh mint
- 1 tablespoon crushed almonds

Put the fruit in a large bowl. Add the lime juice and mint; toss gently to coat. Sprinkle with the crushed almonds.

Good for:

- Digestive health
- Heart health
- Cancer protection

Fruit is bursting with soluble fiber, which helps the body eliminate toxins and promotes weight loss, thereby helping to protect against heart disease. Almonds are rich in vitamin E, which some studies suggest may protect against cervical and prostate cancers.

Makes 2 servings

Per serving: 102 calories, 2 g protein, 21 g carbohydrates, 3 g fat, 0 mg cholesterol, 2 mg sodium, 3 g fiber

Mandarin Cabbage Slaw

What could be easier than this salad? Once you've shredded the cabbage, you basically just throw it together. But oh, what a treat. And check out that calorie count!

- 10 raw cabbage leaves, shredded
- 8 canned hearts of palm, cut into strips
- 10½ tangerine (Mandarin orange) sections, drained
- ⅓ cup fat-free honey Dijon salad dressing

In a large bowl, combine the cabbage, hearts of palm, and orange sections. Toss with the dressing.

Good for:

- Weight loss
- Colon health
- Improving liver function
- Lowering cholesterol
- Cancer prevention

Cabbage is one of the cruciferous vegetables, all of which contain powerful anticancer compounds. Cabbage is also high in fiber, which helps sweep wastes from the body and lower cholesterol.

Makes 4 servings

Per serving: 94 calories, 3 g protein, 21 g carbohydrates, 1 g fat, 0 mg cholesterol, 476 mg sodium, 5 g fiber

Mediterranean Coleslaw

This coleslaw is a refreshing change from commercial coleslaw, which is typically made with mayonnaise and sugar. Enjoy this side dish at your next outdoor barbecue or the next time you bring home a ready-made roast chicken.

1 medium tomato

½ head of cabbage, shredded very fine

½ red bell pepper, sliced into slivers

4 tablespoons olive oil

Juice from ⅓ of a lemon

½ teaspoon salt (or to taste)

Quarter and slice the tomato very thin. The tomato will release a lot of juice as you slice it. Combine that juice, the tomato slices, the cabbage, and the pepper in a bowl. Drizzle on the olive oil and toss. Add the lemon juice and salt and toss again.

You can eat this right away, but it's even better after a couple of hours or even the next day. If you wait until the next day, you may find that you need to add a little more lemon and salt. You can use green bell pepper instead of red, if that's what you have on hand, but the red pepper is prettier in this dish.

Good for:

Detoxifying the colon

Improving liver function

Heart health

Constipation

Cabbage provides enzymes and sulfur that help your liver's detoxification efforts. Tomatoes and red bell peppers are high-antioxidant foods. This slaw is also a high-fiber food that encourages the swift movement of food through the digestive system. It also contains sulphoraphane, a biochemical that the liver needs in order to carry out its detoxification efforts. All the vegetables contain vitamin C, a heart-protective antioxidant. And the olive oil is monounsaturated, a type of oil that helps keep your cholesterol levels under control.

Makes 4 servings

Per serving: 148 calories, 1 g protein, 6 g carbohydrates, 14 g fat, 0 mg cholesterol, 302 mg sodium, 2 g fiber

Garlic-Herb Dip

You'll love dunking raw veggies into this flavorful dip, enlivened with dill and fresh parsley.

½ cup sour cream

¼ cup mayonnaise

2 large cloves fresh garlic, minced

2 sprigs fresh parsley, finely chopped

1 tablespoon Worcestershire sauce

½ tablespoon finely minced onion

½ tablespoon dill weed

½ teaspoon seasoned salt

In a small bowl, thoroughly combine the sour cream, mayonnaise, garlic, parsley, Worcestershire sauce, onion, dill weed, and seasoned salt.

Good for:

Eye health
Cancer prevention

Garlic contains quercetin, an antioxidant shown to protect colon cells from certain cancer-causing substances. Parsley contains terpenoids, compounds that delay the onset of cancer and reduce the number of cancerous tumors. Dill weed is a good source of beta-carotene and a fair source of lutein and zeaxanthin, all of which help protect eyesight.

Makes 6 servings (2 tablespoons each)

Per serving: 111 calories, 1 g protein, 2 g carbohydrates, 11 g fat, 15 mg cholesterol, 285 mg sodium, 0 g fiber

Turkish White-Bean Dip

Serve this creamy dip with low-fat tortilla chips, pita chips, raw vegetables, crackers, or bread.

1 can (16 ounces) white beans such as cannellini or great Northern, rinsed and drained

2 teaspoons extra-virgin olive oil

2 teaspoons lime juice

1 teaspoon ground cumin

1 teaspoon minced garlic

¼ cup chopped arugula or watercress

Salt and ground black pepper

In a food processor or blender, combine the beans, oil, lime juice, cumin, and garlic. Process until smooth.

Transfer to a small bowl. Stir in the arugula or watercress and season with the salt and pepper.

Good for:

Detoxifying the colon
Lowering cholesterol
Heart health
Weight loss

Beans are high in fiber, which speeds waste removal from the colon and helps lower cholesterol. Fiber also provides a feeling of fullness that satisfies the appetite.

Makes 10 servings (2 tablespoons each)

Per serving: 45 calories, 2 g protein, 7 g carbohydrates, 1 g fat, 0 mg cholesterol, 30 mg sodium, 2 g fiber

Minestrone Soup ✗

There's no better way to eat your veggies than by spooning up this rich and flavorful soup.

3 tablespoons olive oil

1 leek, sliced

2 carrots, chopped

1 zucchini, thinly sliced

4 ounces green beans, cut into 1-inch pieces

2 stalks celery, thinly sliced

1½ quarts vegetable stock

1 pound chopped tomatoes

1 tablespoon chopped fresh thyme

1 can (15 ounces) cannellini beans, with liquid

Salt and ground black pepper

In a large saucepan, heat the olive oil over medium heat. Add the leek, carrots, zucchini, green beans, and celery. Cover, reduce heat to low, and cook for 15 minutes, shaking the pan occasionally. Stir in the stock, tomatoes, and thyme. Bring to a boil. Cover and reduce heat to low; simmer for 30 minutes. Stir in the cannellini beans, including the liquid. Simmer for an additional 10 minutes. Season with salt and pepper to taste before serving.

Good for:

Digestion

Cancer prevention

Heart health

Cellular health

Cannellini beans are rich in heart-protective fiber. Olive oil is high in monounsaturated fat, which helps lower cholesterol, and is rich in vitamins A, E, and D. Carrots are rich in carotenoid antioxidants, which disarm free radicals that alter cells' DNA. Celery contains coumarins, compounds that help prevent free radicals from damaging cells, reducing the risk of cells becoming cancerous. A volatile oil in thyme, thymol, has been found to increase the percentage of healthy fats in cell membranes and other cell structures.

Makes 4 servings

Per serving: 267 calories, 10 g protein, 38 g carbohydrates, 12 g fat, 0 mg cholesterol, 1,130 mg sodium, 11 g fiber

Moroccan Carrot Salad with Toasted Cumin

Carrots are a traditional choice for detoxifying the body. Eating more carrots is always a good idea, and when they taste this good, who can resist?

¾ teaspoon ground cumin

¼ teaspoon ground coriander

½ cup (4 ounces) reduced-fat sour cream

4 teaspoons lemon juice

1½ teaspoons extra-virgin olive oil

1½ teaspoons flaxseed oil

¼ teaspoon freshly grated orange peel

¼ teaspoon salt

7 medium carrots, shredded

½ cup currants

2 tablespoons chopped red onion

In a small skillet over medium heat, cook the cumin and coriander, stirring often, for 2 minutes or until fragrant and slightly darker in color. Place in a medium bowl and let cool. Stir in the sour cream, lemon juice, olive oil, flaxseed oil, orange peel, and salt.

Add the carrots, currants, and onion and toss to coat well. Let stand for 15 minutes to allow the flavors to blend.

Good for:

Detoxification from heavy metals

Antiaging

Coriander and cilantro were shown in one small study to help flush heavy metals from the body. Carrots are high in antioxidant vitamins that mop up free radicals—molecules that damage the body and contribute to aging.

Makes 4 servings

Per serving: 185 calories, 3 g protein, 29 g carbohydrates, 7 g fat, 12 mg cholesterol, 201 mg sodium, 5 g fiber

Roasted Vegetable Salad with Balsamic and Basil Vinaigrette

Eating your vegetables has never been this easy. You'll love this hearty salad of eggplant, tomato, and zucchini, dressed with a piquant vinaigrette dressing.

1 tablespoon balsamic vinegar

1 clove garlic, crushed

¾ teaspoon dried basil

1½ tablespoons plus 2 teaspoons olive oil

1 red onion, quartered and the layers separated

1 medium zucchini, cubed

½ small eggplant, cubed

1 red bell pepper, thinly sliced

1 medium tomato, cut into ½-inch wedges

¼ teaspoon fennel seeds, crushed

Pinch of black pepper

In a small bowl, whisk together the vinegar, garlic, ¼ teaspoon of the basil, and 1½ tablespoons of the oil. Set aside.

Preheat the oven to 450°F. Coat a 13" × 9" baking dish with 1 teaspoon of the remaining oil. In a medium bowl, toss the onion, zucchini, eggplant, red pepper, tomato, fennel seeds, black pepper, the remaining ½ teaspoon of basil, and the remaining teaspoon of oil. Place in the baking dish. Roast, stirring occasionally, for 20 to 30 minutes, or until the vegetables are tender. Transfer to a large bowl. Serve warm or chilled. Toss with the basil vinaigrette just before serving.

Good for:

Heart health

Cancer prevention

The vegetables are high in fiber and various antioxidants, which help neutralize and destroy free radicals that can lead to heart disease, cancer, and other diseases. Basil contains monoterpenoids, compounds with antibacterial properties.

Makes 2 servings

Per serving: 252 calories, 5 g protein, 27 g carbohydrates, 15 g fat, 0 mg cholesterol, 14 mg sodium, 8 g fiber

Salted Edamame

Edamame are soybeans harvested while they're still green, just before they've had a chance to harden. Why pop peanuts into your mouth when you can enjoy this low-cal snack that's even better for you?

> 1 pound fresh or frozen unshelled edamame
>
> ½ teaspoon coarse salt

Place a large bowl of ice water on the counter.

Bring a large pot of water to a boil over high heat. Add the edamame and cook until bright green and tender, about 10 minutes for fresh or 5 minutes for frozen. Remove the edamame from the boiling water with a slotted spoon and place it in the ice water. Drain well.

Place the edamame in a serving bowl and toss with the salt. To eat, pop open the shells and slip the edamame into your mouth. Serve with a bowl for empty shells.

Good for:

Cancer prevention
Relieving premenstrual and menopausal
symptoms
Improving liver function
Weight loss

Edamame is rich in isoflavones, compounds that mimic estrogen. Because they take the place of estrogen in the body, isoflavones help prevent conditions associated with excess estrogen, among them breast cancer, PMS, and menopausal discomforts. Edamame also contains a complete protein, which means that it is a good choice for vegetarians looking to support the liver's detoxification efforts. It's naturally low in calories, so it's a good snack choice for those trying to lose weight.

Makes 8 servings

Per serving: 80 calories, 6 g protein, 4 g carbohydrates, 2.5 g fat, 0 mg cholesterol, 140 mg sodium, 3 g fiber

Tortilla Soup with Lime

This soup is satisfying enough to serve as a light meal in and of itself. Have it with a green salad and you've done your body a double good turn.

- 4 corn tortillas (6 inches in diameter), halved and cut into ¼-inch-wide strips
- 2¼ cups chicken broth
- 1¼ cups water
- 12 ounces turkey breast cutlets, cut into ½-inch-thick strips
- 2 large onions, halved and thinly sliced
- 2 large red bell peppers, cut into thin strips
- 1 large jalapeño chile pepper, seeded and minced (wear plastic gloves when handling)
- 2 teaspoons ground cumin
- ¼ teaspoon dried oregano, crushed
- ½ cup frozen corn kernels
- ½ cup cherry tomatoes, quartered
- ¼ cup fresh cilantro, chopped
- 2 tablespoons lime juice
- ½ ripe avocado, diced

Preheat the oven to 400°F. Coat 1 or 2 large baking sheets with cooking spray.

Arrange the tortilla strips on the prepared baking sheets and bake for 2 minutes, or until crisped and lightly browned on the edges.

In a large saucepan, combine the broth, water, turkey, onions, bell peppers, jalapeño, cumin, and oregano. Bring to a boil over high heat. Reduce the heat to medium-low, cover, and simmer for 10 minutes.

Add the corn and simmer for 5 minutes. Stir in the tomatoes, cilantro, and lime juice. Ladle the soup into bowls and top each portion with avocado and tortilla crisps.

Good for:

Detoxifying from heavy metals
Improving liver function
Antiaging
Prostate health

Cilantro and coriander were shown in one small study to help eliminate toxic heavy metal contamination from the body.

Makes 4 servings

Per serving: 258 calories, 25 g protein, 53 g carbohydrates, 6 g fat, 53 mg cholesterol, 419 mg sodium, 6 g fiber

Sunflower-Seed Dressing

Give your tastebuds a thrill! Fresh herbs add zing—and health benefits—to this "sunny" dressing.

1½ cups sunflower seeds

2 cups water

½ cup lemon juice

⅛ cup tamari

⅛ cup honey

1 teaspoon salt

½ green bell pepper, seeds and membranes removed

½ bunch fresh basil, chopped

½ bunch fresh cilantro, chopped

Process the sunflower seeds, water, lemon juice, tamari, honey, salt, pepper, basil, and cilantro in a food processor until creamy.

Good for:

Heart health
Bone health

The sunflower seeds contain linoleic acid, which can help reduce cholesterol deposits on the walls of the arteries, while cilantro contains bone-protective calcium and the antioxidant beta-carotene.

Makes 12 servings (¼ cup each)

Per serving: 110 calories, 5 g protein, 8 g carbohydrates, 8 g fat, 0 mg cholesterol, 415 mg sodium, 1 g fiber

Tahini Dressing

Given bite with garlic, tahini, and red pepper, this intensely flavored dressing will turn dull vegetables dramatic.

½ cup fat-free plain yogurt

1 clove garlic, minced

3 tablespoons tahini

1 tablespoon lemon juice

1 teaspoon ground cumin

½ teaspoon salt

¼ teaspoon ground red pepper

Whisk the yogurt, garlic, tahini, lemon juice, cumin, salt, and pepper in a small bowl until smooth.

Good for:

Digestion

Red pepper stimulates circulation, aids digestion, and promotes sweating, all of which aid the body's detoxification's efforts. Cumin may stimulate the secretion of pancreatic enzymes necessary for proper digestion and the assimilation of nutrients. Tahini is a good source of copper and thiamin, a B vitamin that helps convert food into energy.

Makes 2 servings

Per serving: 167 calories, 7 g protein, 11 g carbohydrates, 12 g fat, 1 mg cholesterol, 625 mg sodium, 2 g fiber

Tomato-Dill Dressing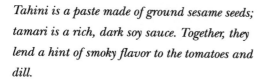

Tahini is a paste made of ground sesame seeds; tamari is a rich, dark soy sauce. Together, they lend a hint of smoky flavor to the tomatoes and dill.

¾ cup tahini

1½ ounces tamari

7 cloves garlic (use less)

4 tomatoes

½ cup water

½ tablespoon dill

Blend the tahini, tamari, garlic, tomatoes, water, and dill in a food processor until creamy.

Good for:

Immune function

Cancer prevention

Garlic contains essential oils and other components that have potent antibiotic, antifungal, and antiviral properties, while dill contains volatile oils that may help neutralize such carcinogens as the benzopyrenes in cigarette smoke.

Makes 8 servings (2 tablespoons each)

Per serving: 153 calories, 5 g protein, 9 g carbohydrates, 12 g fat, 0 mg cholesterol, 311 mg sodium, 2 g fiber

Juices and Beverages
Carrot-Apple Snazz

This juice is sweet, tart, and slightly astringent at the same time. Use this beverage as a meal replacement while fasting or enjoy it as a refresher at any time. It's indescribably delicious!

> 4 carrots, peeled
>
> 1 apple, peeled, cored, and cut into chunks
>
> A handful of parsley
>
> 2 stalks celery with leaves

Alternate feeding carrots and apple chunks into the juicer. Then juice the parsley, followed by the celery stalks.

Good for:

> Fasting and cleansing
> Improving liver function
> Heart health
> Antiaging

The fruit and vegetable juices contain nutrients that can support liver function while you're fasting and cleansing. They are also rich in antioxidants, which protect the heart and have an antiaging effect.

Makes 1 serving

Per serving: 254 calories, 6 g protein, 61 g carbohydrates, 0 g fat, 0 mg cholesterol, 282 mg sodium, 16 g fiber

Fruit Smoothie

Filled with fiber and plant protein rather than animal protein, this creamy treat is as healthy as it is delicious.

> 1 cup fat-free or soy milk
>
> ½ to 1 cup water
>
> ½ cup berries, mashed banana, or other fruit
>
> 1 scoop rice protein powder
>
> 1 tablespoon wheat germ, almond or cashew butter, or honey (optional)

Whir the milk, water, fruit, and protein powder in a blender on high until smooth. Add the wheat germ, almond or cashew butter, or honey (if using).

Good for:

> Breast health
> Improving liver function
> Digestion
> Heart health

Soy milk is high in phytoestrogens (a natural form of estrogen found in plants), which may help protect against breast cancer. The fiber, vitamins, minerals, and plant compounds in fruit support liver detoxification. Rice protein powder is an excellent source of protein, needed by the liver for detoxification.

Makes 1 serving

Per serving: 215 calories, 23 g protein, 18 g carbohydrates, 6 g fat, 0 mg cholesterol, 218 mg sodium, 6 g fiber (Analysis does not include optional wheat germ, almond or cashew butter, or honey.)

Peach, Apple, and Pear Surprise

The surprise is how easy it is to get the benefits of four pieces of fruit in just one glass—and also how just plain good it tastes.

> 2 peaches, pits removed
>
> 1 apple, cored and sliced
>
> 1 pear, cored and sliced

Process the peaches, apple, and pear in a juicer and serve.

Per serving: 240 calories, 2 g protein, 64 g carbohydrates, 0 g fat, 0 mg cholesterol, 0 mg sodium, 12 g fiber

Good for:

> Improving liver function
>
> Fasting and cleansing
>
> Weight loss
>
> Lowering cholesterol
>
> Heart health
>
> Antiaging

Peaches contain carotenes and flavonoids, which support the liver's detoxifying efforts. Apples and pears both contain pectin, a type of water-soluble fiber, much of which is still present when the fruit is juiced. Fiber helps sweep wastes from the colon and lower cholesterol.

Makes 1 serving

Per serving: 240 calories, 2 g protein, 64 g carbohydrates, 0 g fat, 0 mg cholesterol, 0 mg sodium, 12 g fiber

Rice Protein Shake

Protein plays a vital role in detoxification, and this rich shake is full of it, as well as healthy fats and antioxidants.

> 1 scoop rice protein powder
>
> 8 ounces fat-free or rice milk
>
> 1 tablespoon flax oil
>
> ½ cup berries or ½ yam or sweet potato
>
> 1 tablespoon wheat germ, almond or cashew butter, or honey (optional)

Whir the protein powder, milk, oil, and berries or yam or sweet potato in a blender on high until smooth. Add the wheat germ, almond or cashew butter, or honey (if using).

Good for:

> Improving liver function

Flax oil is rich in essential fatty acids, which support liver detoxification, while sweet potatoes contain phytochelatins, chemicals shown to bind to toxic heavy metals like copper, cadmium, mercury, and lead.

Makes 1 serving

Per serving: 365 calories, 17 g protein, 37 g carbohydrates, 17 g fat, 0 mg cholesterol, 265 mg sodium, 3 g fiber (Analysis does not include optional wheat germ, almond or cashew butter, or honey.)

Sparkling Orange, Mango, and Kiwifruit Juice

Mineral water adds zest to this delicious and nutritious fruit juice.

  1 orange, peeled and sectioned

  ½ mango, peeled and sliced

  1 kiwifruit, peeled and sliced

  Sparkling mineral water

Process the orange, mango, and kiwi in a juicer. Pour the juice into a large glass. Fill the remainder of the glass with mineral water and serve.

Good for:

  Fasting and cleansing
  Improving liver function
  Antiaging
  Colds

Oranges contain limonene, a phytochemical that the liver needs in order to carry out its detoxification of the body. Orange, mango, and kiwi are all high in vitamin C, an antiaging nutrient and a powerful antioxidant.

Makes 1 serving

Per serving: 190 calories, 3 g protein, 47 g carbohydrates, 1 g fat, 0 mg cholesterol, 0 mg sodium, 7 g fiber

Vegetable Juice

Start your day with this low-calorie, nutritious juice.

  1 cup water

  Salt

  Black pepper

  1 beet, washed and finely chopped

  2 carrots, washed, peeled, and finely chopped

  3 leaves fresh spinach, washed and finely chopped

  2 tomatoes, washed, peeled, and finely chopped

  Fresh lime juice (add a few drops first and then check to see if you need more)

Process the water, salt, pepper, beet, carrots, spinach, tomatoes, and lime juice in a blender until smooth. Serve immediately.

Good for:

  Fasting and cleansing
  Improving liver function
  Prostate health
  Weight loss
  Heart health

Tomatoes supply vitamin C, carotenes, potassium, and lycopene, which protects the prostate. Carrots have carotenes, as well. The liver needs a variety of carotenes in order to detoxify the body.

Makes 1 serving

Per serving: 150 calories, 5 g protein, 33 g carbohydrates, 2 g fat, 0 mg cholesterol, 490 mg sodium, 9 g fiber

Chapter 5

The Essential Herbs:
Nature's Best Purifiers

WHEN PEOPLE TALK ABOUT DETOX PROGRAMS, herbal medicines always come up. Friends talk about herbs that flush toxins right out of the body. Take a trip to the local health food store, and you'll find 20 or more different herbal products with "Detox" boldly printed on the packaging. TV and radio ads tout "miracle" herbal products that promise to zap every last toxin from your body.

The word is out. Herbs *do* have a role in a detox program.

Though you may have heard about using herbs for detox purposes, you may not know where or how to begin. What herb should you use? For how long should you use it? What dose should you take? As soon as you move from talking about using herbs for detox to actually *using* herbs for detox, things start to get sticky. There is a lot of casual talk about the subject, but not a lot of practical know-how or guidance is available. For the inside story on creating an herbal detox plan, we turned to Doug Schar, Dip.Phyt., MCPP, MNIMH, a Washington, D.C.–based herbalist who was medically trained in Europe. Schar has practiced herbal medicine for 15 years and has written several books on the subject of wellness through herbs.

His advice goes well beyond Herbal Detox 101. Thanks to his guidance, this chapter includes the most important information you need about using herbs for purification. This chapter will help you find the best detox herbs to meet your personal needs and help you create a sensible herbal detox program that will really make a difference in your life.

So where do we start? As is often the case, it is best to start at the beginning, with a little history. You might be surprised to discover that the herbal purification story actually started centuries ago.

ANCIENT SECRETS FOR HERBAL HEALING

Though we are inclined to think of toxins as being something new and using herbs to combat toxicity as being almost space age, this is not the case. For centuries, human beings have used herbs for this purpose. The toxins have changed, but using herbs to get toxins out of the body before they make you sick has been an accepted practice since the beginning of written history.

In Europe, from the earliest days, people combed the woods for tasty mushrooms. Whereas most mushrooms are harmless, some deliver a toxic punch that destroys the liver along with the person who owns it. Long ago, mushroom gatherers learned that if you accidentally ate a bad mushroom, milk thistle (*Silybum marianum*) would help you survive the meal.

Lucretia Borgia and other European nobles resolved more than one disagreement with the aid of poison. In those days, poisoning people who got in your way was standard operating procedure. Are you familiar with the stories of food tasters employed by the European nobility? These unfortunates were not mere status symbols. They risked their lives, one taste at a time, to keep the king safe from malicious poisoning. If a taster was poisoned, Mithradites Treacle was used to counteract the effects of the poison. Concocted from herbs, this counterpoison was used to detoxify the body and ensure survival.

Poisoning was not just a political affair. Gerard, a famous 16th-century European herbalist, tells us that it was also a domestic problem. Gerard cautioned stepchildren to keep a supply of lemons around the house to counteract the poisoning they might expect from their stepmothers. According to Gerard, lemons worked against the diverse poisons at the disposal of the stepmothers of the day.

In North America, Native Americans knew all about toxins. On this continent, the tribes dealt with two sorts. The first sort were toxins injected into the body by poisonous beasts, critters like rattlesnakes and scorpions. The second sort were toxins delivered by the tip of an arrow. In both cases, the Native Americans used echinacea to detoxify the poisons injected into the body by beast or enemy.

Globally, herbs were also used to detoxify toxins of a less-sinister nature: toxins produced by the body itself. Long winters, short on green vegetables and rich in meat and potatoes, meant people felt pretty bad by the time spring rolled around. Folks observed that consuming stodgy food for months on end resulted in the body's producing and storing toxins. These stored toxins made people feel cranky and sluggish. The traditional solution to this seasonal problem was a spring tonic. In Europe, people gathered the spring greens dandelion, watercress, and chicory to help the body rid itself of stored toxins. In North America, folks brewed white pine needles, Douglas fir fronds, and sassafras bark into spring-cleaning teas.

Today, we know more about the ancient detox herbs than the ancient healers did. Researchers have spent years scrutinizing these long-used remedies. In the process, they have discovered the hidden secrets of these herbs. Many of the old remedies' uses have been validated through scientific scrutiny. In some cases, study has even highlighted new uses for these herbs. Empowered by this knowledge, we have the opportunity to use herbal detox agents with unprecedented precision and accuracy.

YOUR PURIFICATION PLAN HERBAL DETOX STRATEGIES

Now that modern research has validated so many of these herbal detox agents, scientists have divided the miracle plants into two basic categories:

⚕ Herbs that increase the body's excretion of toxins (housekeeping herbs)
⚕ Herbs that increase the body's resistance to toxins (resistance herbs)

To use herbs most effectively for safe yet powerful purification, our simple, three-step approach combines herbs from both of these categories and adds a tea made from red sorrel, perhaps Nature's best all-purpose cleaner. Our approach is to:

• Select a "housekeeping" herb and use it for 1 month.
• Select a "resistance raising" herb and use it periodically, when you need special protection.
• Add red sorrel (or another antitoxin beverage) to your shopping list and use it regularly.

Let's have a look at your options for each of these steps. You'll discover the herbs you should consider for your personal purification plan.

Note: Consult with your health care practitioner before adding herbal remedies to your health care regimen.

Step One: Select a Housekeeping Herb

HOUSEKEEPING HERBS: INCREASING YOUR BODY'S EXCRETION OF TOXINS

Your body has the innate capacity to rid itself of toxins. It doesn't matter whether these toxins are produced by your body or you take them in through food, air, or water. Your body knows how to get rid of them. To be more specific, your kidneys, liver, skin, and immune system work together to detoxify your body.

Practitioners of herbal medicine believe in working with the body and never against it. In this light, they use certain herbs to encourage the body to do what it does naturally. This is where the housekeeping herbs come in. These herbs are administered to stimulate the toxin removal system. They encourage the body to do what it already does naturally, just with renewed focus and vitality.

Actually, you already know about certain herbs that have this capacity. You have probably eaten one too many prunes and found yourself spending a few extra minutes on the toilet the next day. Or perhaps you've had a big cup of coffee before hitting the road and ended up desperately looking for the nearest rest stop. Ever eat a hot pepper and break out in big beads of sweat? These are all examples of herbs stimulating the organs of toxin removal into dynamic action. However, that is just the beginning. There are lots of herbs that get these systems cranking.

Though you probably know that your digestive tract, urinary tract, and skin move toxins out of your body, you may not know that your immune system has a role to play. The immune soldier cells patrol the body looking for bacteria, viruses, and cancer, and when they spot trouble, they collect it and dispose of it. The immune cells also pick up toxins. They search the cracks and crevices of your body for toxic substances, and if they spot any, they vacuum them up. You might think of the immune cells as your own microscopic DustBusters. The immune system is the silent star of our natural detox ability. Talk about deep cleaning!

Here, too, herbal medicines can be used to increase your body's efficiency. There are a number of herbal immune system stimulants that have been proven to increase the number of immune cells

Keys to Success with Housekeeping Herbs

HOUSEKEEPING HERBS can be used to boost your body's natural capacity to rid itself of toxins by helping stimulate urination, sweating, and defecation. Here are some tips for using them properly.

- Select one herb that strengthens your weakness. If you don't urinate a lot, use a diuretic herb to increase urination. If you don't sweat much, use an herb that increases sweating, and so on.
- Stick with one herb. Plan to use that herb for a solid month. This will go a long way toward getting toxins out of your system.

- After a month of using a housekeeping herb, discontinue its use, but don't forget about it completely. Detox is not a once-a-year proposition. It's something we need to attend to all the time. So bring back the herb for a full week every month to maintain your detoxification and stay clean.

---

produced by the body and the activity of the existing immune cells. They get the immune soldiers cranked out and into action. Herbs like echinacea, maitake, astragalus, and boneset all give the immune system a kick start.

SELECTING THE RIGHT HOUSEKEEPING HERB

What is the best herb to do this job for you? Simply put, it is the herb that matches your weakness with strength. What does this mean?

Well, for optimal waste removal, we want our digestive tract, urinary tract, skin, and immune system to be functioning at full steam. We want all four routes of waste removal fully functional. However, this is not always the case. Most of us know which of our waste removal systems work really well and which do not. As an example, some will be quick to say that their kidneys are all-too active or that they sweat like a barnyard resident. On the other hand, others will say they rarely urinate or sweat. When looking for a housekeeping herb, look for one that stimulates your weakest waste removal system. Identify your personal weakness, and then select an herb that counters this weakness.

⚬ If you don't produce that much urine, select an herb that increases urination.
⚬ If you have a tendency to be constipated, select an herb that acts as a laxative.
⚬ If you have a tendency toward infection, select an herb that stimulates the immune system.
⚬ If you never sweat, select an herb that opens up the pores and gets sweat running out.

Here are some excellent housekeeping options. Read through these and find one that stimulates your weakest link.

Buchu: The Pipe Flusher (Kidney Stimulant)

Scientific name: *Barosma betulina*

Part used: Leaf

Best For:

Urinary tract infections. Contains compounds that kill the bacteria that cause urinary tract infections and other compounds that soothe irritated urinary tissues.

Kidney stones. Holding urine for too long gives stones the chance to form. This herb gets the urine flowing so the stones can't form.

Infrequent urination. Regular urination means toxins are constantly whisked

When to Consult a Doctor

IN A HEALTHY PERSON, the routes for excreting toxins can be stimulated with no ill effects. In fact, it's a good thing. However, if the kidneys are not working properly to begin with, they should not be stimulated. If you have any chronic disease that affects your organs of excretion, speak to a doctor before adding herbs to your regimen. If you're not sure whether your disease applies, ask your doctor. But in general, anyone with liver disease, kidney disease, or digestive disease should discuss any detox regimen with his or her doctor.

out of your body. Buchu contains oils that increase urine production.

What It Does. Buchu is an aromatic herb rich in volatile oils. These volatile oils give the spicy leaves their fruity, black currant taste. In fact, many fruit-flavored herbal teas rely on buchu for the backbone of their fruit taste. These same oils stimulate the kidney cells to increase activity. The leaves also contain mucilage, resins, and tannins thought to contribute to the diuretic effect. Perfectly nontoxic, buchu is so safe it is used in popular herbal teas.

Using Buchu. The advantage of this kidney stimulant is its great taste. Let's just say detoxing with buchu is nothing short of a pleasure and that adding this remedy to your life will be easy. The best way to use buchu is in the form of a hot tea. Buy buchu leaves at the health food store. Boil water and add 1 teaspoon of leaves to 1 cup of water. Let them infuse for 5 minutes, strain, and drink while still hot. Three cups of this tea per day is the recommended dosage. Remember: It will increase urine output, so plan ahead. For a major detoxification, think about using buchu every day for a month. After this, use buchu several times a month to keep toxins flowing where you want them to flow—down the drain.

R$_x$: One dose, three times a day.
One dose =
1 cup of buchu leaf tea (see above for instructions) OR
1 teaspoon of tincture 1:5 OR
20 drops of tincture 1:1

Origins. Buchu is an aromatic shrub native to South Africa. When the European colonials first arrived on the southernmost tip of that continent, they encountered buchu. Long used by the Hottentot tribe as a cleansing herb and vitality tonic, buchu quickly became traded internationally. It was shipped from Africa to London, and then on to North America to be used as a urinary stimulant. At the beginning of the 19th century, it was one of America's most popular urinary tonics.

Detox Makeover. For people who spend much of their work time in a car, keeping fluid intake down is a matter of survival! For Ernie, a 52-year-old taxi driver in New York City, it became a way of life. "When you drive a cab, you can't stop all the time, and finding a men's room in New York is not that easy. Fortunately, I was never a person who had to make a lot of pit stops." However, there was trouble in paradise when Ernie developed a kidney stone. His doctors said that he was not passing urine regularly enough, and this led to stone formation. "Having a kidney stone was the worst experience of my life. It was so painful I decided I would do anything to avoid a second attack!" Using buchu, he started urinating like a racehorse and hasn't been troubled with kidney stones since. "It hasn't made driving a cab easier, but it's better than the alternative—passing another stone!"

Dandelion: Human DustBuster (Liver Stimulant)

Scientific name: *Taraxacum officinalis*

Part used: Root

Best For:

Sluggish digestion. Increases digestive gland activity. This causes speedy digestion, absorption, and excretion of waste.

Constipation. Increases bile production. Bile has a natural laxative effect, so constipation improves and waste excretion is increased.

Mild liver insufficiency. Activates blood-cleansing liver cells. If your liver is performing suboptimally, dandelion can be used to give it gentle encouragement.

What It Does. The root contains a collection of compounds that stimulate waste removal on several levels. Some compounds increase liver filtration, others kidney filtration, and others still the immune system and the cells that make it up!

Dandelion is a mild laxative. However, its laxative effect is rooted in its detoxifying action. As the liver cleanses the blood, it deposits the waste products into bile. The liver then ships the bile into the gallbladder and the gallbladder in turn ships the bile into the intestine. Out go the toxins. Bile has many physiological actions, including a laxative effect. All this is to say that you get two for the price of one when you take dandelion: increased liver cleansing and a reduction in constipation.

Using Dandelion. If you tend to be constipated, dandelion may be the housekeeping herb for you. Many a case of chronic constipation has been eased with its use. Indeed, if any part of digestion is an issue, think about dandelion. It improves digestion, absorption, and excretion.

Dandelion root is available at health food stores. Add 1 teaspoon of the root to 2 cups of boiling water. Boil the root for 15 minutes to extract all of its medicinal attributes. Take 1 cup three times a day. It is probably easiest to make the day's worth of tea in the morning. You can reheat the tea in a saucepan or in the microwave as the day goes along. For a major detox, think about using dandelion tea every day for a month. After that, use it occasionally to keep your system free of toxins. You may find it easier to take a tincture rather than make the tea. And don't try to use the plant from your yard—pesticides, fertilizers, and the habits of roaming dogs make it not worth the risk. Besides, the herb is quite inexpensive at the health food store.

R_x: One dose, three times a day.

One dose =

1 cup of dandelion root tea (see above for instructions) OR

Two 500 mg tablets of tableted dandelion root OR

1 teaspoon of tincture 1:5 OR

20 drops of tincture 1:1

Origins. Dandelion is an aggressive little plant that has spread itself around the globe. Though in North America it is seen as an enemy to a pristine lawn, elsewhere it is seen as *the* detox herb of choice. In Europe, Asia, Africa, and South America dandelion has long been used to rid the body of unhealthy toxins. The key words here are long used. For thousands of years, people have used it in spring detox regimens and any other time retention of toxins was causing illness.

Detox Makeover. We all get constipated now and then, but for Linna, a 50-year-old office manager in New York, this uncomfortable feeling was her near-constant companion. "For as long as I can remember, I could never take for granted being able to go to the bathroom," she says. Beyond the discomfort, her sluggish digestive tract and infrequent bowel movements concerned her. "Holding onto waste cannot be good for a person. Waste needs to move, and this was not happening for me." Starting with a regular cup of dandelion tea in the morning and eventually adding another cup in the afternoon, Linna found the relief she had been looking for. Not only did her bowel movements become regular within just a week, she credits the tea, which acted as a laxative and detoxifier, with increasing her energy and reducing her feelings of toxicity. "The tea was a little bitter at first, and I didn't really like it. But I'm glad I stayed with it, and I wouldn't think of stopping drinking it. I've never felt better," she adds.

Echinacea: The Deep Cleaner (Immune System Stimulant)

Scientific name: *Echinacea angustifolia*

Part used: Root

Best For:

Recurrent urinary, skin, or respiratory infections. Stimulates the production and activity of white blood cells responsible for keeping infection under control. Echinacea can be used to end chronic infections.

Cancer prevention. Activates the immune system. People with a history of cancer or cancer in their families need to know about this herb. The immune system is responsible for killing cancer cells before they have the chance to take hold.

Exposure to infectious disease. Stimulates the immune system. Schoolteachers, airline attendants, bus drivers, and nurses are regularly exposed to infection. This herb helps these workers stay free of infection.

What It Does. Time and time again, science has proven that echinacea stimulates both the production and activity of immune cells. Its ability to increase immune function was first observed in the 1920s, and this finding has been substantiated many times over. When you use echinacea, you have more immune cells combing the body for toxins, and at an accelerated rate.

Using Echinacea. If you are the person in the office who always gets the cold going around, your immunity might not be the best. If your immune system is letting bacteria and viruses survive, it's also likely to be leaving toxins in place. To increase your immune function, use echinacea.

When you head out to buy an echinacea product, look for a product made of the root of *Echinacea angustifolia*. Many companies are marketing products made from leaves and flowers, and you want to avoid those. Though you can make a tea out of loose dried root (just boil 1 teaspoon of dried root in 1 cup of water for 10 minutes), it's easier to use tablets. One 500 mg tablet three times a day will do the trick. For a big cleanse, think about using echinacea for a month. After that, use echinacea occasionally to keep your body free of toxins.

Rx: One dose, three times a day.

One dose =

1 cup of loose dry root tea (see above for instructions) OR

One 500 mg tablet of tableted echinacea root OR

1 teaspoon of tincture 1:5 OR

20 drops of tincture 1:1

Origins. Echinacea was first used by the Native Americans to treat rattlesnake, scorpion, and tarantula bites. This may seem a bit odd, as we see it as an immune stimulant useful for coughs and colds. However, there is a common thread. When a venomous insect or animal bites, they inject venom into the body. These toxins destroy tissue. The immune system sends in immune cells to vacuum the toxins out before they can do any damage. Native Americans found that echinacea prevented snakebite-caused gangrene. It got the snake venom out before it could destroy the tissues surrounding the bite.

Detox Makeover. "I really love working with kids," says Dave, a 35-year-old Washington, D.C., schoolteacher, "but it comes with certain occupational hazards. Like being around sick kids day in and day out." As a result, he was troubled with regular cases of tonsillitis. Each fall he would catch a minor cold, and it would quickly turn into a dreaded sore throat. "The doctors gave me prescription after prescription for antibiotics,

and they even suggested removing my tonsils. I wanted to give something else a try before resorting to a major surgery." Dave suspected constant exposure to infection was taxing his immune system and that it was functioning under par as a result. Through a little Internet research he discovered that echinacea might give his immune system the jump-start it needed. It did.

"Not only did the tonsil problem go away, but my skin improved. I had always had an acne problem, and this lessened as I used the echinacea." Regular dosing with echinacea meant he stopped getting tonsillitis and his skin looked better than it ever had before.

Elder: Sweat Lodge in a Bottle (Skin Stimulant)

Scientific name: *Sambucus nigra*

Part used: Flower

Best For:

Lack of sweating. Opens up the sweat glands and gets them pumping toxins out of the body. For those who don't sweat, elder is a great addition to their health care regimen.

Poor circulation. Gently increases circulation. It causes a warm glow shortly after a person drinks a hot cup of the tea. This makes it popular among those with cold feet and hands.

Coughs and colds. Can be used to break a fever. More importantly, it stimulates the immune system to nip a cold in the bud or shorten the duration of a cold.

What It Does. The exact mechanism of elder's action is still unknown. The theory is that it contains chemicals that increase circulation to the sweat glands. With blood nourishing the glands, the glands get busy and produce sweat. Practically speaking, when people have a piping hot cup of elder tea, they break out in gentle perspiration.

Using Elder. This is another easy-to-use remedy. Elder flower tea is a treat for even the fussiest beverage connoisseur. Put 1 teaspoon of the flowers in 1 cup of boiling water, allow it to infuse for 5 minutes, then strain, and it will work its magic. If you want to really pump up the volume on its detox effect, add a teaspoon of honey and lemon juice to your cup of hot tea. It's a lovely and powerful combination. For a proper house-cleaning, think about using elder three times a day for a month. After that, use it for occasional cleanup.

R_x: One dose, three times a day.

One dose =

1 cup of elder flower tea (see above for instructions) OR

1 teaspoon of tincture 1:5 OR

20 drops of tincture 1:1

Origins. The elder tree is a European native long used for a wide variety of purposes. The stems and leaves are made into healing salves, while the berries are made into vitality-stimulating syrups. The flowers are used as a remedy for coughs, colds, fevers, and water retention. Officially speaking, the flowers are termed *diaphoretic*, meaning they increase the sweat glands' production of sweat. Historically, lack of sweating was seen as a source of illness, and these flowers were used to correct this physiological problem. Along these lines, elder's ability to increase sweating is the reason it was used to break a fever!

Detox Makeover. Sweating is something most cultures see as a healthy activity. Sweat lodges, saunas, and the like are used to facilitate the process. For Dwayne, a 40-year-old doctor living in Virginia, *nothing* seemed to bring on a good sweat. "You know something is wrong when cutting the grass in August doesn't make you sweat," he says. Dwayne thought it might be a genetic problem.

"My family are all fair-complexioned and of northern European descent. We just don't sweat. The good news is that I don't need to use deodorant or antiperspirant. The bad news is that I always worried that I wasn't getting toxins out of my body the way others did." Clearly he had inactive sweat glands. An elderly aunt suggested he use an old English sweat producer. Dwayne drank hot cups of elder flower tea, and this switched on his sweat glands. "Regular cups of elder tea seemed to be the magic answer. A few cups and I had small beads of sweat forming on my forehead! I feel better and people have even been telling me I look better."

Step Two: Select a Resistance Herb

RESISTANCE HERBS: RAISING YOUR IMMUNITY

Resistance herbs, also known as adaptogens, are herbal medicines that raise resistance to toxins. In thousands of animal and human experiments, researchers have shown that adaptogens make the body less susceptible to toxin damage. In the toxin-laden world we live in, this is very exciting news. We all need increased resistance to toxins. To take full advantage of this type of herbal medicine, you need some background information.

Most everyone knows that lead; preservatives; artificial colors, flavors, and sweeteners; exhaust from cars; and the like are bad for our health. Herbal research has revealed just why that is. Here's part of the story you may not have heard.

Beginning in the 1940s, researchers began studying stress. Specifically, a researcher named Hans Selye took an interest in the subject. Selye found that when a person is exposed to a toxic substance, regardless of the nature of the toxin, a generalized physical reaction occurs. Initially, the body responds with shock. Then the body adapts to the toxin. Selye found that over time, this adaptation fails. The body can resist the toxin for only so long. Once resistance fails, all kinds of physiological abnormalities set in.

What kind of problems did Selye notice? The list included hormone abnormalities (overproduction and underproduction), immune abnormalities (allergies, psoriasis, eczema, arthritis, asthma, and ulcerative colitis), and nervous abnormalities (depression, anxiety, and learning deficits). And these are just a few of the problems that can develop.

The original stress scientist, Selye felt that the solution was to find substances that increased resistance to toxic compounds. Enter Israel Brekhman. This Russian researcher was fascinated with the work of Selye and set out to find substances that raised the body's resistance to all forms of stress, and toxic compounds in particular. He found such substances and called them adaptogens because they help the body adapt to resisting toxins.

SELECTING THE RIGHT RESISTANCE HERB

When we talk about herbal medicine and detoxification, the adaptogen is of primary importance. Our bodies are bombarded with toxins daily. Adaptogens increase our bodies' ability to withstand them.

Adaptogen research began in the 1950s, and a lot has been learned since then. At the moment, we have a host of adaptogens available to us. Once again, the job is to find the adaptogen that most appropriately fits your circumstance. Though all adaptogens raise resistance to toxins, they each have particular strengths. Read on to learn about some specific adaptogens and try to find the adaptogen that most closely matches your needs.

Ashwagandha: For Those Under Par

Scientific name: *Withania somnifera*

Part used: Root

Best For:

The elderly. Used to strengthen the elderly and decrease symptoms of aging.

The ill. Increases the vitality of those suffering from chronic disease and increases their resistance.

Burnout. Bolsters those who have been through a rough patch and find themselves feeling worn out. It raises resistance in those who have been afflicted by stress or serious health problems.

What It Does. Researchers have demonstrated that ashwagandha increases resistance to many forms of stress and limits the damaging physiological effects of stress, including stress-related nerve damage. (Stress can damage both the brain and the nervous system.) One study using rats showed that ashwagandha reduced the amount of damage done to the brain under stressful circumstances.

The herb acts as a powerful antioxidant, neutralizing some of the internal toxins produced by the body itself. It also corrects blood abnormalities associated with toxic chemical exposure, prevents cancer formation, and reduces liver and kidney damage associated with pharmaceutical drugs. It also apparently reduces toxicity associated with heavy metals.

Using Ashwagandha. Ashwagandha is a traditional tonic remedy for the young, the elderly, and the vulnerable, all of whom are less able to resist toxins. It was used to boost the strength and health of those who had suboptimal resistance. This is good guidance for those looking for an herb to boost their resistance to toxins. For those with less-than-robust health, ashwagandha is an excellent choice, and it can be used long-term.

R$_x$: One dose, twice a day.

One dose =

1½ teaspoons of dried root powder, taken morning and night. (Traditionally this is added to boiling milk, though it can be taken just as a powder mixed with some boiling water.) OR

Two 250 mg tablets of standardized extract

Origins. Ashwagandha is native to India, where it is a major player in traditional ayurvedic medicine. There it is viewed as a tonic and aphrodisiac and is used to strengthen the young and the old—in short, the vulnerable—against the stresses of life. It is said to make the weak strong and the strong stronger. Lurking in this history is something the modern person can take forward. If you are in any way compromised in your ability to resist stress and disease, think about using ashwagandha.

Detox Makeover. Stella, a corporate lawyer in Atlanta, had experienced excellent health her whole life. However, when she turned 70, she noticed that something changed.

"The thing about being blessed with excellent stamina is that when it dips, you really notice," she says. She had lost her "bounce back." A late night out, a patch of stress, one too many drinks, or a cold suddenly took a greater toll than it would have in the past. It took her longer to recover from what previously would have been a minor event. "I really didn't want to admit my age was zapping my endurance, but it was. I just did not have the zip I used to have."

Not being a person to take a problem sitting down, Stella looked for something that might help. She discovered ashwagandha and decided it was worth a

Keys to Success with Resistance Herbs

THOUGH YOUR BODY HAS A BUILT-IN ABILITY to resist toxins, it can do so for only so long. At some point, resistance fails and all kinds of health conditions set in. That's when resistance herbs, also called adaptogens, can be used to raise resistance to toxins. Here's how.

- Select an adaptogen that is most appropriate to your particular health needs. (Though adaptogens have similar features, they also have individual strengths.)

- Use adaptogens when you are heading into a toxin-rich time, such as when you are going to paint your house, fly on a plane, or go on vacation where it's likely that you'll overindulge.

- Use adaptogens to raise your resistance to toxin exposure if you are routinely exposed to toxic substances. Farm workers, lawn-care workers, dry cleaners, hairdressers, chemical factory workers, petrochemical refinery workers, commercial cleaners, and hotel maids can all benefit from using adaptogens.

- Use adaptogens to raise your resistance to the toxicity of prescription medications. Over-the-counter and prescription medications, while helpful, also put stress on your body. These compounds were not meant to be in your body, and so your body has to work to get them out. If you regularly take medicine, consider using an adaptogen.

try. "It took a couple of weeks to make a difference, but using it regularly, I felt more like my energetic former self." She regained her stamina and found that she was much better able to handle stresses of all kinds, especially stresses coming from toxin intake. "I have no intention of slowing down, and with ashwagandha, I'm thinking it won't be necessary."

Eleuthero: All-Purpose Resistance Booster

Scientific name: *Eleutherococcus senticosus*

Part used: Root bark

Best For:

Working mothers. Reduces the damage done to the body by a demanding schedule. Stress simply doesn't do its usual damage when this herb is used.

Cancer treatment support. Used to raise resistance to the side effects of cancer therapies and to speed recovery from cancer therapies. Research indicates it also has a role in preventive regimens.

Athletes. Long used by professional athletes to help their bodies recover from the stress of arduous exercise, eleuthero is the jock's best friend. Numerous studies have established that it increases stamina and reduces wear and tear.

What It Does. In one study, when the herb was administered regularly to laboratory animals that were exposed to toxins, the animals did not succumb to disease as often as untreated animals did. Research reveals that eleuthero raises resistance to some specific forms of toxic stress, radiation, and narcotics. Eleuthero has also been widely studied in humans. It has, in fact, been administered to more than 2,100 people in 44 separate studies. In these studies, the herb increased individuals' ability to withstand stressors such as toxic compounds.

Eleuthero may also be the best herbal medicine for people who are exposed to cancer-causing compounds. Early on, researchers found that it reduced tumors that had been caused by chemicals. It was also found to reduce cancer caused by a variety of chemicals. The research has continued to reveal the same beneficial aspects of eleuthero. To date, 18 studies using laboratory animals have demonstrated that eleuthero reduces cancer in animals that have been exposed to cancer-causing compounds.

Oddly, toxic chemicals cause cancer, and toxic chemicals are used to treat cancer. Here, too, eleuthero can help. In scientific studies, eleuthero has been shown to protect against radiation and toxic chemotherapy regimens. In fact, it reduced the toxicity of several lethally toxic chemotherapy drugs.

Using Eleuthero. Eleuthero is a good all-purpose adaptogen. It's an excellent option for raising your resistance to toxins.

Herbs for Super Humans

AMERICA CONCENTRATED ON STAR WARS TECHNOLOGY to protect against nuclear, biological, and chemical warfare. In the Soviet Union, they did the same thing. But they also did something else. They began looking for compounds that made people superhuman. They looked for medicines that would make people better able to resist the toxins of warfare. Where did they look? They looked at the herbal remedies that traditional societies called tonics.

Their search proved rewarding. They found herbs that make the body more resistant to the toxins associated with chemical warfare, pollution, industrial accidents, and the like. They found herbs that helped rid the body of toxins. They found remedies like adaptogens, which could be used to raise resistance to toxins. Russian research left us with a whole slew of herbal remedies that can be used to get on top of the toxin problem. Many of their finds are discussed in this chapter.

It's useful both for those who are occasionally exposed to toxic compounds and for those who are regularly exposed. If you are painting the house, refinishing the floors, or treating the grass, use it for a week following your exposure. If you work with chemicals and exposure occurs daily, use the herb 2 weeks out of every month. If you are going to be exposed to toxins either occasionally or routinely, use the herb to raise your resistance. This is especially important if there is cancer in your family or if it seems to be a particular hazard of your profession.

To make eleuthero tea, add ½ teaspoon of dried bark to 1 cup of water and let it boil for 15 minutes. Strain, then drink.

R_x: One dose, twice a day.

One dose =

1 cup of dried eleuthero bark tea (see above for instructions) OR

Two 500 mg tablets of tableted dried bark OR

One 100 mg tablet of standardized extract containing 1 percent or more eleutheroside OR

1 teaspoon of tincture 1:5 OR

20 drops of tincture 1:1

Origins. Eleuthero is a thorny shrub found growing in Far Eastern Russia, Northeastern China, Korea, and Japan. Throughout Asia, the herb is used to stimulate vitality and to increase a person's ability to withstand the daily grind. Its reputed powers led researchers to investigate whether the herb really increased resistance to stress. Research began in the 1950s and has never stopped.

Detox Makeover. Many jobs require working with chemicals, and that was certainly the case with Majorie, a 55-year-old London chemist who spent her career in the brewery industry. "When you become a chemist, you sort of have the expectation you will spend your time working with chemicals! I study chemistry and love working in my field," she says. In her work life, she was routinely exposed to very toxic chemicals. For many years it did not affect her health. However, at one point in her life, her health started to deteriorate. "The big shocker for me, however silly as it might sound, was that the chemicals would affect my health at all." She developed asthma and eczema, and at the same time she was unable to fight off coughs and colds. "It seemed like I could not get well, no matter what I did. My lifetime of working around toxins seemed to be making itself known. It was a little late in the game to change careers, so I looked around for something that would increase my strength. That's when I came across eleuthero." With daily doses of eleuthero, she regained her health, and her ability to resist toxins was restored. The skin conditions cleared up and she stopped getting monthly coughs and colds. "What I learned was this: If you are going to deal with chemicals all the time, you need to do something to reduce their effects on the body," she says.

Ginseng: For Drinkers, Smokers, and Drug Users

Scientific name: *Panax ginseng*

Part used: Root

Best For:

Smokers. Reduces the toxic effects of cigarette smoking and may reduce the chance of cancer. Studies indicate that ginseng increases resistance to regular toxin exposure, like that experienced by smokers.

Drinkers. Reduces the toxicity of alcohol and reduces the subtle damage done by drinking. Ginseng can even be used to prevent or reduce hangovers.

Drug takers. Increases resistance to toxic drugs. It may have a role in diminishing damage done by both street drugs and prescription drugs.

People addicted to a variety of substances. Your body is constantly exposed to compounds that undermine your health. It has to spend a lot of time getting these really toxic compounds out of your body when it should be attending to other matters. Under these conditions, your body is stressed and needs something that will help it out. History and science both reveal that ginseng may offer the necessary boost.

What It Does. In animal studies, ginseng was shown to increase resistance to radiation, toxic chemicals (carbon tetrachloride and thioacetamide), and narcotic and alcohol intoxication. When exposed to these compounds, laboratory animals were better able to resist the damaging effects and stayed healthier than would have otherwise been expected.

Among other things, chronic exposure to toxic compounds can cause cancer. Smokers develop lung cancer, drinkers develop liver cancer, and the jury is still out on what cancers recreational drug users might develop. We do know for sure that repeated exposure to toxic compounds causes cancer. Here, too, ginseng can help.

Ginseng increases resistance to cancer. It has been found to inhibit the production of tumors caused by toxins, to inhibit the spread of tumors, to increase tolerance of toxic antitumor drugs, and to stimulate the body's natural killer cell activity. Natural killer cells, a part of the immune system, help eliminate cancer cells from the body. One study also demonstrated that ginseng inhibited the cancer development associated with chronic hepatitis and liver cirrhosis.

Using Ginseng. Ginseng should be used to reduce the damage that regular exposure to toxins does to the body. In other words, if you are regularly putting chemicals into your body, use ginseng regularly. If you are occasionally putting chemicals into your body, use ginseng occasionally. If exposure is constant, think about using ginseng 2 weeks out of every month. If exposure is incidental, use ginseng for a week following the exposure.

You can take ginseng in the form of a tea. Just boil 1 teaspoon of dried root in 1 cup of water for 10 to 20 minutes. Strain, then drink.

R_x: One dose daily.

One dose =

1 cup of dried ginseng root tea (see above for instructions) OR

Two 500 mg tablets of dried root OR

One tablet of standardized extract containing 5 mg of ginsenosides OR

1 teaspoon root tincture 1:5 OR

20 drops root tincture 1:1

Origins. In Asia, ginseng has been used for centuries to stimulate the return of health and vitality among the ill and the elderly. Whenever health was challenged by a potentially lethal event, significant injury, or poisoning, people reached for ginseng to increase their resistance. Its reputation was so great that herb researchers started taking this plant apart early on. Between 1969 and 2003, more than 2,300 studies have been conducted on this herb. What's the conclusion? Ginseng really does increase strength and vitality, even when there is something like disease or chronic exposure to toxins undermining well-being.

Detox Makeover. Some habits are hard to break, even when you know you should. This was certainly the case with Bill, a 60-year-old cable television installer living in New Mexico. "I have needed to quit smoking for a long time, but every time I have tried, I didn't make

it. I would end up at the convenience store buying a pack of cigarettes." For a long time, the smoking did not seem to affect his health. He was able to participate in sports and rarely got a cold. "The truth is, for a long time, the smoking didn't reduce my quality of life. However, a couple of years ago I got bronchitis for the first time. Ever since then, it's an annual affair. Yes, it's a problem, but quitting seems to be an even bigger problem!" One of Bill's children suggested he try using an herbal medicine to reduce the damage the smoking was doing. Working with an herbalist, he decided to give ginseng a try. Though he was not successful at quitting, he did manage to add ginseng to his routine. "I feel a lot better since I started using the ginseng. I'm not great, but I am better than I was when I wasn't doing anything. My kids even say my color is better."

Milk Thistle: Chemical Wonder Worker

Scientific name: *Silybum marianum*

Part used: Seed

Best For:

Farmers and lawn-care workers. Agricultural pesticides, herbicides, and fertilizers tax the liver and can damage your body. Milk thistle, with its proven ability to protect the liver, can be used to reduce this damage.

Painters, plumbers, and electricians. Tradesmen are exposed to solvents, lead, and a collection of toxic chemicals. Milk thistle can be used to speed removal of these damaging compounds and protect the liver from damage.

Dry cleaners, photo-shop workers, toll-booth attendants, and professional drivers. These workers inhale toxic fumes that are absorbed through the lungs and removed by the liver. Milk thistle can be used to protect the liver from the damaging effects of these toxins.

What It Does. In 1900, not that many people worked with chemicals. In the year 2004, not many people can avoid working with chemicals. Many workers know they have chemicals landing on their skin and ending up in their lungs. Painters breathe in fumes from paint, and lawn-care workers end up covered with pesticides and herbicides. Not surprisingly, people are concerned about the effects regular toxin exposure is having on their health.

Though it would be nice if people could switch jobs, this is often not feasible. Medically speaking, the liver is largely responsible for getting these compounds out of your system. As such, the livers of these workers are under siege and could use a little help. Milk thistle might be just what the doctor ordered.

Research reveals that milk thistle contains flavolignans that are hepatoprotectant, meaning they protect the liver from damage due to toxic substances. Milk thistle seed contains 3 percent silymarin, which is actually a generic name for the flavolignan compounds that protect the liver. The most active substance is something known as silybin.

The action of these chemicals is simple, and it occurs on the cellular level. Silymarin makes the liver cells less susceptible to damage by toxins. The toxins enter the liver via the blood, but they are not able to do as much damage because milk thistle increases the liver's production of an antitoxin chemical called glutathione, raising it to 35 percent above normal.

Using Milk Thistle. Milk thistle protects your liver from all sorts of chemical damage. Toxins from the workplace and the environment are less troublesome when milk thistle is a regular part of your routine. Painters, lawn-care workers, pool maintenance crews, farm workers, factory workers, hairdressers, and the like are all candidates for regular doses of milk thistle. In these cases, it should be used as a daily tonic. It's easy to make a tea by boiling 1 teaspoon of milk thistle seed in 1 cup of water for 10 minutes. Just strain the seed out and drink.

R_x: One dose, three times a day.

One dose =

1 cup of milk thistle seed tea (see above for instructions) OR

Take a Pass on Purgatives

TAKE A FEW PILLS and purge out all the toxins in your body in one fell swoop—it certainly *sounds* appealing. In fact, it sounds too good to be true. And guess what? It is.

Currently, many eager and enthusiastic salespeople are hyping powerful laxatives as super-detox agents. Herbs like aloe, dock, and senna will make you rush to the toilet feeling like a bullet train is about to arrive. The immediate results are impressive. The problem with these herbs is that you end up losing more than toxins. You can also lose important minerals from your body. What's more, you can end up laxative dependent.

Indeed, if you know anything about the history of these herbs, you know that they have no place in a 21st-century detox plan. More than 100 years ago, doctors used treatments like bleeding, mercury, lead, and strong herbal laxatives. At the time, doctors felt that disease was caused by vitality, and if you could drain a person of vitality, that individual would recover from the disease. As crazy as this may sound, people believed it. People were given laxatives to the point of death, in the aim of returning them to health. Now we find people using these potentially dangerous herbs in detox regimens. The best advice here? Avoid powerful laxatives!

2 tablets of standardized extract containing 100 mg silymarin, going as high as 600 mg per day OR

1 teaspoon milk thistle tincture 1:5 OR 20 drops milk thistle tincture 1:1

Origins. Native to the Mediterranean, milk thistle has been used since antiquity to protect the liver against damaging diseases and compounds. Arabian physicians working in the 9th century were quite aware of liver disease. Hepatitis was a common condition due to sanitation problems, and these doctors dealt with more than their share of the disease. Time and time again, when a person yellowed due to liver failure, the condition was remedied with milk thistle. Later in European history, it was also used to help people survive accidental or intentional poisoning. The ancients knew that ginseng, a classic treatment for mushroom poisoning, would spare the liver if taken early.

Detox Makeover. Farming is a tough job for many reasons, and no one knows that better than Stan, a 48-year-old farmer who has been in the business since he was a child. He inherited his Ohio farm from his father. "When I first took over the farm, we didn't use that many chemicals. But in the last couple of years, the demand is for cheap produce. The only way we can provide people with what they want is to use lots of fertilizers, pesticides, and herbicides," he says. Stan has to support his family, and he felt that the only way he could do this was to jump on the chemicals bandwagon. "I don't know any farmer who wants to use this stuff. We just don't have a choice." He did what he felt he had to do, but he was still concerned about working with dangerous compounds. "I have seen neighbors die of strange cancers, and I don't want to go that way myself. I was reading a health magazine and came across milk thistle. The article said that it could reduce the toxicity of chemicals. I figured it couldn't hurt." He began using milk thistle whenever he had to spray the fields with pesticide or spread fertilizer. "I think of it as an insurance policy. You pay in now and reap the benefit down the road."

Rhodiola: Protection from Toxins and Autotoxins

Scientific name: *Rhodiola rosea*

Part used: Root

Best For:

People under stress and with stress-related diseases. While stressed, your body produces toxic compounds that damage every tissue in your body. Rhodiola reduces the damage done by these body-damaging substances.

People experiencing environmental changes. Increases resistance to this form of stress and makes it easier for your body to adapt. Changes in altitude, temperature, humidity, and water are stressful for the human body. Airline travel, though convenient, is hard on the body. Rhodiola helps the body deal with all of these environmental changes.

What It Does. Stress causes your body to produce toxins, toxins that can wreak havoc on your physical health. There is strong evidence that rhodiola may be the best adaptogen for many a stressed-out individual. Clinical trials have shown that the herb reduced fatigue in physicians working the night shift, reduced fatigue in students studying for final exams, and increased the ability to do physical exercise among individuals doing physical work. It was also shown to decrease levels of psychic fatigue and situation anxiety.

Rhodiola has also been shown to increase resistance to toxins produced by your own body, more specifically, to stress-related compounds like adrenaline. Adrenaline, a hormone produced in stressful circumstances, damages the blood vessels serving the brain and heart. This herb has been found to reduce the damage done by this body-produced compound. In one study using laboratory animals, it reduced palpitations associated with adrenaline.

Rhodiola also acts as a powerful antioxidant, neutralizing heart-damaging free radicals. Free radicals are reactive oxygen molecules that do considerable damage to the body and contribute to both aging and disease. Rhodiola has also been shown to reduce digestive abnormalities associated with excessive adrenaline production. Finally, one study demonstrated that the herb reduced toxicity and liver damage associated with a very toxic antitumor drug.

Using Rhodiola. During stress, your body produces damaging toxic compounds, and rhodiola can be used to increase resistance to these toxins. Indeed, it seems especially well-suited to the person experiencing a tremendous amount of stress. When stress is a big concern, think about rhodiola.

R$_x$: There are many types of rhodiola products on the market. Your best bet is to buy a product made by a reputable company and to use it per the packaging instructions.

Origins. Rhodiola is native to Ireland, Scotland, Scandinavia, and Russia. A traditional remedy, the herb has long been used to improve physical endurance, treat weakness, improve work capacity, and ensure longevity. Interestingly, it was used by the Vikings to enhance stamina and increase strength. Its traditional uses led researchers to screen the herb for adaptogenic activity.

Detox Makeover. The contemporary work environment is harsh, and it is getting harsher. Barb, a 35-year-old C.P.A., works for a major Baltimore accounting firm. At the beginning of her career, her job was stressful. "I thought dealing with tax season and end-of-fiscal-year was exhausting. But, in the age of layoffs, buyouts, and corporate scandals, that is the easy part. Never knowing if you are going to have a job from day to day is the real killer." She found the stress was driving her blood pressure up, upsetting her stomach, and causing anxiety attacks. "I talked to my doctor about all this, and he offered very symptomatic treatments— drugs to bring the pressure down, drugs to calm my nerves. But I knew this was not going to do anything about the real problem. I had to do something about the stress. It was all the adrenaline rushes that were making me sick." Barb used

rhodiola to get her body-produced toxin levels down and to combat the stress she was under. "Using rhodiola, I began to feel better. The stress seems to bounce off me, whereas before it was sticking. Even better, I have avoided blood pressure medication, stomach acid blockers, and antidepressants."

Schizandra: The Liver's Lover

Scientific name: *Schizandra sinensis*

Part used: Berry

Best For:

Drinkers. Protects your liver from chronic exposure to toxic substances, including alcohol. If used regularly, it may prevent liver damage.

Chemical workers. Speeds the process of removing toxic chemicals from your body and protects your liver from damage. Working with chemicals means your liver has to work double time to get chemicals out of your body. This herb helps your liver do this job.

Poor liver function. Improves liver function and thereby speeds toxin removal. When the liver functions under par, toxins remain in your system longer than they should.

What It Does. Schizandra acts as a free-radical scavenger. It contains nine different compounds that neutralize these damaging substances.

When it comes to its antitoxic effect, this herb has a remarkable record. In studies done using lab animals, schizandra was shown to prevent cerebral toxicity in animals exposed to a compound toxic to the brain, to inhibit tumor formation following exposure to tumor-causing chemicals, and to prevent massive liver-cell death after exposure to liver-destroying compounds.

In fact, protecting the liver from toxin damage may be this herb's strong suit. In one study using lab animals, it reduced liver damage associated with an Alzheimer's drug and the very liver damaging compound carbon tetrachloride.

In study after study, both on animals and humans, schizandra reduced the amount of damage done to the body, and in particular, the liver, when toxic compounds were an issue. And, as with all adaptogens, researchers found that this herb increased general resistance and energy levels while doing its magic.

Using Schizandra. Beyond its general antitoxin effects, this herb has some fairly specific uses. First, schizandra has a role in reducing the toxicity associated with drug therapies. In the study that demonstrated schizandra's ability to protect the liver from toxicity associated with one Alzheimer's medication, the efficacy of the drug was not affected. If prescription medicines you need to take are also causing liver damage, think about using schizandra.

Second, the herb has a role in raising liver resistance to toxic compound exposure in workers. Anyone exposed to toxic compounds, either routinely or incidentally, should think about using this herb.

Lastly, schizandra's ability to protect the liver from damage suggests that it's a must for those who have a problem with alcohol. Excessive alcohol intake is notoriously damaging to the liver. Once the liver has been damaged, it can't get toxins out of the body efficiently. If alcohol is an issue, schizandra may be the best adaptogen available.

You can take schizandra by drinking a beverage made from the berries. Boil 1½ teaspoons of berries in 1 cup of water for 5 minutes. Strain and drink each morning.

R_x: One dose daily.

One dose =

1 cup of schizandra berry tea (see above for instructions)

Origins. Native to China, schizandra has been used as a tonic for thousands of years and is one of the fundamental herbs in Traditional Chinese Medicine. Many parts of the plant are used medicinally. For detoxification purposes, the berry is of the greatest interest. Traditionally, it is considered to be an astringent, aphrodisiac, stimulant, and tonic. It has been used primarily for night sweats but also for amnesia, asthma, coughs, diabetes, diarrhea, dysentery, insomnia, premature ejaculation, and tuberculosis. Though this seems like a diverse list of conditions, there is a central theme here: The herb raises resistance to whatever is taxing the body.

Detox Makeover. Some people like a drink more than others do. Stan, a 70-year-old hard drinker from Boston, is one of those people.

"I'm not stupid, I know drinking is not the healthiest of hobbies," he says. But despite being continuously encouraged by friends and family to quit drinking, Stan has not been able to change his lifestyle. However, when his drinking began to affect both his digestive tract and his skin, he took some action. "A couple of years ago I noticed my face had turned red and that I could no longer eat oily foods. It seemed like everything I put in my mouth soured my stomach." At that point, he was advised

to start using schizandra. "I had heard that this Chinese remedy made the drink easier to handle. I figured I had nothing to lose, and it was worth a try."

The herb has been very effective in providing some relief and protection to Stan while he continues to struggle with his addiction to alcohol. "My skin is not as red as it used to be, and my stomach is not bothering me as much."

Step Three: Add Red Sorrel

RED SORREL: THE ALL-PURPOSE PURIFIER

Whatever people drink, they tend to drink routinely. Coffee drinkers drink coffee, beer drinkers drink beer. If you drink toxin-laden beverages (those containing caffeine or alcohol) all the time, you flood your body with toxins all the time. Alternatively, if you drink antitoxin beverages regularly, you regularly fill your body with toxin-neutralizing refreshment. Getting in the habit of drinking good-for-you beverages goes a long way toward taking care of the toxin problem.

If you have ever been subject to some of the medicinal-tasting herbal brews some people concoct, this may sound like an unattractive proposition. Who is going to trade in their cola for a vile-tasting herbal brew? The answer to that is "no one." However, what if there were an antitoxin beverage that was a delicious addition to any meal or relaxing moment? That's where this next herb really shines. It's not only a good-for-you antitoxin, but it's also just plain good.

Red Sorrel

Scientific name: *Hibiscus sabdariffa*

Part used: Flower

Best For:

Everyone. Contributes to your body's regular detox efforts. We all drink beverages. Red sorrel produces a beverage that undermines the negative effects of many of the toxins we encounter. And this medicine is a pleasure to take.

Junk food eaters. Even though the medical research has not yet conclusively proven its usefulness in this regard, red sorrel is thought to speed the removal of the chemicals found in junk food and prevent those chemicals from damaging your body.

Party people. This is to help people who use alcohol, not to recommend that they overdo it. The regular intake of alcohol or drugs can cause toxin-related diseases. Red sorrel can offer your body some protection from this abuse and serve to prevent or cure a hangover.

Other Delicious Antitoxin Beverages

RED SORREL IS NOT THE ONLY ANTITOXIN coming from the plant kingdom. If you don't care for red sorrel tea or would like even more cleansing power, you can also get detox benefits from adding these refreshing drinks to your diet:

Apple juice
Cranberry juice
Douglas fir frond tea

Grape juice
Green tea
White pine needle tea

What It Does. Have you ever tasted one of those zippy fruit-flavored herbal teas? They have become increasingly popular among the health conscious and even the not-so-health-conscious. Peach, apple, and cinnamon-pear are some of the flavors you can find at the grocery store. If you read the fine print on the labeling, you will find that they are all loaded with red sorrel. In fact, red sorrel gives these teas their fruity flavor. More than an ingredient, red sorrel is a phenomenal detoxifier all on its own. And it comes with boatloads of history and science.

Red sorrel has been the subject of a whole bunch of intriguing studies. Though researchers began investigating its traditional uses, their work revealed it to be the perfect antidote to bad food. Time and time again, researchers have found it to be active in reducing the effects of both the toxins in bad food and the toxins our bodies produce after we eat bad food.

We now know that the free radicals circulating in our bodies cause heart disease, cancer, arthritis, and aging in general. Five separate studies found protocatechuic acid (PCA), a compound found in red sorrel, to be a powerful free-radical scavenger. It is, in fact, a more powerful free-radical neutralizer than vitamin E. It has been shown to prevent free radicals from damaging the body, inhibiting their ability to turn normal cells into cancer cells.

In another study, the colon cells of lab animals exposed to cancer-causing chemicals did not become cancerous when pretreated with red sorrel. In fact, red sorrel reduced mutation by 60 to 90 percent. Other researchers found that skin-cancer-causing chemicals did not cause skin cancer in test animals who were first bathed in red sorrel tea. Again, the conclusion was that red sorrel inhibited the transformation of normal cells into cancer cells. Even more importantly, red sorrel was found to encourage human cancer cells to self-destruct rather than replicate.

Free radicals cause chemical changes in low-density lipoproteins (bad cholesterol) that in turn result in atherosclerosis, the leading cause of heart disease. PCA has been found to neutralize free radicals before they have a chance to cause these chemical changes. Additionally, red sorrel reduced bad cholesterol levels in test animals fed high-cholesterol diets.

What's more, red sorrel tea was also found to reduce blood pressure in both lab animals and humans. In a human clinical trial, 54 people with high blood pressure experienced a 10 percent reduction in blood pressure levels while taking red sorrel tea. Could it get any better? Yes. Red sorrel was also shown to inhibit many body-produced heart and blood vessel damaging enzymes (angiotensin converting enzyme, elastase, trypsin, and alpha-chymotrypsin).

As if all of that isn't enough, red sorrel also protects the liver. In Jamaica, tradition has it that red sorrel keeps a hangover at bay. Once again, a folk tradition has been validated. Red sorrel's famous red color is due to compounds known as *Hibiscus anthocyanins*. It has been established that these compounds prevent liver damage in animals. Lab animals, treated with liver-destroying chemicals, did not develop liver damage when pretreated with red sorrel.

Using Red Sorrel. Red sorrel can be used to reduce the toxins in our bodies. And it's a healthy beverage you and even your fussiest friend will enjoy. Serve it up at a dinner party and you will hear nothing but praise. Looking for something sweet and brightly colored to give the kids? Look no further. Red sorrel is as popular among children as the most toxin-laden fruit punch. It goes well with whatever you are serving or eating.

The traditional way of using sorrel may be the best way. Add 2 cups of dried red sorrel blossoms to 10 cups of water. Boil the mixture for 15 minutes, and then add turbinado sugar. Then pour yourself a cup of one of the healthiest, tastiest beverages ever known.

R_x: You can drink as much of this as you like, but to get the medicinal benefits, try to have 3 cups a day!

Origins. Native to Africa, red sorrel's spicy red flowers have long been used to remedy coughs and colds, inflammation, cancer, heart disease, and liver disease. Although it clearly has great medicinal benefits, the reason it has been carried to the four corners of the earth is for other, slightly less noble reasons: It makes a great punch. A favorite cooling beverage in Ethiopia, red sorrel made its way to the Caribbean early in colonial history because it is an excellent beverage. Once there, it became popular and still is. A trip to Jamaica gives tourists a chance to sample a local tradition, red sorrel and rum punch. It's a good combination, as the red sorrel goes a long way toward mitigating the damage done by the rum!

Keys to Success with Herbal Detox

HERE'S HOW TO MAKE HERBS YOUR MOST TRUSTED ALLIES in your detoxification efforts.

⊚ Create a detox regimen that you can maintain. Think long term and try to avoid Herculean efforts. It's better to add one herb to your regular program and stick with it than to go overboard and quit in a few weeks.

⊚ Think ahead. If you know you are going to paint the house, fertilize the yard, overindulge, or in some way be exposed to toxins, use a resistance herb to raise your resistance to chemicals. When the exposure is over, use a housekeeping herb to speed the removal of toxins.

⊚ Know that your body has the capacity to deal with toxins. Your liver, kidneys, sweat glands, and immune system are all in place to get toxins out of your body. Work with your body, using herbal medicine to increase this capacity.

⊚ Use a resistance herb to increase your body's ability to resist the damaging effects of toxins. Chronic exposure to toxins wears your body out.

⊚ Choose to drink an antitoxin instead of a beverage that contains toxins. Making this simple change will make an enormous difference in your health.

⊚ Make herbal detox a regular part of your life. Like exercise, it's something you should think about every day.

Detox Makeover. Working women have a lot on their plates. They may have to manage a career, household, and kids, and they rarely get assistance. Gloria, a 43-year-old woman, works full-time and mothers three kids. "Most days I feel like I have two full-time jobs—probably because I do!" Though she likes the idea of feeding her kids organic foods, for her it just isn't realistic. She lives in rural Pennsylvania and getting to the organic market is a day's trip. "Organic food ap-

Tea versus Tincture

FOR DETOX OR ANY OTHER PURPOSE, the key to success is using your selected herbs regularly. As such, the best way to take herbs is the way that is most convenient for you—the manner in which you are most likely to keep using them. If you enjoy making and drinking tea, then plan to use herbal teas. If you live life on the run, then tinctures may be a more viable option. Tinctures are easy to transport in a purse or briefcase. Be realistic and come up with a plan that you can actually live with.

Using teas. The herbs listed in this chapter can be purchased in natural food stores, health food stores, and with increasing frequency, in drugstores and supermarkets. They're available both loose and in tea bags. There is no difference between these two options. Which one you use is simply a matter of personal preference. Tea bags can be tossed into a teapot or mug. Loose tea needs to be strained out of the tea before you drink it.

Using tinctures. Tinctures are water/alcohol extracts of herbs. A mixture of alcohol and water is passed over the herbs and the herbs' healing principles are thus captured in the liquid. Importantly, any tincture worth buying will have a ratio on the bottle. It will say Tincture 1:4, Tincture 1:3, or something similar. These ratios indicate the strength of the tincture. Pay attention to these numbers. A 1:1 tincture is 10 times as strong as a 1:10 tincture! If you have been directed to take a 1:10 tincture, take a 1:10 tincture; do not assume that more is better. You can take tinctures straight from the bottle or mix them with tea, juice, or water. The choice is yours.

peals to me, but with my schedule, it is not a reality. With the best of intentions, I find myself at the local grocery in the frozen prepared-food section," she says.

"Even though I can't always get the food thing right, I do make a huge effort to make sure the kids drink healthy beverages. A couple of years ago I discovered red sorrel and decided that it was a good beverage choice. The kids love it and don't give me any grief when they see it coming," she says. Gloria always has a pitcher in the icebox, and, when the kids squeal for something sweet to drink, out comes the red sorrel tea.

Chapter 6

Detoxercise:
Building a Better, Cleaner Body

IMAGINE YOURSELF AS A BODY OF WATER. Given the choice, would you rather be a stagnant pond, sitting and collecting debris, pollution, and bacteria, or a mountain stream, energetically trickling through rocks and flora, filtering out dirt and impurities? Though the analogy may be somewhat of an oversimplification, your body works much like these two waters. It collects disease-causing toxins when you're sedentary, and it runs itself clean when you move.

As you've already learned, the environment is rife with toxins, which is a fancy term for any elements that your body has no use for and that may be harmful. They include thousands of foreign substances ranging from heavy metals like lead and mercury to pesticides and PCBs to everyday food colorings and preservatives.

We also make our own "toxins" in the form of cellular waste and excess hormones, such as estrogen. Left unchecked, all toxins can poison the body. Some signs of accumulating inner "gunk" are everyday woes like fatigue, sluggishness, headaches, digestive problems, and assorted skin conditions. But toxins that the body does not throw off can also lead to bigger worries, such as cancer, heart disease, and arthritis.

"Even diseases that we've typically blamed on genetics and aging may have a connection to toxins like heavy metals," says Frederic J. Vagnini, M.D., who runs the Heart, Diabetes, and Weight Loss Center of New York in New York City. "Lead has recently been associated with hypertension. Cadmium is linked to arteriosclerosis. Mercury and other metals wreak havoc on our health in ways we're just beginning to understand."

PURIFICATION IN MOTION

Exercise cleanses and protects our bodies in ways that we're just beginning to comprehend. We've known since the age of Hippocrates that exercise can keep us healthy. Modern research shows that regular exercisers have half the number of colds as those who are sedentary, and they are at a significantly decreased risk for many cancers, especially breast and other reproductive-system cancers. But experts have only recently begun linking the detoxifying power of exercise with these important health benefits.

Just as there's more than one way that toxins infiltrate your system, there's more than one way that exercise helps flush them out. The following are the most well-documented ways physical exercise helps you detoxify.

The Purification Patrol

A healthy lymphatic system is key to keeping your immune system in top working condition. Disease-fighting white blood cells are stored in your lymph nodes, which are located under your arms, at your neck, and around your spine and groin. These cells are carried by lymphatic fluid through thread-like "veins" throughout your body.

In his studies on immunity, researcher David Nieman, Ph.D., professor of health and exercise science at Appalachian State University in Boone, North Carolina, likens immune cells to cops. When you're sedentary, they hang out in the station, or lymph tissue, where they are fairly inactive. Soon after you start exercising, however, and for a few hours afterward, they pull out of the station and patrol your body, seeking and destroying invading bacteria and viruses. In one of his studies, Dr. Nieman found that when 150 people walked regularly for 12 weeks, they had about half the number of sore throats and colds as their sedentary peers.

Lymph also pulls double-duty as trash collector. While sweeping through your system, lymph fluid filters out and carries away cellular waste and other toxins, so they can be processed and removed from your body.

You have two to three times as much lymphatic fluid in your body as you do blood. Yet unlike blood, which is pushed through your body at the amazing rate of 1.3 gallons per minute by a pump (your heart) that stops only when you're dead, your lymphatic system moves very little until you do, relying mostly on muscle compression on the lymphatic vessels to keep the fluid circulating. What's the best way to keep your lymph flowing freely?

Exercise every day. Regular physical activity not only keeps the lymph circulating on a regular basis, it also improves your general range of motion and body posture—both of which also help keep the lymph moving freely and easily throughout your body.

Replenish. On the flip side, if you don't exercise, the lymph becomes like a backed-up sewage system—the toxic waste spills over into your body and causes problems.

"Letting the lymphatic system become stagnant leads to impaired immunity and a degenerative process because the body is not able to properly cleanse and replenish," says holistic medicine expert Martin Dayton, M.D., D.O., of the Dayton Medical Center in Sunny Isles Beach, Florida.

The Dreaded Obesity-Cancer Connection

THE STATISTICS LINKING OVERWEIGHT AND OBESITY WITH CANCER ARE STAGGERING. If you're overweight, your risk for cancers of all kinds is raised significantly. The more overweight you are, the greater your risk. According to the Mayo Clinic, compared to women of a healthy weight, obese women have:

- Up to 1½ times greater risk for breast cancer after menopause
- 2 to 4 times the risk of endometrial cancer
- 2 to 4 times the risk of kidney cancer
- 2 times the risk of pancreatic cancer
- 46 percent higher risk of developing colon cancer

Burning Your Trash

You've likely heard the warnings about mercury buildup in fatty fish. Well, like our aquatic counterparts, we too accumulate waste in our fat stores. "Fat is a great repository for toxic material," says Dr. Dayton. "And naturally, the more fat you have, the more waste you can collect."

What's more, once you have excess fat stores, they become metabolically active themselves, pumping out excess hormones that wreak as much internal havoc as any environmental toxin does. "Estrogen is created in fat tissue," says Dr. Vagnini, "and too much estrogen appears to have a strong connection to cancer, especially breast cancer."

Exercise helps reduce your risk by burning fat. When you burn fat, you not only release stored toxins into the bloodstream, where they can be filtered and excreted by your liver, kidneys, and lungs, but you also eliminate the storage space where toxins hide.

As you lose fat, you also produce less estrogen. Researchers at the Fred Hutchinson Cancer Research Center found that women doing aerobic exercise for 45 minutes a day, 5 days a week, were able to lower their estrogen levels 4 percent after just 12 weeks. "This general release and lowering of toxins is likely one of the reasons exercise is connected with a reduction in cancer risk," says Dr. Dayton. (Remember, estrogen itself is not a toxin; excess estrogen definitely is.)

As a bonus, as you continue to exercise and become more physically fit, you become a more efficient fat burner in general, meaning that your body is better able to burn dietary fat (as opposed to carbohydrates, your body's preferred fuel during exercise) when you work out. That's important because then you'll be less likely to store toxins in the first place, says Andrew Rubman, N.D., founder of the Southbury Clinic for Traditional Medicines in Connecticut. "Being able to successfully metabolize fat as fuel puts you at an advantage, because if you're leveraging the fat you eat for energy, daily assaults from pesticides and pollutants will just pass right on through."

Drink lots of water. If you're exercising regularly, you're burning lots of fat and releasing stored toxins. So be sure to flush them from your system faster by also drinking plenty of fluids. "Water helps dilute and eliminate all those toxins," says Dr. Dayton, who suggests drinking 8 to 10 glasses of filtered water per day, every day, but especially when you're exercising.

Sweating It Out

You are literally wrapped in one of nature's finest waste-removal systems: your skin. The average adult has 18 to 20 square feet of skin. It weighs over 5 pounds, and though it doesn't look like a liver or a kidney, it is an excellent eliminative organ.

Like the liver and lungs, the skin can help transform toxins from fat into water-soluble forms that can be removed by the kidneys. The skin itself also excretes great amounts of metabolic waste and pollutants. Hence the phrase, "sweat it out."

"Sweating is an excellent way of eliminating toxins," says Dr. Dayton. "As you heat the body and perspire, you release heavy metals like lead and mercury, organic toxins like pesticides and insecticides, and various pollutants—many of which we haven't even identified yet."

Though any heart-pumping aerobic exercise will work, there are special exercise regimens designed to promote profuse sweating and detoxification.

Try hot yoga. Bikram yoga, for example, is practiced in heated rooms with temperatures ranging from 85 to 105 degrees. This balmy environment, combined with a vigorous routine that consists of 26 challenging poses, raises your heart rate and elicits sweat by the bucketful. It's so effective for purification that the Bastyr Center for Natural Health in Seattle now recommends it as a regular part of the treatment regimen for hepatitis C, a chronic viral liver infection.

Bake a little. "Sitting in a sauna after exercise encourages even more elimination," says New York City–based exercise physiologist Shari Lieberman, Ph.D., author of *The Real Vitamin and Mineral Book*. (You wouldn't want to do this right after Bikram yoga, however. That would be too much of a good thing.)

Don't soak in your own toxins. It's a good idea to wear workout clothes made from absorbent, wicking fabrics (like CoolMax) to pull the sweat away from your skin, says Dr. Lieberman. "And take a shower as soon as you can when you're done exercising," she says. "You don't want those toxins sitting on your skin or absorbing back in."

A Clean Sweep

Jack LaLanne once described our bowel functions as "Nature's broom." Another big benefit of exercise is that it speeds metabolism and assists our natural peristaltic action, which is a fancy way of saying that it keeps you "regular," allowing for consistent waste removal.

"Many people think you need enemas

and colonics for detoxification," says Dr. Rubman. "But I would argue that in most cases, regular exercise is all the stimulation that your GI tract needs."

Physical activity also promotes increased circulation in general, which increases perfusion, or healthy bloodflow, through important detoxifying organs like the kidneys and liver, says Dr. Vagnini.

"The key here is moderate exercise, which brings plenty of oxygen-rich blood to the organs and helps with the transfer of waste," Dr. Vagnini says. "Intense exercise won't have this same effect because blood tends to be shunted away from the abdominal area and into the working muscles during hard physical activity."

Both moderate and vigorous exercise help blow out the cobwebs and clear your blood vessels and lungs, however. Sedentary people use only about one-third of their lung capacity. The other two-thirds contains stagnant air that is rich in toxins and metabolic waste. This not only prevents your lungs from doing their job properly, but it also limits the amount of oxygen-rich blood the rest of your body receives.

When you get your lungs huffing and puffing through physical activity, you literally blow the toxins from your lungs and allow more oxygen into your bloodstream. "Many toxins can be broken into exhalable forms and expelled through increased respiration," says Dr. Vagnini.

Building Your Immunity Team

One of the most important ways exercise helps detoxify the body is by stimulating the immune system to build its arsenal of disease-fighting cells. These metabolic warriors (such as natural killer T cells and macrophages) patrol your body and neutralize harmful invaders before they can do their dirty work.

"There's an entire new field of medicine called exercise-immunology that focuses heavily on how exercise directly affects the immune system," says exercise physiologist Laurie Cullen, N.D., of the Bastyr Center for Natural Health in Seattle. "We know regular, moderate exercise like walking, jogging, cycling, and swimming has a positive effect on many immune functions."

In a study looking at immune cell production, researchers at Texas Christian University found that exercisers who rode a stationary bike for 1 hour twice a day not only had significantly higher counts of important immune system cells than those who didn't exercise, but their immunity was even higher after the second daily bout of exercise. The researchers concluded that you didn't necessarily need to pedal away for 2 hours each day to reap those benefits, but that repeated bouts of activity throughout the day is likely good for stimulating immune activity.

A robust immune system is not only essential for keeping your system free from infection-causing viruses and bacteria, but it also plays a role in preventing cancer. "Our immune system is in constant surveillance mode, whether we exercise or not," says Dr. Cullen. "But if you add exercise, it works even harder, and you're that much less likely to get sick."

Curbing Your Stress

Lastly, but no less importantly, exercise helps with purification by purging toxic emotions. If it sounds "new agey" to talk about emotional pollution, consider this: Stress—a runaway emotion in our society—causes a cascade of physical reactions including accelerated heartbeat, a rise in blood pressure, an increase in blood sugar, and a boost in stomach acid. That potent physical stress response may actually help you if you're gearing up to punch out a foe or flee from a fire. But chances are you're neither fighting nor taking flight, but rather sitting on a desk chair, stewing in that toxic environment.

Common symptoms of stress include muscle tension; upset stomach; head-aches; compulsive eating, drinking, or smoking; fatigue; and insomnia—all of which not only hamper detoxification, but also pour more poison into your already-addled system. Making matters worse, hormones like cortisol and adrenaline, which are associated with stress, promote fat (and thereby toxin) storage, particularly in the abdominal area.

"Stress, hostility, and anger are well-established, serious risk factors for heart disease," says Dr. Vagnini, "and they likely contribute to other degenerative conditions as well."

Exercise provides stress relief by burning off stress hormones and lowering blood pressure. Regular physical activity also makes you more stress resilient.

In a recent study, researchers measured the physical fitness of 26 men and women, ages 19 to 38. They then tested their responses to emotional and physical stress by first giving them a difficult math problem to solve and then dunking their hand in ice water for 2 minutes. They found that many of the physically fit participants had less of a spike in blood pressure during the tests than their less-fit counterparts. Experts say the rigors of physical activity help the body respond to all types of stress and ultimately protect the heart.

Exercise R~x~

There are as many different types of exercise as there are ways you can imagine to move your body. Whether you run, dance, play sports, hop up and down on one foot, or even just lie on the floor and do ab crunches, it's all considered exercise. Though all types of exercise will help you detoxify, some are clearly more beneficial than others. The following are what works best.

Walk This Way

Generally speaking, aerobic exercises like walking, jogging, cycling, and swimming are the most detoxifying, says Dr. Lieberman. "You move the lymphatic system, you sweat, and you increase blood circulation and respiration. It does it all," she says.

Aerobic exercise—sometimes known as cardio—is simply any physical activity that raises your heart rate for a prolonged period of time, like a 45-minute Spinning class or a 30-minute jog, as opposed to anaerobic activity, like lifting weights, which requires only short bursts of energy. Of the wide array of aerobic activities you can choose from, walking is hands-down the most popular. It's also something almost everyone can do, regardless of his or her fitness level, to get a daily dose of detoxification.

In her book *Our Toxic World*, Doris J. Rapp, M.D., recommends walking energetically, planting on your heel and rocking up and pressing off of your toes with each step for about 20 minutes a day, as one of the easiest ways to stimulate your lymphatic system. She also recommends walking as a way of cleansing the muscles and the lungs.

"Moderate-intensity aerobic exercise is also the exercise regimen recommended to prevent cancer," says Dr. Cullen. "In all the studies, sustained aerobic exercise like walking and jogging stimulates the protective effects."

Jump for Joy

Want the inner sparkle of a child? Jump up and down like one. Bouncing on a trampoline, such as a minitramp or "rebounder," is one of the least-appreciated exercises for cleansing and strengthening every cell of your body. It's also one of the best workouts for activating the lymphatic system.

Your lymphatic system is filled with millions of one-way valves that allow lymph to flow in one direction, usually upward. The change of speed and direction with each bounce opens every valve and gives your lymphatic system a super squeeze, so all your cells are completely flushed of their metabolic waste and then saturated with incoming fresh oxygen and nutrients.

What's more, bouncing strengthens your cells. When you start bouncing up and down, your body is subjected to the force of acceleration and deceleration plus gravity, or G Force. As you continue bouncing, every cell, including those of your muscles and bones, responds to the increased force by getting stronger.

Many fitness facilities have mini-tramps available for general use. Or you can buy one at a sporting goods or department store starting at about $40 or via the Internet at fitness sites like www.bodytrends.com.

Let Your Body Flow

Few forms of exercise can boast 5,000 years of faithful practice by millions of people across the globe. Yoga can. For centuries, yoga has been prescribed as moving medicine for the immune system. Yoga helps lower stress hormones that compromise immunity while stimulating the lymphatic system to purge toxins and bringing fresh, nutrient-filled, oxygenated blood to each organ to ensure optimum function.

Yoga even includes specific poses that are known to clear toxins from specific body regions and that support specific body functions and organs. For instance, inverted poses like Downward Facing Dog, which position your head and torso lower than other parts of your body, help flush out your lungs and sinuses, so your body can oust bacteria and toxins caught in your mucus.

"Whole-body stretching and strengthening exercises like yoga and tai chi are fantastic detoxifiers because they stretch out the areas surrounding the lymph nodes through their full range of motion, and they encourage lymphatic drainage," says Dr. Lieberman.

The gentle twisting, turning, bending, and reaching of mind-body exercises like yoga also put light pressure on your digestive system, which aids in the expedient expulsion of toxins through your bowels.

Pick Up the Pace

There's a longstanding myth among exercisers that you need to exercise at a lower intensity for a longer duration to maximize fat burning and thereby release toxins. Not true. To really rev your metabolism, burn more calories, and keep your fat-burning switch turned on for a longer time after you're done exercising, try picking up the pace.

Research shows that not only do you burn more calories when you exercise vigorously, but following the workout you get a robust hormonal charge that causes your body to burn more fat when you're at rest. What's more, your metabolism stays revved up five times longer after a spirited workout session than after an easy one. Over time, this can add up to burning an additional 100 to 200 calories, many of them from fat, a day.

Slip in some fast time. We're not talking about imitating Flo Jo around your high school track, of course, just sneaking brief spurts of intensity into the aerobic workouts you already do. For instance, if you walk now, try picking up your pace and power walking or jogging just enough so your breathing becomes heavy (but you're not gasping for breath) for 2 or 3 minutes. Then walk easy for 2 or 3 minutes. And so on. Before long, the higher-intensity segments will feel easier, and you'll be a speedier walker, too, so you'll be burning more calories each time you exercise.

Make Some Muscle

Sometime in our mid to late thirties, due to hormonal changes and generally decreasing activity levels, we start losing lean muscle tissue at the rate of about ½ pound a year—a loss that can accelerate to 1 pound a year in women once they hit menopause. That's important because muscle tissue burns about 15 times

as many calories each day, even when you're just sleeping or reading, as fat tissue does.

When you lose muscle, your daily calorie burn drops. If you do nothing to stem the loss, by the time you're 65, you could have lost half of your lean body mass and doubled it with body fat. As you know, the more fat you have, the more room there is for toxins to hide out.

The best way to solve this problem is strength training. Strength training boosts natural muscle-making chemicals such as human growth hormone and preserves the muscle we have, while also replacing the muscle tissue we've lost.

Lifting weights also helps you shed fat by simply burning calories. A 140-pound woman can burn off almost 200 calories during a challenging 30-minute strength-training routine. What's more, your calorie-burning metabolism can stay elevated for up to 48 hours after you've finished lifting.

In one study, researchers had 15 sedentary men and women in their sixties and seventies perform two sets of 10 to 12 strength-training exercises 3 days a week for 6 months. At the end of the study, the group boosted their resting metabolism—the calories they burned just by living and breathing—by 7 percent, or 88 calories a day. They increased the total number of calories they burned on an average day—including their workouts and cooldown period—by more than 230 calories.

Start lifting. The key to maximizing your fat-burning metabolism is challenging the most muscle fibers possible. That means starting a strength-training routine if you've never lifted weights before, or changing your routine to a new, more challenging one if you're already a regular lifter.

Target as many muscles as you can. The more muscles you recruit in your lifting routine, the more lean tissue and the less toxin-trapping fat you'll have. A woman who targets all her major muscle groups twice a week can expect to replace 5 pounds of muscle—5 to 10 years' worth—in just a few months of strength training.

Take It Outside

Whenever possible, infuse your exercise routine with some fresh air by exercising outdoors, ideally going somewhere beautiful like a park, along a river, by the ocean, or into the mountains.

Even if you just walk down a tree-lined street, however, you're still helping your body detoxify and heal. Human beings have a natural affinity for the outdoors. One much-cited study from the mid-

1980s demonstrated that people recovering from abdominal surgery with a view of nature from their windows had significantly shorter hospital stays, required less pain medication, and made fewer complaints than those whose rooms faced a brick wall. And, of course, plants and trees help detoxify us by filtering our air and cleansing our environment of carbon dioxide and other environmental pollutants.

When exercising outside, however, it's important that you not add to your toxic burden by walking or jogging along crowded roads or highways where you're breathing exhaust. This is particularly important in warm-weather months, when the pollution tends to get trapped in the atmosphere, bogging down the air we breathe with heavy metals and other dangerous elements. It's even more important if you're doing a spirited exercise like jogging or cycling that increases your breathing rate. When exercising vigorously, your air intake increases tenfold. And most of the air is getting pulled right through your mouth, which, unlike your nose, isn't lined with fine hairs that filter the air before it reaches your lungs.

You can avoid nullifying your detoxifying exercise with environmental pollutants by exercising at the right time and place. Some simple tips:

Avoid the rush. Motor vehicles are a major source of air pollution. Avoid exercising when they're out in great numbers, such as during the afternoon rush hour. By that hour, pollution has been accumulating all day and is getting even heavier. If you must exercise at that time of day, get as far away from the roads as you can to avoid direct exposure.

Shed and scrub. Pollutants and pollen (a natural toxin for allergic people) collect on your clothes when you exercise. Change clothes and hop in the shower (or at least towel off) as soon as possible when you're done exercising to avoid breathing in the pollen and pollutants trapped on your clothes.

Check the index. Most major newspaper and online weather reports print smog and air pollution levels in what is called the Air Quality Index (AQI) or Pollution Standards Index (PSI). When the numbers creep above 100, pollution is high. If they skyrocket above 200, stay inside and write your congressman to support stricter clean air controls.

What the Experts Do

IF THERE'S ONE THING all the experts do, it's that they don't do just one thing. They hike, play basketball, lift weights, swim, and run, often going days without repeating an activity.

"I was obese once, so I know how important daily activity is," says Frederic J. Vagnini, M.D., who runs the Heart, Diabetes, and Weight Loss Center of New York in New York City. "But I also know that no matter how good exercise is for you, you won't do it if you're bored. That's why I'm a firm believer in cross-training and always trying a new activity," he says. Andrew Rubman, N.D., founder of the Southbury Clinic for Traditional Medicines in Connecticut, agrees. "Physical activity not only helps you enjoy life more, but it also should be enjoyable in and of itself. I ski, sail, and hike, among other things. The body responds best if you present it with different types of stimulation that challenge your muscles in unique ways."

THE PURIFICATION PLAN DETOXERCISE ROUTINE

The best exercise detoxification routine blends the right dose of fat-burning aerobic exercise, muscle-toning strength training, and range-of-motion enhancing stretching. "By performing a variety of types of exercise, you ensure that your detoxification efforts are well balanced and that you cover every body region," says Dr. Dayton.

See The 7-Day Plan below for your complete 1-week detoxercise plan. It includes 30 minutes of activity a day, but feel free to add more cardio (heart-pumping aerobic) activities like walking, cycling, and swimming, if you like. (Remember, jumping on a minitrampoline is an excellent cardiovascular and detoxifying workout.)

You also can do more yoga or other flexibility and balance exercises. It's best to limit strength training to 2 or 3 days a week, however, so your muscles have a chance to rest and rebuild between sessions. On days when time is crunched, you can break down your 30-minute exercise session into two 15-minute or even three 10-minute chunks.

The 7-Day Plan

Day 1	Day 2	Day 3	Day 4
Gentle cardio of your choice (walking, bicycling, swimming) for 25 minutes	Warm up with gentle cardio for 5 minutes	Warm up with gentle cardio for 5 minutes	Gentle cardio of your choice (walking, bicycling, swimming) for 25 minutes
Cleansing Yoga Series (see page 128)	Detox Tone-Up Plan (see page 132)	Detox Tone-Up Plan (see page 132)	
	Cooldown for 5 minutes	Cooldown for 5 minutes	
	Cardio with a Kick (see page 142)		

Day 5	Day 6	Day 7	
Cleansing Yoga Series (see page 128)	Rest	Cardio with a Kick (see page 142)	

Cleansing Yoga Series

Perform each position twice, moving slowly and deliberately, stretching into position only until you feel a comfortable stretch. Hold at that point for 30 seconds. Return to your starting position, rest for a few seconds, and repeat.

DOWNWARD FACING DOG

Benefits: Reduces stress, relieves constipation and indigestion, cleanses sinuses and lungs

(A) Position yourself on the floor on your hands and knees, feet flexed, toes to the floor.

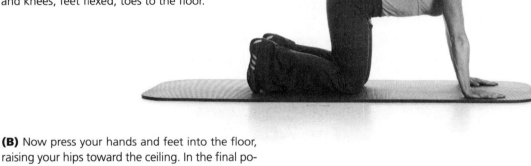

(B) Now press your hands and feet into the floor, raising your hips toward the ceiling. In the final position, your body should look like an upside-down V. Keep your back and legs straight, and keep lifting your tailbone toward the ceiling as you lower your heels to the floor as far as is comfortably possible. (NOTE: This can be difficult if you are overweight or have wrist problems.) If you have trouble performing the full position, try keeping your knees slightly bent, or place your hands on something slightly higher than the floor, like an aerobic step or the first step of a staircase.

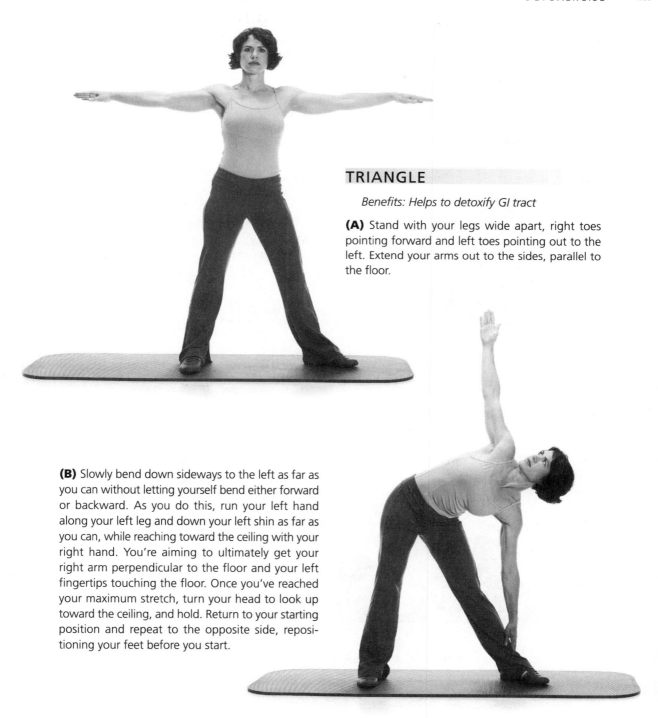

TRIANGLE

Benefits: Helps to detoxify GI tract

(A) Stand with your legs wide apart, right toes pointing forward and left toes pointing out to the left. Extend your arms out to the sides, parallel to the floor.

(B) Slowly bend down sideways to the left as far as you can without letting yourself bend either forward or backward. As you do this, run your left hand along your left leg and down your left shin as far as you can, while reaching toward the ceiling with your right hand. You're aiming to ultimately get your right arm perpendicular to the floor and your left fingertips touching the floor. Once you've reached your maximum stretch, turn your head to look up toward the ceiling, and hold. Return to your starting position and repeat to the opposite side, repositioning your feet before you start.

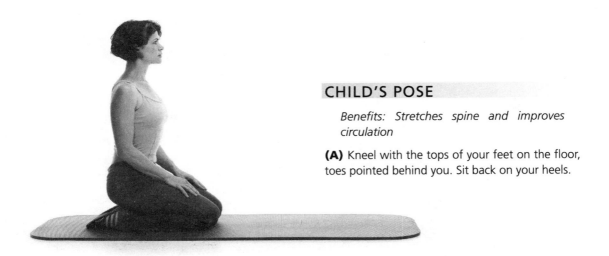

CHILD'S POSE

Benefits: Stretches spine and improves circulation

(A) Kneel with the tops of your feet on the floor, toes pointed behind you. Sit back on your heels.

(B) Slowly lower your chest to your thighs as you stretch your arms overhead and rest your palms and forehead on the floor (or as close to it as is comfortable). If you are overweight, you can spread your legs to make space for your abdomen. Hold.

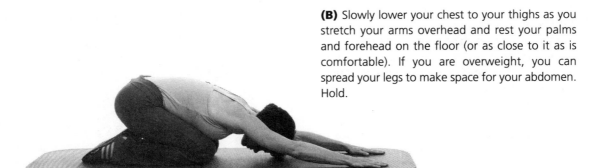

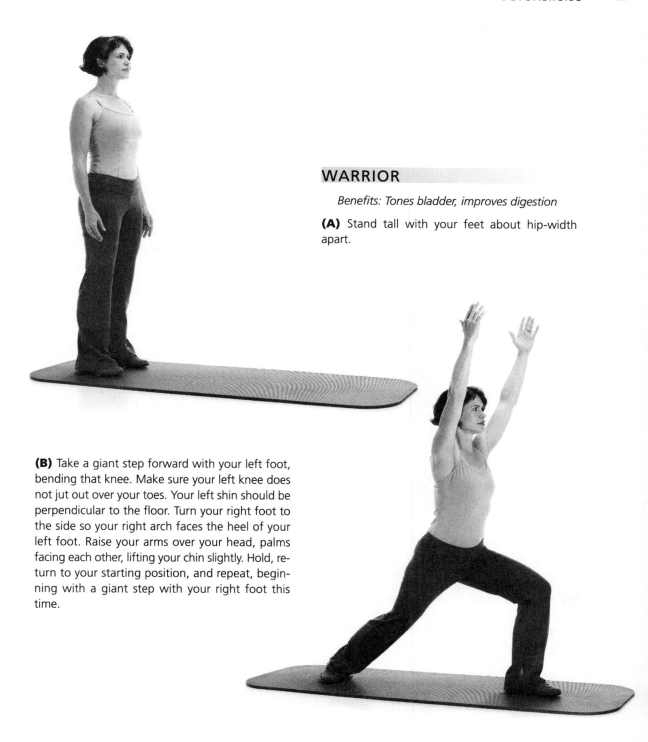

WARRIOR

Benefits: Tones bladder, improves digestion

(A) Stand tall with your feet about hip-width apart.

(B) Take a giant step forward with your left foot, bending that knee. Make sure your left knee does not jut out over your toes. Your left shin should be perpendicular to the floor. Turn your right foot to the side so your right arch faces the heel of your left foot. Raise your arms over your head, palms facing each other, lifting your chin slightly. Hold, return to your starting position, and repeat, beginning with a giant step with your right foot this time.

DETOX TONE-UP PLAN

Perform two sets of 10 to 12 repetitions of each exercise. Use dumbbells that are heavy enough so the final 1 or 2 repetitions are challenging.

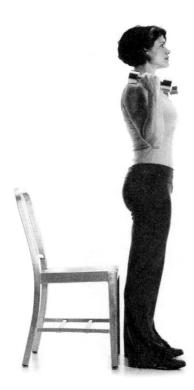

DUMBBELL SQUATS

(A) Stand with your back to a chair and your feet about shoulder-width apart. Hold dumbbells up at your shoulders, palms facing in.

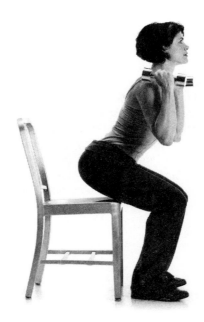

(B) Keeping your back straight, bend from your knees and hips as though you are sitting down. Don't let your knees move forward over your toes. Stop just shy of touching the chair, then stand back up.

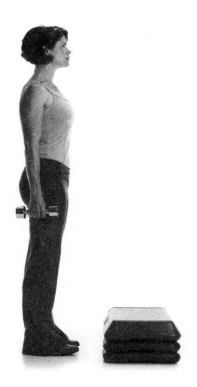

STEP UP

(A) Stand facing an aerobic step or regular step holding dumbbells at your sides. Step up with your right leg, followed by your left leg, so both feet are on the step.

(B) Then, step down with your right foot, followed by your left. Repeat, alternating legs, to perform a full set with each leg.

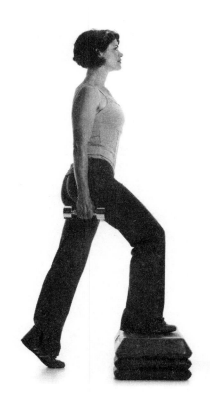

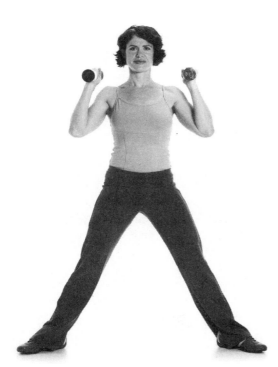

SIDE TO SIDES

(A) Hold dumbbells at your shoulders with your palms facing in. Stand with feet wide apart, toes pointed out.

(B) Bend your left knee down until your left thigh is nearly parallel to the floor and your right leg is extended. Straighten back up. Then bend your right knee. Repeat, alternating legs to perform a full set with each leg.

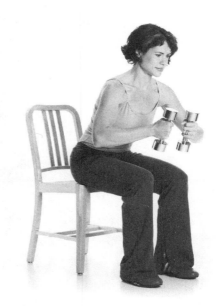

BACK FLY

(A) Sit in a chair with your feet flat on the floor and about hip-width apart. Hold a dumbbell in each hand so the weights are at about chest level and are 12 inches from your body, palms facing each other and elbows slightly bent, as if you were holding a beach ball. Bend slightly forward from your hips (about 3 to 5 inches).

(B) Keeping your back straight, squeeze your shoulder blades together and pull your elbows back as far as is comfortable. Pause, then return to start.

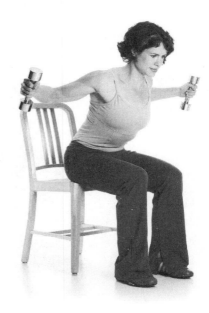

CHEST PRESS

(A) Lie on the floor (or a bench, if one is available) and hold dumbbells end to end just above your chest; your elbows should be pointing out.

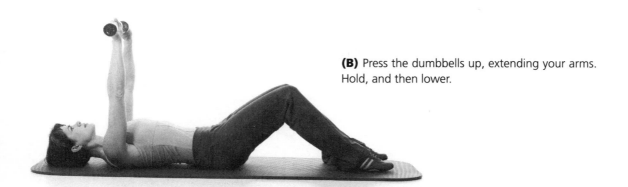

(B) Press the dumbbells up, extending your arms. Hold, and then lower.

CURL AND PRESS

(A) Sit on a supportive chair (preferably one without arms), feet flat on the floor and about shoulder-width apart. Hold a dumbbell in each hand, arms extended down to your sides and palms facing out.

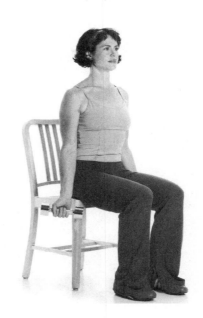

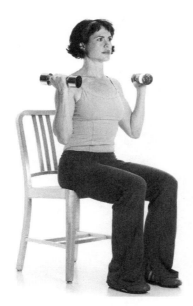

(B) Slowly bend your elbows and curl the weights up toward your shoulders.

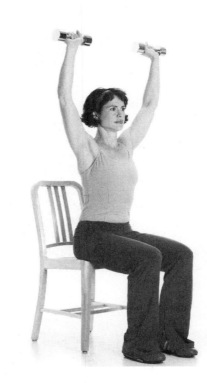

(C) Without stopping, rotate your wrists so your palms are facing forward and press the weights overhead. Pause. Slowly reverse the move back to the starting position.

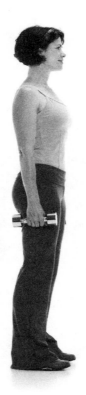

CALF RAISE

(A) Stand with your legs about hip-width apart and hold dumbbells at your sides, palms facing in.

(B) Slowly rise up onto the balls of your feet while keeping your torso and legs straight. Hold, and then lower.

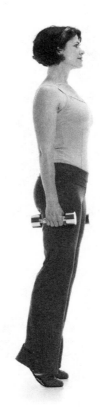

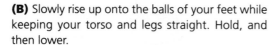

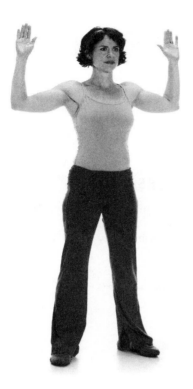

STANDING CROSSOVER

(A) This move is performed without dumbbells. Stand with your feet a few inches apart. Raise your arms to your sides and bend your elbows to form right angles, pointing your fingers toward the ceiling and your palms forward.

(B) Now contract your abs and pull your right knee and left elbow toward one another. Pause, and return to start. Complete a set, and then switch sides.

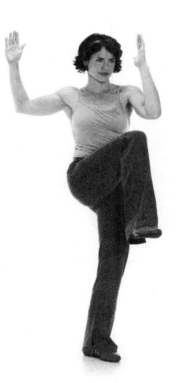

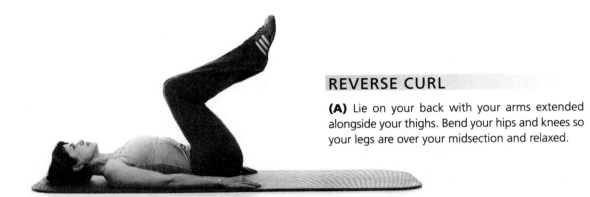

REVERSE CURL

(A) Lie on your back with your arms extended alongside your thighs. Bend your hips and knees so your legs are over your midsection and relaxed.

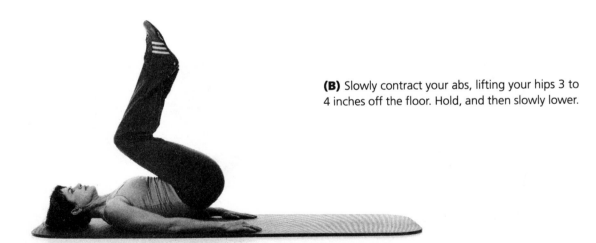

(B) Slowly contract your abs, lifting your hips 3 to 4 inches off the floor. Hold, and then slowly lower.

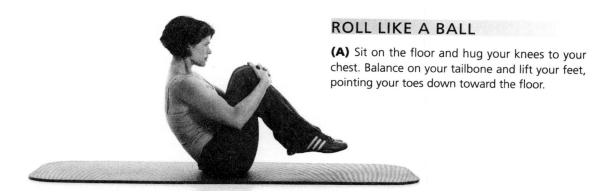

ROLL LIKE A BALL

(A) Sit on the floor and hug your knees to your chest. Balance on your tailbone and lift your feet, pointing your toes down toward the floor.

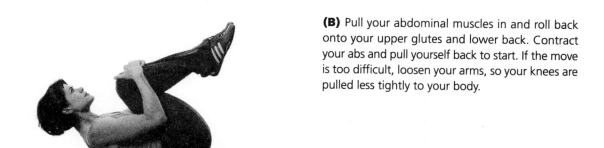

(B) Pull your abdominal muscles in and roll back onto your upper glutes and lower back. Contract your abs and pull yourself back to start. If the move is too difficult, loosen your arms, so your knees are pulled less tightly to your body.

CARDIO WITH A KICK

This program introduces light speed work into your usual aerobic (cardio) routine. Though it specifies walking, you can do the same thing on a bicycle or even in a pool. Simply increase your effort to the specified intensity for the prescribed duration.

The number in parentheses indicates the intensity on a scale of 1 to 10, with 1 being the absolute easiest (almost snoozing) and 10 being the most intense (full-out effort).

This whole routine should take you about half an hour:

◎ Begin with an easy walking cadence (3): 4 minutes

◎ Increase tempo to a brisk pace (6): 5 minutes

◎ Walk like you're trying to catch a bus (7): 10 minutes

◎ Walk as fast as your feet will carry you (9): 3 minutes

◎ Reduce your pace to a brisk walk (6): 5 minutes

◎ Cool down at an easy pace (3): 3 minutes

Chapter 7

Fasting and Cleansing: Lightening Your Body's Toxic Burden

NO MATTER HOW WELL YOU EAT, if you live on planet Earth in the 21st century, you are exposed to and you take into your body a variety of chemical toxins that the human body never before had to deal with during its millennia-long evolutionary journey. So it's no surprise that our bodies get gummed up. Toxins build up in the liver, kidneys, and blood; they get stored away in the adipose tissue (that's fat), and they end up causing awful degenerative diseases like cancer and heart disease. They also contribute to the aging process. Why wouldn't you want to get rid of as much of your toxic overload as you possibly could?

That leads to one of the main concerns that need to be addressed up front, before we look at the benefits of fasting and cleansing and how to go about it. Practitioners of alternative medicine have prescribed fasting and cleansing therapies for decades—actually for centuries, if you consider the traditional practices of India and the Orient. As alternative medicine becomes more widespread and people learn about the outstanding benefits that fasting and cleansing can provide, they've responded with enthusiasm—sometimes with too much enthusiasm.

They reason that if a little fasting is good, a lot must be better. If a little cleansing is good, why not really ream things out all at once and be done with it, and then go for a good, long fast? For a lot of reasons, that's not a good idea—at least not if you're contemplating doing this on your own, without medical supervision.

"I get people who come to me and say, 'I want to do a 2-week water fast,' and I say, 'No,'" says Carrie Demers, M.D., director of the Himalayan Institute's Center for Health and Healing in Honesdale, Pennsylvania. "Why would you want to do that? What is this, some kind of macho, Mount Everest of fasting?"

Health practitioners at the Center for Health and Healing use fasting as one of many healing modalities that also include nutrition, meditation, massage, and exercise. Dr. Demers has supervised numerous clients safely through fasts that serve to cleanse and detoxify the body.

FASTING FOUNDATIONS

"Most people are nutritionally deficient," explains Dr. Demers. "And when they fast, they send their body into freak-out mode."

Alternative health care practitioners concur with Dr. Demers's assessment. If your regular daily eating habits are not already healthy, you'd be better off concentrating your efforts on improving your daily diet, and putting off any thoughts of fasting until you've cleaned up your act, says Geoff Lecovin, D.C., N.D., L.Ac., a chiropractor, naturopath, and acupuncturist practicing in Kirkland, Washington. Among the many healing modalities that are part of his regular practice, Dr. Lecovin supervises therapeutic fasting. "If someone just wants to cleanse, I'd say look at lifestyle first," he says. "Clean up your diet, exercise."

If you're not properly prepared before you fast, your body will not only not detoxify, it will think it's starving and respond by clutching for dear life onto everything it has—including the toxins. You'll feel irritated, headachy, and exhausted. And your metabolism will slow down. Then, once you start to eat again, you'll feel compelled to gorge and will likely gain weight. And, after all that work you've done, you'll still be carrying the toxic load that is stressing your body and threatening your health.

It's not a pretty picture, and it's not likely something you want to do to yourself. But if you make the mistake of aligning yourself with a misguided so-called health care practitioner who urges excessive fasting on you, you could end up harming yourself. You could go through the unpleasantness of a long fast and end up very much the worse for wear.

"My personal schtick is trying to teach people how to live well all the time," Dr. Demers says. "Don't just pollute yourself, then do a cleansing a couple of times a year. Support your cleansing organs every day. Breathe deep, eat right, sweat, take liver-cleansing herbs. Get your lifestyle together."

If you do all of these things, she says, your body will be ready to benefit from its first fast. If you don't do these things on a regular basis, there's a good chance that fasting will be not only unpleasant, but also not particularly helpful.

It's not hard to understand what happens with the body as it's faced with its first fast. "Your body is animal," explains Dr. Demers. "Your body has the same instincts as an animal. It feels threatened. That fountain of self-preservation kicks in."

PREPARING TO FAST

You can get your body used to the idea of fasting by using the same kinds of techniques that you would use when trying to train a wild animal: Be gentle and convince it that cooperation brings rewards, says Dr. Demers.

In fact, one beneficial regime that gets your body used to fasting is doing a small fast every single day.

"Every evening at 7:00, stop eating and fast until breakfast," says Dr. Demers. "Let your body do its cleanse and repair."

That's why the first meal of the day is called breakfast. Ideally, you've been fasting for a good 12 hours before you eat that first meal. And why is this a good thing to do? It's a good practice for the same reasons that somewhat longer mini-fasts are good for your body.

Your body uses an incredible amount of energy (and nutrients) digesting its food. If you spend the entire evening snacking in front of the TV, continually throwing more food on top of partially digested food from the evening's meal and previous snacks without ever giving your body a chance to empty your stomach and move things along, you're adding considerably to your toxic load.

On the other hand, you can give your body a daily opportunity to cleanse itself by eliminating your evening snack fest. That way, each evening, once your food is digested, your body can turn its energy to cleanup activities, such as eliminating toxins. By the way, that's one reason that the French tend to be beautifully slim. They might indulge in cheese and wine and other high-calorie delights during regular meals, but mindless snacking is not a part of their culture.

It's okay to have a cup of herbal tea while you're watching TV or reading in the evening, says Dr. Demers, but you really should train yourself to stop eating after dinner. That will accomplish more detoxification on an ongoing basis than fasting a couple of times a year will.

FASTING BASICS

If you want to further enhance your body's cleanup efforts, a certain amount of fasting is helpful, provided the fasts are short, supported by adequate nutrition, and conducted safely, says Dr. Demers. Here's an overview of the basic procedure for conducting a fast, no matter what its length:

⚬ Prepare your body to fast.
⚬ Leave stress behind.
⚬ Start slowly. Don't try a longer fast until your body has learned how to benefit from shorter fasts.
⚬ Unless you're conducting a longer therapeutic fast under medical supervision (more about this later), give your body adequate nutrition to support the fasting process.
⚬ At all times, listen to your body. Put safety first.
⚬ Come out of your fast carefully and with the right kind of nutritional support.

Before going into detail about how each of these rules works in practice, it should be noted that some people should not fast at all. These include:

⚬ Women who are pregnant or nursing.
⚬ Young children.
⚬ People who are extremely thin or who have eating disorders.
⚬ People who have diabetes, cancer, heart disease, or any other serious illness. These people should not do even short fasts on their own. While they may benefit from fasting, they should do so only under the close supervision of a health care professional experienced in supervising therapeutic fasts.

GETTING STARTED

To begin, be very clear about the benefits that you hope to gain from fasting. If you know what you hope to gain from this process, you will not find it difficult to stick to your resolve and forgo your normal dietary routine for even a short period of time. If you're not clear on what you hope to gain, you'll find that your resolve will disappear at the first hunger pang. Some people find themselves getting hungry within minutes of beginning a fast—a sure sign that they are not yet emotionally ready to begin a fast.

Here are some other steps you need to take to prepare for a fast:

Adjust your diet. Before you fast, set a date a week or so away, and begin to lighten up your diet. Assuming that you already eat a healthy diet on a daily basis (you shouldn't be fasting if you don't), you should clean up your diet even further.

Focus on fiber. Make sure you eat plenty of high-fiber foods, fruits, and vegetables in the days leading up to your fast. Have a green salad and enjoy plenty of fresh juices every day for several days before you fast.

Get hydrated. Drink plenty of water. Aim for at least eight 8-ounce glasses a day.

Be a little more strict with yourself. If you haven't already done so as part of your regular diet, now is the time to cut way back on meats, sugar, and fatty foods. Spend a week or two being especially vigilant about what goes into your mouth.

Keep moving. Get plenty of exercise. At the very least, go for a walk every day.

EASE IN SLOWLY

Don't just jump right into a 3-day fast. If you've never fasted before, try skipping an occasional meal, replacing what you'd normally eat with a glass of freshly prepared (not canned or bottled) fruit or vegetable juice.

Do a couple of "practice" fasts. After you've tried skipping a meal a few times, try fasting for just 1 day a few times. If you ease into the fasting experience, says Dr. Demers, your body will "get it." Instead of panicking during a longer fast and holding on to everything, including toxins, your body will understand on its own that you're not starving it, that you will begin eating again, and that it's just been given an opportunity to use all the energy and enzymes that would have gone into digesting food to clean house, instead.

Give your body time to "get" it. As your body—your trained animal—learns to benefit from a short fast, it will cooperate by starting to release its toxic overload as soon as it feels the fasting routine that you've established get underway.

Pick up the pace. After you've done a couple of 1-day fasts, you can try implementing a longer fast, anywhere from 2 to 3 days, on your own. Fasts that are any longer than that really fall under the category of medical therapy and should be undertaken only under the supervision of a trained health care professional.

Seek professional support. "Anyone who's doing a longer fast should be under the care of somebody," says Dr. Lecovin. "Your health could be compromised, as could your ability to think clearly. Have someone at least monitor what you're doing. Don't self-treat."

Pamper yourself. If you've never fasted for a day or 2 or 3 before, you probably don't want your first time to be during your workweek. Pick a weekend, or better yet a 3-day weekend, when you can pamper yourself. Spend some time writing in your journal, going for walks in beautiful surroundings, and introspecting.

Take advantage of this special time. Many spiritual traditions use fasting as part of spiritual discipline, and many people find that even a fast of a few days proves to be a time of unusual mental clarity and alertness. That's not a contradiction, by the way, with Dr. Lecovin's concern about thinking clearly that was mentioned earlier. If you're not ready to fast or you're overdoing it, fasting can have an unpleasant side effect—mental fog.

In general, even if your fast is entirely for physical, detoxification reasons, this can be a special time to relax and turn your thoughts inward.

NUTRITION WHILE FASTING

Are we going to suggest that you eat while fasting? Not exactly.

By strict definition, a fast means doing without food entirely and subsisting on just water. But the word "fasting" has come to be used to cover a whole continuum of dietary regimes that eliminate regular meals. This can mean "fasting" on just one food, or fasting by skipping a couple of meals and replacing them with a simple food like dry toast or juice. Even in ancient times traditional fasts often included taking in some nutrition. In centuries past, for example, Christians who did not eat meat during Lent referred to those meatless days as fasting.

Many health fasting experts now recommend doing exactly that—taking in a modest amount of nutrients while otherwise fasting. Both Dr. Demers and Dr. Lecovin recommend that variety of fast.

Here's how to give your body a reasonable amount of nutritional support while fasting:

Limit yourself to a simple dish. Dr. Demers recommends fasting either on fresh juices or, for people who find that too rigorous, limiting your meals to one simple, nutritious dish. She especially favors a simple Indian dish of beans and rice known as kichari. (See the recipe for Fenugreek Kichari on page 55.) For most, she recommends using freshly made juice as the alternative that's best for the body.

One technique that works nicely for many people is to have fresh juices for breakfast and dinner and have kichari for lunch.

"If you give your body simple nutrition, it's easier to release toxins," she says. "The purpose of a fast is to help your body unburden itself. It increases your digestive fire."

Get juiced. For people who are accustomed to fasting, Dr. Demers recommends drinking freshly made fruit and vegetable juices every couple of hours during the day or days of fasting. Have orange juice in the morning, she advises, then later in the day switch to other kinds of juices—carrot, celery, parsley, tomato, or cucumber.

Enjoy taste and variety. There are a number of juicing recipes beginning on page 78, and there are also great recipes for fresh juices both online and in books devoted solely to juicing recipes. And if you're fasting during the winter, when good fresh produce is hard to come by, you can make hot vegetable broths. Simply use your favorite vegetables to make soup, then strain. You drink the liquid and either compost the vegetables or let your family members enjoy them. Carrots, cabbage, parsley, and onions are all good choices. "Juices are absorbed readily, easily, with very little effort, and are an easy source of nutrition," Dr. Demers explains. They're low in calories, but they provide enough nutrition to both support the detoxification process and to help your body understand that it's not starving, so it can begin to release its toxic load.

HAVE AN EXIT STRATEGY

After you've been fasting for a few days, it's understandable that you'll be salivating at the thought of that first solid meal. So what'll it be? Pizza? Steak and eggs? Maybe you can make it a special occasion by digging out your grandmother's favorite recipe for coconut cake . . .

Whoa! Back off a little. When you fast,

your body closes down its production of the enzymes and other biochemicals that you need to digest your food. And unless you return to eating in a slow and methodical manner, you could end up with a mass of undigested food plugging your digestive system and, yep, releasing toxins right back into your cleaned-up body.

You need to back out of fasting on juice only as carefully as you eased into it. On the day you choose to end your fast, have a little fresh fruit for breakfast and lunch and dinner. The next day, have some steamed vegetables or a salad for lunch and dinner. The next day, you can add a cereal or a meal made with whole grains. The idea is to let your body get revved back up before it has to deal with solid meals. (If you've been fasting for several days under medical supervision, your post-fast meals will be carefully watched as well.)

LISTEN TO YOUR BODY

All of this has probably left you with the impression that fasting is a piece of cake, so to speak. And for many people it is. But let's face it, when your body begins throwing off its excess toxins, they have to come out somewhere. They leave their places of storage via your bloodstream,

your liver, your kidneys, your lungs, and the very pores of your skin. And depending upon how much comes out and how fast, they can create unpleasant symptoms. These include:

- Abdominal discomfort
- Anxiousness
- Assorted body aches
- Bad breath
- Body odor
- Dizziness
- Headaches
- Insomnia
- Irritability
- Mental fogginess
- Nausea

You can safely put up with a mild level of discomfort. You can pretty much be the judge of how much discomfort you're willing to experience in order to give your body a chance to detoxify. But there are a couple of symptoms that should automatically signal the end of a fast:

- Abdominal pain
- Delirium
- Emotional or psychological distress
- Fever
- Heart palpitations or irregularities
- Vomiting
- Watery diarrhea

Watery diarrhea can cause the body to lose electrolytes, important minerals that the body needs in order to perform certain functions, such as keeping the heart beating. In general, pay attention to how you feel and respect what your body is trying to tell you. If you're feeling so uncomfortable that you're questioning the wisdom of fasting in the first place, feel free to end the fast.

Fasting is not an endurance test or a test of willpower. This should not be a cause for suffering. The kind of gentle fasts we're discussing here are for the purpose of detoxifying and cleansing your body. If you're carrying a heavy toxic load and you're cleaning out the toxins a little too swiftly, you're going to feel downright lousy. The answer is to slow down. Respect the wisdom of your body. Go ahead and end the fast. Continue eating a healthful diet for a time. And, if you're so inclined, try a shorter fast at some point in the future.

Don't feel guilty. Don't feel like you've failed. Simply acknowledge that you've listened to your body and move on.

ENDING A FAST QUICKLY

If you're in the middle of what you thought was going to be a 3-day fast and you find that you can't go on, what do you do? It's easy to end a fast; you just eat something. Have a piece of fruit. Or, if you're really uncomfortable, make yourself a bowl of oatmeal or a baked potato. Your unpleasant symptoms should disappear almost immediately.

One thing you should not do at this point is either overeat or reach for an unhealthy food. If you grab a bag of greasy chips or a candy bar, your body will not thank you, and you could end up feeling even worse.

This is a good place to pause and reiterate what we called attention to earlier. Fasting and cleansing have become so trendy that a great many well-meaning, enthusiastic, but inadequately trained people have jumped on the bandwagon and are happy to supervise your fast for a fee. If you're going to try a longer fast under supervision, you might want to look for an M.D. or an NPLEX board certified naturopathic physician (N.D.) who has experience in supervising therapeutic fasts.

And use your best judgment if someone is telling you that your unpleasant fasting symptoms are a "healing crisis." It is possible to have a healing crisis while you're detoxifying your body. But do you really have to suffer to move toxins out of your body? No. There are ways to detoxify that do not involve nausea or delirium. It's okay to end a fast any time your body and your best judgment tell you that you've had enough. Don't ever let someone bully you into fasting longer than your inner wisdom tells you is right for you.

LONGER FASTS: SERIOUS THERAPY

Given everything we've said about the body needing to have nutrients while fasting, why would anyone want to undertake a longer fast of a week, 10 days, or even longer?

The answer is simple. Fasting over an extended period of time can be an effective healing therapy, according to Joseph Pizzorno, N.D., author of *Total Wellness;* coauthor of *Textbook of Natural Medicine* and *Encyclopedia of Natural Medicine;* and founder of Bastyr University in Seattle. Both extended modified fasts and fasting on just water have been used for centuries as healing modalities. And people keep on using fasts for healing purposes because they work, he says.

In his own books, Dr. Pizzorno goes into a great deal of detail about providing nutritional support both for the liver and for the other detoxifying systems of the body. If all of these systems need nutrients in order to do their jobs, then how can extended fasting or fasting on just water for any length of time be effective? How could detoxification, not to mention alleviation of disease symptoms, even take place?

"That," says Dr. Pizzorno, "is the $64,000 question. I don't know. We don't understand why it works. Research is clearly needed. But it does. It could be that the body is implementing other detoxifying processes."

There's no disputing the fact that people with chronic illnesses who have not been helped by anything else frequently experience dramatic improvements when they fast for extended periods of time, Dr. Pizzorno says. To be effective, these fasts can be on just water and they can last for many days. And they absolutely must be under medical supervision.

Research clearly shows impressive results, he says, with a wide variety of conditions. Among them are:

◎ Arthritis
◎ Asthma
◎ Depression
◎ Diabetes
◎ Fibroids
◎ Heart disease

◎ High blood pressure

◎ Irritable bowel syndrome

◎ Lupus, as well as many other autoimmune diseases

◎ Mental illness, including schizophrenia

◎ Obesity

◎ Skin conditions, including acne, eczema, and psoriasis

◎ Ulcers

Some health care professionals who use water fasting as a healing modality recommend fasts that last a month or even longer. Dr. Pizzorno has supervised a number of extended fasts himself. While he has supervised water fasts that have lasted for as long as 30 days, the best results he's personally seen have come from fasts of approximately 1 week.

Following the fast, he typically has clients do a "food challenge"; that is, he has them reintroduce suspect foods one at a time in order to determine which foods are problematic. Foods that an individual is allergic or sensitive to are the main culprits in a whole host of chronic and painful conditions.

People who are looking to detoxify as a means of dealing with chronic diseases should not try fasting on their own, he says. This is really important. People with diabetes or heart disease, for example,

could quickly get themselves into serious trouble. In fact, people with serious diseases should be supervised 24 hours a day in a clinical setting when they do even short fasts, he says.

If you have a chronic condition that might respond to fasting and you'd like to try it, you need to find a health care professional who is experienced in conducting therapeutic fasts. One good source for finding such a person is the International Association of Hygienic Physicians (IAHP), a group of physicians and other health care professionals who use fasting as therapy. You can find them online or contact them at 4620 Euclid Boulevard, Youngstown, OH 44512.

HERBAL CLEANSING KITS

No matter what kind of fast you're on—short, long, mono-diet, juice, water only—there are herbs that can help support and expedite your cleanse. Many of these herbs were described in detail in chapter 5 on page 81.

There are also numerous kits that you can buy, either in health food stores or online, that can prove helpful. These typically consist of a bulking agent, usually psyllium; herbs that encourage bowel

Detox Makeover

FRANCES STARED DOWN INTO THE TOILET. She could not believe that matter so voluminous, foul smelling, and gross had come from her body. Again. Just 3 short weeks into her cleanse, and the products were obviously doing their job. (Ugh!) The bright side, of course, was that this stuff, which had been inside of her, was now outside. "No wonder I've been feeling so toxic," she thought, as she flushed.

Frances, a 48-year-old editor in Des Moines, Iowa, had researched herbal cleansing kits carefully, poring over everything from prices to promises for dozens of products. She'd selected Arise and Shine products because she appreciated all the detail provided in *Cleanse and Purify Thyself (Book 1.5)*, a book written by Richard Anderson, N.D., the developer of the product line. She appreciated that the author viewed cleansing as a spiritual procedure—purifying the body temple—while at the same time paying such scrupulous attention to safety issues.

Ultimately, Frances followed the cleanse program for just under the recommended 4 weeks. During the process, she felt irritable, deprived, and even irrationally angry at times—symptoms she had expected based on her precleanse reading. On the positive side, she successfully put caffeine addiction behind her, lost 11 pounds, and dropped her total cholesterol reading by 56 points. Subjectively, she felt her eyes and skin looked clearer. Certainly, she was experiencing a much higher level of energy.

Bottom line? Frances felt the hard work and discomfort, not to mention the cash outlay, were a small price to pay for the results.

movements and support your liver and other cleansing systems of your body; and possibly probiotics, strains of friendly bacteria intended to prevent the toxic kind from taking up residence in your cleaned-out gut. While these kits are fairly expensive—often upwards of $100—it's convenient to have all cleansing supplies packaged together along with a schedule and dietary recommendations.

People who use these packaged kits need to be wary, though, according to Dr. Lecovin. Because some of the herbal kits contain harsher laxatives, it's easy to overdo it. Overdoing it can lead to headaches, dehydration, and the loss of essential vitamins and minerals.

If you opt for a kit and experience watery diarrhea, muscle spasms, or both, back off. Use less of the product, and discontinue its use altogether if the unpleasant side effects don't disappear.

FLUSHING THE TOXIC COLON

We can't leave the subject of fasting and cleansing without taking a look at the whole area of enemas and colonics. Both techniques involve physically flushing the colon with warm water. Enemas are self-administered, using an inexpensive piece of equipment—a bag that looks like a hot water bottle, with a tube and nozzle attached. Colonics are administered in a clinical setting by a professional. The difference is that the apparatus that delivers the colonic makes it possible to refill and flush several times for a more thorough cleansing.

The jury is still out on whether a colon washing during and following a fast is necessary or even useful.

"You don't need to do this to yourself," says Dr. Pizzorno. "You can detox without them."

Others—Dr. Lecovin, for example—feel that these techniques have their place. "It's a tool," he says. "It's not a tool for everyone."

Enemas and colonics do have enthusiastic proponents who feel that these techniques are an important part of fasting.

"I feel they're essential," says Gaia Mather, N.D., who offers colonics in a clinical setting and teaches about both colonics and enemas at National College of Naturopathic Medicine in Portland, Oregon. "There's a time and a place for both."

Most of us could use some help with colon cleansing anyway, she says, especially if bowel movements are sluggish. But during a fast, the body is throwing off lots of toxic material. This comes out through the lungs, through sweat, through urine, and through stools.

Toward the end of a fast, your GI tract kind of "goes to sleep," Dr. Mather explains. If you don't give it a thorough cleaning, you can reabsorb some of the toxic material that you've just thrown off and lose some of the benefits you've gained by fasting.

She advises a daily self-administered enema during a fast. She also advises having a couple of colonics toward the end of a fast. "It's important to keep all the channels of elimination open," she explains.

If you choose to do this, Dr. Mather suggests keeping a few things in mind for your safety:

Don't overdo it. You really shouldn't administer more than one enema a day. If you do, you could absorb too much water and throw your electrolyte balance off. (Electrolytes are important minerals that your body needs.)

Use standard equipment. Don't try using a bigger container, for example. It is possible to do damage with too much water pressure. And follow *to the letter* the directions on the package that the enema equipment comes in.

Keep it to yourself. Don't share equipment with other family members. You wouldn't share toothbrushes, and this equipment is potentially even more germ-laden. Make sure you clean the nozzle thoroughly after each use. Soak it in bleach and water to properly clean it.

Don't use tap water. You don't want to absorb things like chlorine and other toxic substances found in water direct from the faucet. Use bottled, filtered, or distilled water, instead.

Put safety first. Enemas can make you feel depleted. If you are elderly or have certain chronic diseases, such as diabetes, uncontrolled high blood pressure, or congestive heart failure, never self-administer an enema. In these cases, enemas can be safely used only under the advice and supervision of a health care professional.

And here's what to look for if you're opting for a series of colonics:

Find the right professional. Your best bet is to get a referral from a doctor, naturopath, or other health care professional whom you know and trust. If you can't do that, inquire about the training and experience of the person who will be administering the colonics.

Insist on cleanliness. Make sure that the clinic uses disposable speculums and tubing. And if anything about the premises does not look completely clean to you, turn around and walk out the door.

Ask about the water. If the clinic uses tap water rather than filtered water in their machines, go elsewhere.

Don't get taken for a ride. It's fine to have a series of colonics over several weeks, but don't let someone talk you into coming back week after week on into the future.

Finally, we should take a look at a

couple of cleansing techniques that are a lot easier to use and are quite effective. You'll benefit greatly by adding these into your daily routine for the rest of your life.

SAY HELLO TO NETI

You clean your teeth every day, no questions asked. If you grew up in a different culture—India's, to be exact—there's a good chance you'd clean the inside of your nose as well. And if you regularly have problems with things like sinusitis or allergies to pollens, dust, mold, pet dander, and so on, or if you're the first in your office to catch a cold, you might want to consider a daily nasal wash with a neti pot, no matter what culture you come from. Actually, even if you don't have these problems, you should consider implementing this helpful technique, according to Dr. Demers.

"There simply isn't a downside. It's good for everyone," Dr. Demers says. "Every day we breathe in particles, dirt, germs, and pollution. They stick to the mucous membranes in the back of the throat. If you wash the particles away, you have less of a chance of getting sick or reacting to them."

Using a neti pot also helps clear up sinus problems and prevent colds, she maintains.

Your nose is lined with tiny hairs that serve to block particles. And the mucous membranes at the back of your throat are made of cells covered with tiny hair-like structures. These living hairs (cilia) work in unison to push any pollutants down your throat to your stomach, where the dirt is eliminated.

In a dry climate (including everyone's heated house in winter) or in a dusty or polluted environment, the mucous membranes get dried out, or the mucous thickens and builds up. Then these tiny cilia are easily overpowered and can't do their job of protecting you. Hence plugged-up sinuses, often followed by sinus headaches.

You can clear up sinus problems by using a neti pot (which resembles a small teapot with an elongated spout) to pour warm, salty water through your nose. It takes only a minute or two each day for the neti pot to draw excess mucus out of your nasal passages and cleanse them thoroughly of accumulated dust and pollutants. In a pinch, you can also try using a paper cup and squeezing it to narrow the opening. When you pour out of the squeezed cup, the water can dribble a little, so you'll want to get a real neti pot once you start doing this regularly.

You're not likely to find a neti pot

at your local drugstore, but you can order one inexpensively online at www.HimalayanInstitute.org or by calling (800) 822-4547 or (570) 253-5551. Your local health food store may also carry them.

Here's how to use a neti pot:

1. Get inspired. The first time you see someone use a neti pot, you'll be amazed that it's possible to pour water into one nostril and have it come out the other. The key is to position your head correctly. You'll need to read through the directions and get a sense of how it works. The water simply pours right through without causing any discomfort. It won't go down your throat unless you raise your head and let it go down. You could even sing, talk, or whistle a tune while it's pouring through, if you're so inclined.

"When I first did that, I thought I was going to die," laughs Dr. Demers. "But once people get over feeling 'eeuuuwww, it's a weird thing,' it becomes so routine it's like brushing your teeth. People become evangelical about it. I had one client who gave a neti pot to each family member for Christmas."

2. Prepare the pot. Dissolve ½ to ⅔ of a teaspoon of sea salt or kosher salt in 1½ cups of warm water. This is enough water to fill the pot twice and do both nostrils. You use sea salt because it's pure; if you're using kosher salt, make sure it has no additives. You don't want to stick the typical additives in table salt—iodine or anti-caking agents such as sodium silico-aluminate—up your nose. And the water should be about as comfortably warm as bath water. Now fill the neti pot. (If you don't salt the water or if you use cold water, it will be as unpleasant as it was when you were a kid and you got pool water up your nose.)

3. Position your head. Stand over your bathroom sink with your face looking directly down into the sink. Then tilt your head so that your right nostril is higher than your left. Now insert the spout of the pot into your right nostril and pour. Amazingly enough, the water will pour directly through and come out of your left nostril, bringing with it excess mucous along with any dust and pollutants that have lodged inside your nose.

4. Expel excess water. Blow your nose gently, directly into the sink. You could also use a tissue, but be gentle as you blow. There's a lot of liquid to get rid of and if you use excessive pressure, you could end up with liquid in your eustachian tubes—the little internal tubes that connect your throat to your ears. If you do this, you'll have a clogged sensation in your ears. The water will drain out of its own accord after a while, but you can avoid this unpleasantness by blowing gently.

5. **Repeat on the other side.** Tip your head so your left nostril is higher than your right, and pour a second pot of salted water through in the other direction.

6. **Adjust your recipe for comfort.** The water pouring through your nostrils should create a pleasant sensation. If you feel any discomfort, it's for one of two reasons:

- The water temperature isn't right. The water really needs to be pleasantly warm. If you pour cold water or water that's too hot into your nose, it hurts. The idea is to use body-temperature water. Your nasal passages deal with warm liquids all the time.
- The salt content isn't right. Try adjusting the salt content up or down slightly the next time you mix the solution.

After a while, you'll get a sense of the right temperature and the salt concentration that's best for you. For a short video that demonstrates the technique, you can visit the Neti Pot Company Web site at www.bytheplanet.com/Products/Yoga/neti/Netipot.htm.

DON'T FORGET TO FLOSS AND SCRAPE

You probably don't view brushing and flossing your teeth as an important way to detoxify your body, but you should.

You can think of your mouth as a flophouse for bacteria. It's a nice, warm, moist environment with plenty of food. This is a perfect setup for bacteria that want to raise a family. And that's what they do all the time: They multiply. You brush your teeth in the morning and just a few hours later, when you run your tongue over your teeth, you feel slime. That's not spit; that's the slimy, toxic outer coating (glycocalyx) of bacteria that multiply in your mouth.

Bacteria that grow in your mouth don't just cause bad breath. The kinds that are responsible for gum disease have been implicated as one possible cause of heart disease, as well. So you really do want to brush and floss them out daily.

There's one more mouth-cleansing implement to add to your brushing and flossing routine—the tongue scraper. These come in all kinds of shapes and are readily available in drug stores and health food stores. You don't have to get a fancy one. A little plastic device that looks like a shaver (without the razor, of course) will do quite nicely. Once you've finished brushing and flossing, swipe the scraper over your tongue a couple of times and you'll dislodge a few million more toxic bacteria.

Chapter 8

Pure Mind, Pure Heart: Detoxing Your Emotions and Moods

ONE OF THE FAMOUS PECULIARITIES ABOUT SKYSCRAPERS is that many of them have no 13th floor. We all know why, don't we? The number 13 is notorious for bringing "bad luck." Building owners and landlords—yes, even Donald Trump—recognize that the mind is a powerful weapon. If people even think that 13 is bad luck, they're going to avoid renting or buying any apartment or office space that's on the 13th floor. So even in the most modern of cities, the 13th floors have been expelled.

We all have our 13th floors—certain habits, ways of thinking, moods, dilemmas, and negative emotional moments that seem to bring us bad luck. Worse, the "bad luck" can become pervasive, affecting not only how we feel but also our physical health, mental outlook, relationships with others, families, careers, even digestion and sleep patterns. That's why it's so important to identify our private, personal 13th floors—the "bad luck" areas of our emotions—and get rid of them.

At first it may seem a bit superstitious to detoxify yourself of the moods and emotions that cause trouble. But once you begin using the detoxification methods described in this chapter, you'll soon discover that you really do have the mental power to change how you feel and act—and even the state of your health. The techniques of emotional detoxification discussed here come from many different religious, cultural, and scientific traditions. And the myriad benefits of these detoxification techniques have been extremely well established in recent years by medical and psychological research.

IT'S TRUE—BAD MOODS CAN HARM YOU

Take stress, for instance. We are all familiar with the day-to-day stresses caused by tight schedules, lines of traffic, rude people, and pressures at work and home. Even brief psychological stress can produce changes in your heartbeat and adrenaline levels while reducing your immune response, according to research at the department of psychology at Ohio State University. In a study of 22 women, psychologists found that even after short periods of stress, these women had increased heart rates, reduced immunity, and an overabundance of hormones like epinephrine that cause increased muscle tension.

You might assume, as many people do,

that we get used to stress. But that doesn't seem to be the case. In fact, sustained high levels of stress seem to lead directly to a decline in health. In a large study of 73,724 people in Japan, researchers found that over a 2-year period, people who were highly stressed had significantly increased risks of heart attack, stroke, and related heart problems. The trial included both men and women, ages 40 to 79, who had no prior history of stroke or coronary heart disease.

There's also a link between stress, depression, and common illnesses like colds and flu. Researchers in Ohio State University's department of psychiatry found that a group of 69 highly stressed caregivers were far more likely than others to have depression. The group, studied over a 13-month period, was made up of spouses who had to provide constant care for a partner with Alzheimer's disease. By the end of the study, about 32 percent of the overstressed caregivers were diagnosed with symptoms of depression. They were also more susceptible to infection, particularly upper-respiratory problems, so many more were getting colds, flu, and pneumonia as compared to a control group that didn't have the constant worry of being caregivers.

Songs, Psalms, Hymns, and Poems of Prayer

IN MOST RELIGIONS, there are customary prayers that have poetic or musical form. Here are some helpful prayers that come from four different spiritual traditions:

I will lift my eyes to the hills—
From whence comes my help?
My help comes from the Lord,
Who made heaven and earth.

—**Psalm 121:1**

Wisdom, free from the clouds of the two
*   obscuring veils*
Altogether pure and shining brightly like
*   the sun*
Waking us up from the sleep of our
*   disturbed emotions*
And the chains of mental habit
Scattering the darkness of not knowing.

—**Ancient Tibetan prayer**

Earth teach me freedom
As the eagle which soars in the sky.
Earth teach me resignation
As the leaves which die in the fall.
Earth teach me regeneration
As the seed which rises in the spring.
Earth teach me to forget myself
As melted snow forgets its life.
Earth teach me to remember kindness
As dry fields weep with rain.

—**Ute prayer**

Let my life force be linked to my Heart.
Let my Heart be linked to the Truth within
*   me.*
Let this Truth be linked to the Eternal.
That Eternal which is Unending Bliss.

—**Yoga prayer or chant in Vnandamaya practice**

PRAYER FOR HEALTH AND HEALING

Fortunately for us, many researchers have been studying the power of a variety of spiritual, religious, psychological, and mental experiences to improve our outlook and our health. In an overview of a vast array of experiments relating to the power of prayer, Larry Dossey, M.D., author of *Healing Words: The Power of Prayer and the Practice of Medicine* and cochairman of the Panel on Mind/Body Interventions at the Office of Alternative Medicine, National Institutes of Health, has mustered decades of evidence showing that people who pray can help alleviate conditions such as high blood pressure, headaches, and anxiety. What's more, prayer has been shown to speed the healing of wounds and even recovery from heart attacks. Even the level of red blood cells in your body can be affected by prayer, according to Dr. Dossey.

Prayer, of course, is universally practiced in many different kinds of spiritual traditions, including Christian, Judaic, Islamic, Hindu, and Buddhist religions. The positive results, in terms of detoxifying the emotions, alleviating stress, and providing health benefits, seem to be universal, according to Herbert Benson, M.D., president and founder of the Mind/Body Medical Institute and associate professor of medicine at Harvard Medical School and the Deaconess Hospital, and author of *The Relaxation Response*.

Dr. Benson notes that many of us have a fight-or-flight response to numerous experiences in everyday life. We react as if we are almost constantly in emergency situations—with pumping adrenaline, soaring blood pressure, and accelerated breathing.

RELAX TO DETOX

As a counterbalance to these fire-alarm moments, Dr. Benson advocates what has come to be known as the relaxation response. There are many ways to induce the relaxation response, including peacefully watching a sunset, listening to calming music on the radio, meditating, focusing on a single word, or praying. But whatever you choose to do, your body's response is positive. You become less frenetic, so your metabolism (the rate at which you burn energy) decreases. So does muscle tension. Your blood pressure, heart rate, and breathing rate all become modulated.

As Dr. Benson describes this experience, "When you focus for a short time, gently brushing aside any intrusive thoughts, your mind and body suddenly become a five-star resort in which all the service personnel make your restoration and health their priority. . . . This great team of stress-busters and body-relaxers emerges when everyday thoughts and worries are put aside."

One of the most remarkable things about this mind-body-mood connection is that you can actually improve your body's immunity by experiencing feelings of love or having compassionate thoughts, what David McClelland, Ph.D., of Harvard Medical School, has called the Mother Teresa effect.

Dr. McClelland showed students a documentary film about the late Mother Teresa caring for sick patients in India. The film was shown to groups that included both believers and nonbelievers. Irrespective of their attitudes, all of the students had elevated levels of the antibody IgA after viewing the film. Since IgA is one of the body's natural antiviral agents (it helps fight colds, for instance), Dr. McClelland demonstrated that the students had increased their immune response simply by watching a film about a compassionate healer.

If you regularly attend religious services, you're also doing your health a favor. In a study at Duke University, medical researchers measured the concentration of a blood component called interleukin-6 (IL-6) among people who were regular churchgoers. (For comparison, the doctors kept track of a control group of people who went much less frequently.) When IL-6 is high, it's a sign of a weakened immune system. What they discovered during the course of the study was that the concentration of IL-6

was far lower in people who attended church more often than in those who were infrequent churchgoers.

No one could say, of course, which aspect of churchgoing had the beneficial effect—the prayers, the hymns, the sermon, the ritual, or perhaps just the act of gathering together for worship. But the study supports other research showing that regular practice of a religious faith can help us to keep our toxic emotions in check and better our health.

DETOX YOUR STRESS

Even if you're absolutely convinced that you're overstretched and overstressed, you may feel that there are insurmountable barriers to destressing your life. The key, according to Benjamin H. Natelson, M.D., author of *Facing and Fighting Fatigue,* is to reduce your emotional response to stress. One way to do this is by using your imagination—that is, by imagining a peaceful, soothing setting, then putting yourself in the scene for 10 minutes or so. You may surprise yourself with how much more tranquil or relaxed you feel afterwards.

By discovering the destressing technique that works best for you, you can detoxify your stressful moods and emotions. As you begin to reap the rewards, you'll find yourself with more free time because these techniques help you to concentrate and focus while reducing unnecessary activity. Here are some of the most effective methods of reducing stress when you're at home, at the office, running errands, or doing everyday chores.

Face it, lift it, commit it, release it. In their work on the healing power of prayer, Chester L. Tolson, Ph.D., executive director of the Churches United in Global Mission, and Harold G. Koenig, M.D., founder and director of the Center for Study of Religion, Spirituality, and Health at Duke University, have identified four steps of prayer that help people face situations that involve pain, suffering, loss, and grief.

1. **Face it.** That is, realistically state the problem you need to solve, whether you're fearful of the outcome, unwilling to believe it, or embarrassed by what has happened.
2. **Lift it.** Name your needs one by one, and lift those needs to God in prayer. In so doing, you admit to yourself that you can't solve all your own problems, and you're asking God for help.
3. **Commit it.** This means unreservedly handing over your needs and prob-

lems to God's will, with faith that God will see you through.

4. **Release it.** While you can't just pray and forget about your problem, as you release it you will find that your worries diminish. Having faced it, lifted it, and committed it through prayer, releasing the problem is the final stage as you raise the burden from your own shoulders and ease the pressure that you've been feeling.

Assume a prayer posture. If you attend religious services, there's probably a position that the congregation uses when they worship together. But even when you are alone, Pastor Tolson and Dr. Koenig point out, you should find a posture that works for you, one that helps you keep your attention focused on God. You may get in the habit of bowing your head and closing your eyes to create an attitude of quietness and help block out visual distractions. Or you might first want to focus on a religious symbol—a star, a cross, a mandala, Buddha, or a lighted candle. Then close your eyes for further reflection and contemplation.

CLEANSING BREATHS

In addition to prayer, many spiritual traditions make use of a variety of breathing techniques. These can help you focus, reduce stress, and cleanse yourself of unnecessary fear and agitation.

"If breath is the movement of spirit in the body—a central mystery that connects us to all creation—then working with breath is a form of spiritual practice," observes Andrew Weil, M.D., associate director of the Division of Social Perspectives in Medicine, director of the Program in Integrative Medicine at the University of Arizona in Tucson, and author of *Spontaneous Healing*. Dr. Weil describes many ways you can directly affect your health by changing the rhythm and depth of your breathing. The following steps will help you discover how breathing can improve your mental state and your health.

Observe your breath cycle. Sitting in a comfortable position with your eyes closed and clothing loosened, breathe normally as you pay close attention to your breathing. Even if your breath changes, try to follow the cycles of inhalation and exhalation and see where one changes into the other. Do this for about 3 minutes.

Focus on exhalation. This will help you deepen your breathing. Every time you exhale, try to squeeze more and more air out of your lungs. Your inhalations will also deepen, but that happens automatically, because the more air you force out, the more you have to take in.

Let yourself be "breathed." Lie on your back, staying as restful as possible. You will get this sensation if you can imagine you are passively receiving the breath that passes through you. With each exhalation, air is being sucked out of you, and with each inhalation, the breath is being blown into you.

"As the universe breathes into you," suggests Dr. Weil, "let yourself feel the breath penetrating to every part of your body, even to the tips of your fingers and toes." Try to hold on to this perception for 10 breaths. It's an exercise you can do nightly before you fall asleep.

THE PURIFYING POWER OF LAUGHTER

You just know that laughter has to be a good thing. After all, we laugh when we are happy, when we're enjoying good company, when we've been told a great joke, when we've seen a hilarious movie, or when we've enjoyed an adventure. What's not to like about laughter?

But what you know instinctively has also been proven scientifically. Consider the study conducted at Indiana State

University Sycamore Nursing Center. The participants, 33 healthy adult women, were shown two types of videos. Some laughed their way through a humorous video while others (in the control group) simply enjoyed a tourism video. At the end of the viewing period, they were tested for a number of reactions, including stress arousal, humor response, and immune function.

Consistent with many other experiments of this kind, researchers found that stress decreased among those who had the strongest humor response. And the women who saw the funny video also had the greatest jump in immunity, which was determined objectively by measuring the activity of infection-fighting, cancer-fighting natural killer (NK) cells.

Given results like this, it makes sense to find some good reasons to laugh every day. But as we all know, humor is a very personal quality. A joke that makes one person laugh could be too silly or raunchy for someone else. A book, movie, or video that's funny for one person and gets thumbs-up reviews could leave you completely cold.

Paul McGhee, Ph.D., a humor researcher, speaker, and author of *Health, Healing, and the Amuse System: Humor as Survival Training* recommends the following steps to help you develop your own humor library and keep it up to date.

Find your funny bone. The idea is to get a good handle on your own sense of humor. In general, become less serious and cultivate a more playful attitude in life.

Let laughter happen. Go ahead and develop a more hearty and healthy belly laugh. Don't be shy about it. Everyone loves the sound of genuine laughter.

Work on sharing laughter. Improve your joke-telling skills. Create your own spontaneous verbal humor.

Expand your sense of what's funny. Find humor in everyday life. Laugh at yourself. Laugh with others at the events and circumstances you find yourself in.

Put laughter to work. Start applying all these skills to cope with stress.

MANAGE YOUR TIME AND TERRITORY

Some people can endure a level of upheaval and confusion that others find enormously stressful. "I find that people, particularly women, place too much pressure on themselves to perform in too many roles," observes Carolyn Dean, M.D., N.D., author of *Dr. Carolyn Dean's Natural Prescriptions for Common Ailments.*

Explore the World of Laughter

"SOME PEOPLE ARE GOOD LAUGHERS, other aren't," observes Paul McGhee, Ph.D., a humor researcher, speaker, and author of *Health, Healing, and the Amuse System: Humor as Survival Training.* "In general, people who are more outgoing and more expressive are better laughers."

So, what should you do if you're not a naturally big laugher? Dr. McGhee recommends a "fake-it-till-you-make-it" approach. That is, put yourself in situations where you're expected to laugh, then force yourself (if necessary) to laugh harder than you normally would.

Here are some of Dr. McGhee's other suggestions to help you along the road to bigger, better laughing.

Make it a priority. For at least a couple of weeks, go out of your way to laugh as hard as you can. "It may be a phony or artificial feeling at first when you try laughing harder," says Dr. McGhee. "But then you realize that people aren't paying that much attention to you, and it becomes easier."

Give yourself a rating. While you're trying to laugh harder, rate yourself on a scale of 1 to 10. "If it's a 1 or 2, push yourself to a level 6, 7, or 8," says Dr. McGhee. "After a couple of weeks of doing this consciously, you'll find yourself laughing at a 3 or 4 level without thinking about it."

Invite hilarity. Ask people to share their funny stories with you. Go ahead and tell people you're looking for a good laugh. Once you invite the stories, you'll find that people think of you first when they have a funny story to tell. And why wouldn't they, when they know their stories will be greeted with your great laugh?

More laughter is particularly needed in the workplace, says Dr. McGhee. That's because more is being demanded of employees than ever before, and people become frustrated and angry. "If you try to build your sense of humor on the good days," he says, "you'll find it's easier to carry over to the bad ones."

"They take on a full-time job while maintaining a family and caring for both partner and children."

If you feel as if you are in a state of constant disorganization and confusion, stress can take a heavy toll. Here are two ways that experts recommend to help you get your family organized, your activities on schedule, and your papers in order.

Create a family calendar. Once a week, get together with everyone in your household and go over the weekly calendar, suggests Bonnie McCullough, a professional home manager in Lakewood, Colorado, and author of *Totally Organized: Easy-to-Use Techniques for Getting Control of Your Time and Your Home*. The best calendar is a big one, the size of a desk pad, where everyone has room to write.

If there are children in your family, this is an opportunity to find out about their after-school and social activities, to coordinate rides, work out mealtimes, and assign responsibilities. If it's just you and your partner doing the calendar, you can quickly resolve scheduling conflicts so you don't have any surprises during the week. Post the calendar in a prominent place, and encourage everyone in the household to check it every morning.

Assign a purpose to every piece of paper. At home and at work, paper tends to pile up. Often it's because we can't figure out whether to keep it, throw it away, or file it somewhere. It's certainly stressful to lose an important bill, letter, or reminder, but it's just as stressful to watch the piles mount higher and higher as you try to decide what to do with them.

According to Barbara Hemphill, past president of the National Association of Professional Organizers and author of *Taming the Paper Tiger at Home,* you can simplify the process if you put every piece of paper (or the information it contains) into one of several places.

- A "to sort" tray
- The wastebasket
- Into your calendar
- On your "to do" list
- Into an action file
- Into a personal phone book or file of telephone numbers
- Into a reference file

Once you have this paper-management system set up, all your paper can be handled in just a few minutes every day. In working with dozens of clients, Hemphill says she discovered that this system can be adapted to meet anyone's personal style. "You will discover not only that it is possible to control the paper in your life," says Hempill, "but that the rewards greatly enhance the quality of your daily life."

OFFICE TACTICS FOR STRESS RELIEF

One of the big disadvantages of working in an office all day is that you may feel compelled to stay at your desk or computer and look busy, even when you really need a stress-relieving stretch break or even a good little nap. But there are unobtrusive ways you can get some relaxation without announcing that fact to your colleagues or office mates. In fact, the best policy is to do some progressive relaxation beginning first thing in the morning and continuing at regular intervals throughout the day, according to L. John Mason, Ph.D., of the Stress Education Center in Cotati, California, and author of *Guide to Stress Reduction.*

If you make a habit of doing these exercises every hour or so, after 2 weeks they will become habitual. Then you can actually prevent stress, rather than react to it. Here are some simple progressive relaxation techniques recommended by Dr. Mason that you can do without stirring from your seat. Try to remain focused during the brief periods when you're doing these exercises. (It helps to close your eyes.)

Trigger some relaxation. Sitting relaxed in an upright position, take three deep, slow breaths while you relax the muscles of your head and face. Let your shoulders drop and release the tension from your neck muscles. These breaths are the "trigger" to get you in the mood for relaxation. (After the initial three deep breaths, resume breathing normally.)

Give tension an outlet. Ball up your fists and tense the muscles all the way from your wrists up your arms to your biceps and shoulders. Hold the tension for a count of five, then release. As you release, visualize the blood smoothly flowing down into your arms, into your wrists, and all the way to your fingertips.

Pay attention to your legs and feet. If you can, slip your feet out of your shoes and curl your toes. If that's not possible, just press on the balls of your feet. Tighten all the muscles of your lower legs, flexing your calves. Again, hold for a count of five, then release and visualize the blood flowing all the way down to the tips of your toes.

Hunch your shoulders high. "Become a no-neck," suggests Dr. Mason. Hold for a count of five, then release and relax.

Save face. Finally, tighten and release

the muscles of your face and forehead to ease the tension all around the facial area.

Be sure to start early in the day to make the most of the preventive effects of progressive relaxation. As you're doing these exercises, focus on the quality of the tension you create when you tighten your muscles, then on the "letting go" that you feel when you relax. Creating a mental image of the blood-flow to your extremities is an important way to increase your sense of relaxation. To practice, you might want to begin by doing these exercises every 20 minutes or so. When you're in the office, do them about once an hour until they be-

---

Defusing Road Rage

IN MOMENTS OF ANGER, blood pressure rises, metabolism increases, and we're at increased risk of heart attack and stroke. But apart from the physical cost, anger can lead to life-threatening behavior, particularly if you happen to be driving a car.

Jerry L. Deffenbacher, Ph.D., of Colorado State University, has spent nearly 2 decades studying ways to deal with anger. The most effective, according to his studies, involve two basic types of approaches: relaxation exercises and what's called cognitive relaxation therapy. In a study of 57 college students, Dr. Deffenbacher found that both approaches were effective, especially when used in combination. Here's how you can deal with road rage before it happens.

Extend your breathing. Suppose someone just swerved in front of you, nearly causing an accident. Internally, you experience this incident as a life-threatening situation, and your body reacts as if you have to fight for your life. (That's the fight-or-flight reaction.) Immediately you start to breathe faster, as if you had to jump into battle. But stop right there! Concentrate on expelling all the air from your lungs, then take a deep breath. No matter what you're thinking or how angry you're feeling, just concentrate on your slow, deep breaths.

come a regular part of your daily work habits.

GETTING THROUGH LIFE'S CHANGES

In studies of stress, researchers have learned that any kind of significant change in life, positive as well as negative, can raise stress levels. Not surprisingly, losing a job is very stressful, and so is a traumatic event like getting a divorce or having someone fall sick in your family. But stress is also produced by events that, it seems, should make us happy—like getting a new job, moving to

Tense and relax your body. If you're driving, you can't jump up and down to help dispel anger. But you'll get a similar effect if you consciously tense and release the muscles in different parts of your body, particularly the areas that tense up when you're angry. This can be done without moving very much at all. Tighten the muscles around your neck and shoulders, hold for a moment, then relax. Then tighten and relax your arm muscles. Then do your stomach muscles. As you move through your body, progressively tensing and relaxing, you can still concentrate on driving. But you'll find that when you're done, the nervous energy generated by your anger has been dispersed.

Have a chat with yourself. If you want to, you can consciously change your thinking. In his work with students, Dr. Deffenbacher told them how to do it, then worked with them to develop techniques that would help control road-rage reactions. For instance, if a car is on your tail, you might have an angry impulse to speed up ("Okay, buddy, let's see how fast you want to go!") or slow down ("If you insist on tailgating, I'll just stay in your way."). You can actually replace these thoughts if you talk to yourself and say, "I'm going at the right speed, and I'll continue at this speed. I hope you don't take the risk of passing me, but if you decide to do that, there's nothing I can do to prevent you." If you can change your thought pattern, Dr. Deffenbacher points out, you can prevent a bad situation from becoming worse.

a different home, getting married, or having a baby. To face such events, it helps to be prepared with some strategies to release the stress you feel. Here are some methods.

Count your blessings in prayer. Whether you're going through times of great hardship or on the brink of something new and different, you can help your physical and emotional well-being if you essentially "count your blessings."

In a study reported in 2002 in the *Journal of Personality and Social Psychology*, researchers from Southern Methodist University and the University of California, Davis, reported that people who make a habit of giving thanks for life's benefits feel more vital and satisfied than those who just see the dark side.

One of the ways to keep your blessings in mind is by making a conscious effort to give thanks in prayer. "Surround your prayers of thanksgiving, in which you name your personal blessings, with the affirming love of God directly accessible to you," suggests Pastor Tolson. He recommends that prayers of thanksgiving include words of gratitude such as, "Lord, I thank you for all the benefits of my body, my mind, and my spirit. I thank you that you made me just as I am. I accept myself through your grace."

Smooth your move to a new home.

Whenever you make a move, you are likely to encounter unexpected surprises. First, there are all the demands of preparing yourself and your household for the move. Then, suddenly, you're in a completely new place where old friends are farther away and nothing feels familiar.

One way you can purge that stress is by immediately arranging one area of a room to feel and look familiar, suggests Cathy Goodwin, M.B.A., Ph.D., author of *Making the Big Move: How to Transform Relocation into a Creative Life Transition*. In a new house, for instance, you might set up your bed and nightstand before anything else. Make the bed just the way you like it and turn on some of your favorite music. You'll feel better about your new home, and far more relaxed, if you know you can retreat to that familiar area.

Change your answering machine message. For some people, a ringing telephone is both demanding and distracting. If you jump to answer every time it rings, each interruption distracts you from what you were doing. So let your machine take the calls, and try this recommendation from University of North Carolina professor Melissa Stöppler, M.D., who suggests a solution that helps new mothers to keep friends and family up-to-date. "Record a friendly, outgoing message with info about how you and the baby are doing," says Dr. Stöppler. "Then let your callers know you'll get back to them when you have the time and energy."

Of course, you don't need to be a new mother to use this strategy. If you have been sick or have recently returned from the hospital, you can let your callers know that you're on the mend but resting, and you would like to return their calls later. Or, if you need to focus on a project, record a message to let callers know when you'll get back to them.

REMOVING FEARS AND PHOBIAS

After the 1994 earthquake that shook San Francisco, doctors reported a fivefold increase in the incidence of cardiac death. Of course, this was no coincidence. Millions of people were awakened at 4:31 in the morning by the rumbling and shaking of an earthquake that Californians had been dreading for decades. Alarm, panic, and terror—these emotions were felt throughout the city as strongly as the earthquake itself. Studies of similar disaster situations point to the conclusion that fear has a physical effect. To protect our bodies as well as our minds from the stress of fear,

we need coping mechanisms. Here are some of the best.

Tap for relief. Using a technique that combines physical distraction with mental prompting, you can help yourself dispel fear and restore calm almost immediately, according to Roger J. Callahan, Ph.D., former associate professor of psychology at Eastern Michigan University and author of *Tapping the Healer Within: Using Thought Field Therapy to Instantly Conquer Your Fears, Anxieties, and Emotional Distress.* First think about the fear that you have to deal with, while you try to evaluate (on a scale of 1 to 10) how fearful you're feeling. Then, using two fingers, tap firmly five times on the following points on your body:

- About 1 inch under the eye, high on the cheek
- About 4 inches directly below the armpit
- About 1 inch down and 1 inch to the left or right of the center collarbone notch

Each of these points corresponds to an acupuncture or acupressure point in Chinese medicine, where the energy (chi) is particularly concentrated. By tapping repeatedly at these points, you help release the energy and distract yourself from fear.

Meditation to Renew Your Mind

STOP WORRYING . . . buoy your spirits . . . boost your pleasure!

While these may sound like promises of a magic elixir or an illegal drug, they are actually the benefits of something we can all learn—meditation.

"The purpose of meditation is simply to train your awareness to be in the moment," says Daniel H. Gottlieb, Ph.D., a psychologist and family therapist who is the host of Philadelphia's public radio show "Voices in the Family" and author of *Voices of Conflict: Voices of Healing*. "When you're lost in thoughts and emotions, you're dealing with the past and the future," he observes. By meditating, you can observe those thoughts and emotions instead of experiencing them.

Meditation teachers recommend that you focus on something very arbitrary and specific—your breathing, a phrase, or a single word. For instance, you might try to focus on the single area of your nostrils where you feel the intake of breath. While maintaining that focus, your mind will naturally wander, but that doesn't matter. "Gently bring your mind and your attention back to your breath," says Dr. Gottlieb. "Do that without judgment. Don't beat yourself up when your mind wanders."

In the more than 7 years that he has practiced meditation, Dr. Gottlieb says he has learned to do it in many different situations—even between seeing patients. "What it has done for me personally," he says, "is teach me how to devalue my thoughts and emotions. Thoughts are just electrical impulses to the brain, and they're 90 percent wrong. Emotions follow or create the thoughts, so I devalue them, too."

If you think someone is angry with you, for instance, observe how anxious or uncomfortable that makes you feel and how much you want to fight back, make amends, or do something that will win over the other person. If, instead of acting or continuing to feel bad, you meditate, you can simply observe your thoughts and feelings and see how they generate those impulses.

Hum from the right side of your brain. Agoraphobia is a particularly severe, sometimes debilitating type of fear that occurs in people who are afraid to leave their homes or other familiar territory. While most people don't have fears that are that powerful, a technique used to deal with agoraphobia can be used by anyone in any situation. When you start to feel fearful, just hum or sing to yourself, suggests Dr. Dean.

As Dr. Dean points out, there is a valid psychological reason why this quick therapy is helpful. The left side of your brain is the center of emotions that create worry and escalate fear. When you hum or sing, you activate the right side of your brain, which helps to overwhelm and replace some of the nerve-jangling alarms that come from the left.

Have faith that it will end. Associated with fear and anxiety is the dread that you might not survive what you're feeling or "make it through." For people who have these feelings, it can be reassuring to dwell on the fact that you've survived the fear before and you can do it again.

For anyone who prays, this reassurance can become part of the act of prayer. Pastor Tolson recommends a number of Bible phrases that help support the feeling that life goes on and faith is a support. In the New Testament, for in-stance, the first letter of John says, "Perfect love casts out fear." From the Psalms of the Old Testament comes the reminder, "Cast your burden on the Lord, and He shall sustain you." As Pastor Tolson suggests, repeating these phrases or keeping them in mind can help get you through difficult times of fear and stress.

Whatever you do, keep breathing. A typical part of the fight-or-flight reaction is hyperventilation. Without even knowing that it's happening, you tense up and restrict your breathing when you feel fear. As your body becomes oxygen-deprived, it sends more warning signals ("Give me more oxygen!"), so the original fear is compounded by an almost primal fear of suffocation. It's important to break this cycle and avoid hyperventilation, says Bert A. Anderson, M.Div., Ph.D., author of *How to Treat Your Own Panic Disorder.*

Dr. Anderson notes that practitioners of what's called respiratory psychophysiology can help you identify some of the things that you may be doing unconsciously to start the hyperventilation cycle, as well as demonstrate techniques to prevent it. But if you want to learn to prevent it yourself, just be aware of when fear is making you breathe more rapidly. Then slow down your breathing and try to pace yourself. This concentration on your breathing can also help distract you from other sources of fear or anxiety.

DETOX YOUR NEGATIVE THOUGHTS

Many of us are subject to what psychologists call automatic thinking. When something bad happens, you may have a tendency to exaggerate the negative event so it becomes bigger in your own mind than it actually is in reality. Psychologist Aaron T. Beck, Ph.D., professor of psychiatry at the University of Pennsylvania School of Medicine in Philadelphia and president of the Beck Institute, has observed that some people just automatically think that bad things are bound to happen to them again and again. Positive events, on the other hand, are often ignored.

People who are instinctively pessimistic tend to jump to negative conclusions based on very little evidence. This can have social consequences. If someone becomes distracted while you're talking, for instance, you may ask yourself, "Why does he or she think I'm boring?" instead of thinking more objectively, "I wonder what's distracting this person's attention."

But as Dr. Beck and others have shown, there are ways you can turn around this type of thinking with a process called cognitive restructuring. Essentially, you need to challenge the set of beliefs that leads you to form negative conclusions. Here are several steps from Martin Seligman, Ph.D., author of *Learned Optimism*, that you can take.

Dispute negative beliefs. The next time you criticize yourself, jot down the criticism to discover your beliefs. For instance, if you lose your keys, you might write, "I'm always losing things" or "I'm very disorganized." Later on, look at the statement you wrote down and challenge it. You might realize that you've lost your keys only one time in the past 4 weeks. That means there were 27 days when you kept track of your keys, and only 1 day when you lost them.

Exercises like this can remind you of the unreality of your thoughts, identify exaggerated criticism, and help you realize when you're making a mountain out of a molehill.

Say "Stop!" and distract yourself. When you notice that your negative beliefs may be running away with your emotions, a simple distraction can help get your mind off a negative track and onto a positive one. Dr. Seligman suggests putting a rubber band around your wrist. If you start having thoughts like "I'm no good at . . ." or "I always make the same

Yoga Routine for Detoxing Your Emotions

ACCORDING TO YOGA TRADITION, many of your emotional responses are centered or focused in one particular area of your body—what's called the anahata chakra. Symbolized in drawings by a six-pointed star, this is the area that needs to be treated if you become excessively insecure, nervous, anxious, or angry. The following is a simple yoga exercise recommended by Gary Kraftsow, founder of the American Viniyoga Institute and author of *Yoga for Transformation*. This exercise helps bring awareness to the anahata chakra, producing a greater sense of well-being.

Assume the position. Kneel on a rug or mat with your knees together, your shins flat on the floor, and your feet under your buttocks. Bend forward as far as you can. If possible, try to rest your stomach and chest on your thighs and your forehead on the floor, with your hands placed palms-down on either side of your head. If you are overweight, it's okay to let your knees come apart to allow space for your abdomen.

Move with your breath. Inhale deeply and rise up, spreading your arms. At the height of the inhalation, your upper body should be straight and your gaze toward the ceiling. As you look up, raise your arms with your palms open.

Lower your arms. Do this on the exhalation, bringing your palms down to cover your heart while you chant "Yam." This is a traditional chant word that allows for varied expression and intonation. When chanting, repeat the sound as often as you like, drawing out the "a" sound in Yam, then closing your lips to produce a long, humming "m" sound.

Coordinate your movements. As you inhale again, raise your arms again to the open position. Exhale and return to the crouched, kneeling starting position.

Repeat one to eight times. Chant "yam" every time you change from the upraised-arms position to the hands-on-heart position.

mistake . . ." or "I can never . . . ," give that rubber band a good, hard snap. At the same time, say "Stop!" (Say it out loud, if you have to!)

That gives you a timeout from your runaway thoughts. You can focus, instead, on what you have to do next. Later on, you can come back to what's bothering you, and you'll be able to think about it more clearly, with less feeling of catastrophe. To return to the example of the lost keys: If you can say "Stop!" to the negative feelings, you're more likely to figure out a way to get a duplicate set of keys, to get by without them, or to think clearly about where you might have left them.

Enjoy the rewards of disputing your beliefs. One of the problems of pessimism, identified by Drs. Beck and Seligman, is that negative beliefs really can produce negative consequences. If you think, "I'm the type of person who always loses his keys," then you are less likely to forgive yourself ("Everyone does this sometime!") and to think clearly about action-oriented solutions ("Well, I'll have some duplicates made, just in case."). So it helps to remind yourself about your successes whenever you dispute a belief and solve a problem. If you count how you reap the rewards ("I got by without my keys; I made a duplicate set; the next time, there was no problem"), you're more likely to get into the habit of disputing your negative beliefs and moving on to positive responses.

DETOX YOUR RELATIONSHIPS

Disagreements and disputes—even the ones that seem inconsequential—can cast a long shadow. Whether you're in conflict with a spouse, child, parent, friend, or colleague, it's hard to feel good about a discussion that turns into an argument or a dispute that reaches the boiling point. But do you know how to avoid the dynamics that lead to this kind of escalation? Believe it or not, there really are some rules that will help prevent anger and defensiveness from poisoning a relationship.

Start with "I" messages. If you point a finger at someone and declare, "You are to blame for . . . ," that person's knee-jerk response is, "I am not to blame," or "That was not my fault."

It is far more effective and less likely to cause conflict if you use "I" statements to get your point of view across, according to Larry Alan Nadig, Ph.D., a clinical psychologist and marriage and family therapist in Glendale, California.

Dr. Nadig suggests that there are four important parts to an "I" statement. The first part is a nonaccusative "when" statement. This is followed by "the effects are," "I feel," and "I would prefer." For instance, suppose a member of your household always leaves dirty dishes in

the sink. You can address the problem by saying, "When I come home and see a pile of dirty dishes, the effects are that someone has to clean up before dinner. I feel tired at the end of the day. I would

The Food-Mood Connection

MANY OF US HAVE A PERSONAL LIST of "feel-good foods," ranging from mom's spaghetti sauce to a favorite chocolate bar. But is there anything to this? Can certain foods actually make you feel better? The answer may be yes, but the feel-good foods may not be the ones you think they are.

In a study of 200 men and women in southwest England, nearly 9 out of 10 said they used dietary and nutritional strategies to help improve mood—and a significant number reported success. People who cut down on sugar, caffeine, and alcohol said their moods definitely improved. (Unfortunately, they also reported mood-improvement when they cut out chocolate.) The participants in the study said they also experienced improvement when they increased the vegetables, fruit, and oil-rich fish in their diet. And nearly 80 percent said they felt better when they drank more water.

Based on these results, study author and nutritional therapist Amanda Geary created an "ideal meal" designed to lift your mood. The meal would include salmon, mackerel, or tuna along with a salad of lettuce, avocado, and pumpkin seeds. To finish it off, Geary recommends stewed fruit with dried apricots and bananas on an oatmeal biscuit topped with walnuts. She also advocates whole wheat pasta as a mood-lifting addition to the meal. As for traditional mood-lifters like coffee and chocolate, Geary says to avoid them. They do give a momentary lift, but it's followed by a dip in mood and energy.

prefer that everyone in the family wash their own dishes during the day."

Attack the problem, not the person. To resolve conflicts amicably, focus on the issues and work together toward a solution, suggests Dr. Nadig. In the initial stage, you need to identify both what you and the other person want. Working together, generate a number of possible solutions, evaluate the alternative solutions, and then decide on the best one.

You have to acknowledge from the beginning that both of you won't get 100 percent of what you desire. But if you're in a long-term relationship, the other person's interests are as important to you as your own. "You both should be open, honest, and remain respectful, not deceptive, manipulative, or disrespectful," says Dr. Nadig. "Mutual trust is a necessary, core issue in a healthy, long-term relationship, and neither partner should do anything to weaken it."

Mirror the other person's point of view. Misunderstandings happen all too easily, especially when we feel as if we are being attacked or defied. One way to avoid mistaking a message is with a process called mirroring, according to couples therapist Harville Hendrix, Ph.D., cofounder and president of the Institute for Imago Relationship Therapy

in Winter Park, Florida. That is, make sure you understand what the other person is trying to say, and let that person know you are listening before you try to respond. For instance, if your child wants to play with his friends on a school night, you might say, "You must feel left out when your friends are playing together, and you aren't allowed. Is that why you're angry with me for not letting you go with them?"

Of course, once you've started the "mirroring" process, it's important to stay with it until you hear what the other person has to say. By doing that, you begin to understand the other person's point of view and build empathy.

DETOX YOUR NEW HOME

Your emotions are definitely affected by your home environment. If you move into a new house, office, or apartment, you might feel as if it really isn't yours at first, and that creates uneasiness and anxiety. Even if you've lived in the same place for a long time, the atmosphere can begin to feel wrong if something unpleasant has occurred there. How do you get rid of the "old energy" so you can begin to feel better about the place where you live, work, or both?

Traditional practices of feng shui can

be extremely helpful when it comes to detoxifying a space and replacing bad feelings with positive energy. In the practice of feng shui, the objective is to create an environment that allows the maximum flow of positive energy—what is called chi in Eastern healing traditions. Many factors are involved, from the positioning of doors and furniture to the arrangement of plants, pictures, light, crystals, and wind chimes. Because emotional energy is considered such a critical component of health and lifestyle, practitioners of feng shui pay special attention to areas of the home that can contribute to negative emotions such as betrayal, anger, and despair.

Many important feng shui teachings come from Grandmaster H.H. Lin Yun, who recommends the following "scent cure" for a home or office as a way to purge stale or negative energy. Nancy SantoPietro, a feng shui consultant and author of *Feng Shui and Health,* says the scent cure is particularly useful if you have just purchased a house or moved into an apartment that was previously rented. The scent cure essentially clears away the energy of the previous inhabitant or owner and makes the house or room ready for you. You will need an orange, a small bowl of water, and a paring knife. Here are the steps:

1. **Pick your place.** Select a quiet area of the house, and have a seat.
2. **Begin peeling.** Slice off a small, round disk of orange peel and place it in the water bowl. As you do so, think about the positive energy that you would like to have all around you. At the same time, consider the negative thoughts or emotions that have bothered you, and release yourself from them.
3. **Create more disks.** Repeat the peeling ritual eight more times. (When you are done, there should be nine small disks of orange peel in the water.)
4. **Purify your space.** Now stand and take the bowl to the front door. Sprinkle some water by the door, using the traditional "ousting mudra" hand position. Hold out your hand with the forefinger and little finger extended straight ahead and the two middle fingers tucked under. Dip the middle fingers in the water, tuck them under your thumb, then release them, flicking water drops into the room. (In traditional feng shui, women should do the ousting mudra with the right hand, men with the left.)
5. **Add the power of words.** As you do the ousting mudra, recite a mantra (a repeated phrase). One school of feng shui, called Black Hat Feng Shui, teaches the use of the six-word mantra

Om Ma Ni Pad Me Hum, a reverential phrase sometimes translated as "I bow to the jewel in the lotus blossom." Repeat the mantra nine times.

6. **Visualize purification.** With each repetition of the mantra, visualize nine steps toward the positive results that you would like to achieve in your new home. Think of the best possible outcome of your prayers and wishes, and the steps required to get there.

7. **Heal your whole house.** Go through each room repeating the ousting mudra as you sprinkle water, spreading the scent cure throughout the house.

RITUALS FOR PURIFYING MOODS AND EMOTIONS

In every religion and culture, people follow rituals that carry special meaning. Some are purely religious, intended to make us feel closer to a god or an all-encompassing spirit. Others are specifically intended for physical or emotional healing.

In your own detox program, you may have discovered that your daily activities can be enhanced by introducing ritualistic or ceremonial qualities. For instance, food tastes better (and you are more attentive to what you eat) if you approach each meal as a significant moment when you provide life-giving nourishment to your body and mind.

Washing your hands is a very ordinary activity, but it takes on a different quality if you are mindful of the warm water, use a soap with a pleasant fragrance, and gently massage the tension out of your hands while you're washing. There are many ways you can be more attentive to daily activities, becoming more mindful of their worshipful, religious, or magical qualities.

Of course, many ceremonies are deeply rooted in cultural traditions and require the presence of a traditional healer or a whole group of people who are familiar with the myths, chants, masks, music, or dances associated with the ritual. The following are some traditional ceremonies with special meaning within the culture they come from. Though they aren't from our culture, it is still possible to learn from them and adapt them to your own daily life.

A Mayan Purifying Bath

In Mayan tradition, ritual baths helped rid the soul of the diseases associated with human suffering. Spiritual bathing practices were used to deal with fright, trauma, sadness, envy, grief, and many other emotions. Certain herbs, used in the bath water, were associated with spiritual illnesses. If an adult suffered from envy or jealousy, for instance, basil might be added to the bath.

There was additional significance in the number of plants that were used and the prayers that were spoken. The herbs needed to be collected in the correct manner. In the tradition of Mayan healers, collectors should give thanks to the spirit of the plant and its power to make a healing, purifying bath, explain Rosta Arvigo and Nadine Epstein, authors of *Spiritual Bathing: Healing Rituals and Traditions from Around the World.*

Many of the fresh herbs used by the Mayans are not readily available today. But Arvigo and Epstein describe a winter bath using dried herbs that can have the purifying effect of the ritual Mayan bath. You can use either a single dried herb or a combination of different herbs, including basil, rosemary, sage, thyme, oregano, and dried roses. While we don't know the healing properties that the Mayans associated with each of the herbs, the scent of rosemary is traditionally used to improve memory and relieve sorrow; the scent of sage helps reduce fatigue; and rose is commonly used to treat stress and insomnia.

Conducting spiritual bathing at home is rewarding and easy. Here's how.

1. **Prepare ahead of time.** Add 1 cup of dried herbs to a gallon of water, bring to a boil for 5 minutes, then turn off the burner and let the herbs steep for 1 hour.
2. **Strain out the herbs.** When the herbal mixture has steeped and cooled, pour it through a strainer into a second 1-gallon container, filtering out the loose herbs. Squeeze the contents of the strainer with your hands. (To follow the Mayan tradition, you should pray for the healing or purifying effect of the bath while you inhale the aroma of the herbs.)
3. **Prepare the bath.** Fill your bathtub with warm tap water and pour the gallon of herbal "tea" into the tub.
4. **Luxuriate in your bath.** Soak, meditate, and pray for at least one-half hour, staying as relaxed as possible. Purists recommend that you let your body air-dry after your bath to get the greatest benefit from the herbs.

A Native American Talking Circle

In their studies of healing ceremonies among Native Americans, Carl A. Hammerschlag, M.D., and Howard D. Silverman, M.D., discovered that the ceremonial Talking Circle is still a powerful ritual in modern times. In the traditional ceremony, the shaman opens the ceremony by burning sage and touching each participant with an eagle feather. The objective of that ritual is to remind each person that they are in a special place and should shed whatever clings to them from the outside world. The ritual beginning also includes a song or prayer. Then the leader talks about the intention of the ceremony—why the participants are gathered at a certain time in this place.

During the ceremony, an object is passed from hand to hand. It could be a feather, a lighted candle, or some talisman that has special significance. As the object comes around, each person is allowed to speak without time limit, but must stop speaking as soon as the object is passed along. No one else is allowed to speak until the object comes into his or her hand.

In their experience as facilitators, Drs. Hammerschlag and Silverman discovered that the Talking Circle ceremony could be used in many different situations to create a therapeutic group experience. For instance, at a parent and family meeting of the Foundation for Blind Children, Dr. Silverman and his wife formed the participants into four Talking Circles. Each of the groups received a lighted candle and began with a statement of purpose: "to describe one negative and one positive aspect of being the parent of a visually impaired child." In this environment, where they felt understood, supported, and safe, the parents found that when the candle came to them, they were able to open up and share some of the deeply emotional feelings they had about themselves and their children.

If your family has an important issue to discuss, you might try creating your own version of this ritual. Have each participant in turn hold an object that has meaning to the family and speak while others remain silent. As the object makes the rounds of each family member, all of the aspects of the issue will gradually emerge.

A Parting Ritual

Another ritual often observed among Native American tribes was the traditional practice of smudging or smoking to honor the dead, according to E. Barrie Kavasch and Karen Baar, authors of *American Indian Healing Arts*. This ceremony honors the Earth and Creator and, at the same time, helps to drive away trouble, inspire love and caring, and release stress from the body.

To begin the ritual, relatives and members of the tribe gather in a circle. Herbs are placed in a smudge pot or woven into braids tied with cotton string. Someone lights the herb, then blows out the flame. As it continues to smoke, the smoke is not inhaled, but the smudge pot or stick is carried in and out around the circle. With cupped hands, each person draws in some of the smoke toward his head, face, or torso. As the smoke drifts away, it also carries the prayers that mourners send to their ancestors.

Herbs for smudging are available at many natural foods stores. If you want to try this ritual yourself, many different kinds of herbs can be used. Wild white sage (*Artemisia ludoviciana*) is said to drive away bad spirits and prevent negativity. It can be crumbled up in a smudge pot or bundled up with fragrant-smelling woods such as cedar or juniper. Fragrant sweetgrass (*Hierochloe odorata*) encourages good spirits and positive thoughts to come to the gathering. This aromatic herb is usually braided. A mourner lights one end of the braid, blows it out, and as the prayers begin, the first offering of smoke goes up to the Creator. Then the person who carries the sweetgrass waves it toward North, South, East, and West, and finally to the Earth.

According to tradition, as the smoke passes over different parts of the body, it has a variety of effects. Drawn toward the heart, it increases love. As it weaves around the face and head, it brings clearer vision. Swept over the limbs and torso, it has a relaxing effect, stripping away anger and stress.

Chapter 9

Relaxing Home Treatments: Setting Up Your Home Spa

Aннннннннннн!

Slowly and deeply you breathe the freshest of air as the sweet scent of jasmine puffs away all thoughts, transporting you to blissful contentment. Your muscles, one by one, release and relax in a head-to-toe cascade as your body soaks in the powerful detoxifying nourishment from the cozy, moist cocoon embracing your body. You are surrounded by a quiet so total that it heightens your senses, opening you to awareness of your incredibly luxuriant, healthfully intoxicating surroundings.

Detoxification never felt so good.

Stepping from the healing waters, eyes still closed, you are greeted with warm, baby-soft towels that buff away the moisture. You slip into a feather-light silk robe and tissue-soft slippers as you are led to a massage table, where gentle hands warmed with cypress and juniper oils nudge the remaining toxins from your body.

It is a mind and body experience that is totally sensational—the perfectly purifying, delightfully detoxifying spa experience.

At one time the rituals of a first-rate spa were the purview of fortunate individuals who had both the money and the time to escape for a week or two of pampering and detoxifying in some luxuriant locale. Not so anymore. Day spas can be found just about anywhere, making access to a spa experience easier than ever.

The cost, however, is far from spartan. But now, even that can be overcome. Thanks to the Internet and health-minded consumers, the companies that furnish spas with their "magic formulas" have made it possible to have a spa experience in the privacy of your own home.

In addition to online sources, spa-type treatment essentials can be found any-where from high-line cosmetics counters and natural product boutiques to ordinary supermarket shelves and health-food stores. What's more, some of the magic found in certain spa formulas can even be found on your kitchen shelves, if you know where to look. The result is a plethora of options that leave you with only one big question: Where to begin?

SPA SECRETS

If you've ever spent time at a spa or know someone who has, you know that people return looking, well, just "spa-tacular." And they feel great, too. Sure, the buffing of nails and skin and the deep conditioning of hair help. So does dropping a couple pounds due to encouraged exercise and scrumptious spa cuisine. But the real reason for the healthy glow and exuberance is what took place beneath the skin.

"The ultimate benefit of a spa experience is the nature-based therapies that detoxify and purify the body," says Patricia Schneider, director of the Arizona Biltmore Resort and Spa in Phoenix.

Simple everyday living makes the body a magnet for toxins. They are really impossible to avoid. "Most things that touch the skin have the ability, to some degree, to be absorbed by the skin," says Schneider. "Pollution, dust, dirt—anything that lingers in the air can get into the body. Makeup and chemicals in many common products can build up toxins in the skin. Smoking, sickness, chronic conditions, sugars, and processed foods also contribute. Spas use special ingredients from nature that are rich in minerals that have the ability to pull impurities and toxins out of the body."

For example, the Arizona Biltmore Resort and Spa offers a 50-minute, $155 mud wrap using a clay extract from the red mud found in the renowned red-rock region from nearby Sedona. This wrap purifies the body by pulling out built-up toxins. "The extract contains lots of minerals but must be used carefully because it could take out the oils as well, which is something you don't want," says Schneider.

Of course, a Sedona Mud Wrap is hardly the kind of treatment you can expect to do yourself at home. But specialists agree that a spalike experience that is equally beneficial, luxurious, and relaxing can be accomplished in your own home. In this chapter, we'll tell you how.

CREATING NATURE'S AMBIENCE

The common denominator in any spa experience, whether you're getting a pedicure or a mud bath, is the expulsion of stress. "Stress in itself is toxic," says Schneider. "Getting rid of stress is the end goal of a spa experience." And, to this end, spas go to great lengths to create a stress-free atmosphere—an environment of tranquility and total relaxation. In other words, it is an environment that replicates the simplicity and balance found in nature.

In the home, the focal point of the personal spa is the bathroom. If money were no object and you could remodel your bathroom to be the perfect spa room, what would it be like?

Picture this: A large, open room with an expanse of windows and skylights to flood the room with natural light.

Double French doors or, better yet, a movable wall that opens onto a meticulously kept, green-grass manicured garden centered with a statuesque fountain framed by mountain vistas. A decor of earth tones with blue and green accents evocative of water and nature. Walls with built-in speakers to provide soft music. Fixtures and flooring crafted from earthy sandstone and limestone, and space for a comfortable recliner, books, plants, and possibly a fireplace. And for the ultimate relaxing element, an oversize soaking tub concealed behind a waterfall that flows over a glass wall and that turns on with the flick of a switch.

Now, back to reality. Most bathrooms are not big enough to accommodate a chair, let alone a recliner, and tubs and commodes are not exactly like furniture when it comes to rearranging. Yet there is much you can do to create enough ambience for a genuine "spa" feel.

Bring nature indoors. Depending on the size of your bathroom, bring a plant or two into the room. Make sure it is a plant you enjoy looking at because you'll want to enjoy it during your bathing ritual. Or, if you prefer fresh flowers, keep a vase of your favorites close by so you can pick the petals and float them in your bath.

Enhance the detoxifying effect of your

spa by growing plants that help take toxins out of the air. These include bamboo palm, spider plant, mums, peace lily, and mother-in-law's tongue.

Dim the lights. Even if your bathroom gets plenty of natural light, it's likely that many of your home spa rituals will take place at night, so artificial lighting is im-

Detox Makeover

AS A TEENAGER IN OKLAHOMA CITY, Pat S. had eczema so bad that she wouldn't go anywhere without camouflaging her arms and legs, even on the hottest summer days. For 15 years she struggled with the malady until, somewhat by accident, she found her cure: seaweed.

"I was reading about seaweed and how powerfully loaded it is with minerals, so I wanted to try it," she recalls now. "I was especially intrigued by spirulina because it is said to be such a perfect food source."

Because seaweed comes in so many varieties, she decided to keep it simple and stick with the basics. She bought a package each of powdered seaweed and powdered spirulina, which also goes by the name blue-green algae.

"Twice a week I poured the seaweed in my bath and just soaked as long as possible," she says. "Each day I mixed a teaspoon and a half of the spirulina in some apple juice and blended it with bananas and strawberries to make a smoothie. I drank it every day."

The result, to use her word, was "incredible." "Within 2 weeks my eczema was almost totally gone. It went from being so bad to being almost totally gone." That was 15 years ago, and to this day she has never had another outbreak.

Pat says she has kept up her home spa ritual ever since, though she doesn't drink a spirulina smoothie every day. "I drink it a lot, but not daily. However, if I start to see a blotch on my skin, I get right back to it. It goes right away. It's like magic."

A Spa Night Out

STEPHANIE K. IS A DIEHARD PARTY GIRL—spa party, that is. The 35-year-old stay-at-home mom is well known among family and friends for her "pamper party" weekends. In fact, some of her friends have flown all the way across the country just to attend. But who wouldn't? Stephanie lives at the foot of the scenic McDowell Mountains in Scottsdale, Arizona, the spa capital of the United States.

"It all started when I was working and pregnant with my first baby," says Stephanie, a tall, thin blonde with glowing skin and three immaculately groomed children ages 1, 5, and 6. "My husband is out of town on business a lot, and it didn't help that on this upcoming weekend he was going to be away on a big golf outing. I was really stressed, so I thought, why not do something I totally enjoy?"

She called a few friends and her sisters-in-law (who were also going to be golf widows for the weekend). She also called her favorite area spa and put in a special order: a massage table, a masseuse, spa robes, slippers, exercise mats for yoga, towels, sea salts, and someone to organize a spa lunch and

portant. Light should reflect the mood you are setting. Recessed lighting is beneficial because it produces pools of soft light. Dimmer switches are a must because they allow you to lower the lighting for relaxation.

Candles are an excellent way to set the mood. A few candles, whether votives or pillars, create illumination that is ideal for a soothing bath. You can even buy floating candles manufactured for use in a tub. Aromatic candles add to the ambience. Just make sure that the aroma is "set" for the kind of outcome you want (relaxing or energizing) and that it is a scent you enjoy. Check the list of mood-altering aromatics and essences in "Add Oils to Boost the Bath" on page 196.

Find something lovely to look at. You may not have a real garden or ocean out-

dinner at her home. She went to the store and stocked up on spring water, lots of fresh flowers, and ingredients to make fruit smoothies.

"I didn't want to do the nails and hair thing," says Stephanie. "I wanted it to be a 'good things for the body' occasion. When my friends asked me what they could bring, I told them to bring something healthy—and their bathing suits."

The spa party started at 10:00 A.M. with Stephanie leading an hour of yoga. After a light lunch, the women took turns at the massage table while the others gave each other facials, lounged by the pool, or sat in the Jacuzzi that Stephanie had sprinkled with sea salt and relaxing lavender essential oil. They dined on Alaskan salmon, broccoli, salad greens, and fruit.

The event was such a success that it turned into an annual event—and a sleep over. "We sleep outside under the stars, which are so bright in Arizona," says Stephanie. The chaise lounges in her outdoor living room are plenty comfy, and she has an outdoor fireplace should the evening get too cool.

"It is such a great way to do a girls' night out," she says, "and everyone goes home feeling refreshed and renewed."

side your door, but you can mentally put yourself in your favorite outdoor space by hanging a favorite painting or picture in your bath.

Keep the cozies close by. Soft, cozy fabrics like terry, chenille, and silk are part and parcel of the spa experience. Invest in a luxurious robe that wraps generously around you. Purchase extra-plush, extra-large bath towels and keep them in a basket nearby. Buy a package of spa slippers. And in keeping with the spa experience, make them all white.

Pipe in some music. If you have extra income for a home spa splurge, some spa regulars suggest spending it on speakers so you can pipe soothing sounds into the room. Whether it's piano, sitar, or the sound of the tide lapping the beach, the selection is purely personal. Just make sure it is something gentle.

Fill a basket with spa toys. Boutiques and Internet stores offer just about everything you can get at a spa. Browse around and find what suits your fancy. Popular items include a loofah, a long-handled bristle brush for your back, a sea sponge, gel eye masks, bath oils, lotions, and French-milled soaps.

Put water on ice. Fill your favorite ice bucket with bottles of spring or mineral water. Set a dish of detoxifying freshly sliced lemons next to it.

SOAK SOME WEED

So what have spas found that is so heavenly perfect that it can pamper all impurities out of the body? The answer: seaweed. When it comes to whole-body detoxifiers, this common ocean vegetation is believed to be the most potent.

The therapeutic use of seawater and sea vegetation goes back to the time of the ancient Greeks, who used them to treat everything from arthritis to hemorrhoids to infections. Research has shown that sea vegetables contain high amounts of antibacterial, antiviral, and antifungal agents. In addition, they are abundantly rich in vitamins, minerals, and proteins.

"Seaweed," explains Schneider, "is the closest thing in nature to human blood plasma." When combined with the heat of bathwater, the minerals in seaweed penetrate the skin through the pores to the deepest levels and literally draw out the impurities. The heat promotes perspiration that draws the impurities to the surface. A special kind of seaweed called spirulina, or blue-green algae, has the ability to purify to the deepest levels of the body.

Seaweed comes in thousands of species and in a variety of colors and textures. Kelp, dulse, wakame, nori, and kombu are all types you may recognize. All seaweed contains large amounts of minerals such as calcium, phosphorous, magnesium, iron, iodine, and sodium, though the amounts can vary among various types. They also contain acids that bind with toxins and expel them from the body. However, when you're getting started, these nuances aren't important. All seaweeds are potent detoxifying agents. You also do not need to go to the ocean in search of fronds and mess with them in your bathtub. (But if you do, make sure to gather them from the ocean waters and don't take those washed up on shore.) Therapeutic seaweed comes in both powder and dried forms. For a more realistic "feel," you can purchase a gel that you can rub directly on your skin. Just make sure to follow the product directions. Before you take your first plunge, here are a few things to keep in mind.

Experiment. If you have an adventurous nature, consider going the dry route, where you can experiment with several varieties to find the ones that you find most appealing. And before you do, here is some seaweed trivia: About 3 ounces of dried seaweed is equal to about 2½ pounds of wet seaweed.

Contain yourself. You don't want the remnants of your seaweed bath to go down the drain, so you'll need to steep dried seaweed as you would a tea. Using an infusion ball or muslin bag, steep the seaweed in hot water for 20 to 30 minutes. As you are drawing the bath, toss the infusion ball or bag into the tub along with the hot water. Just make sure to discard it before you drain the tub.

Make it hot. Because toxins exit the body through perspiration, you should make the bath as hot as you safely can stand it. A slight film will form on your skin as the seaweed coats it. Once your skin absorbs the seaweed, the film will disappear. This is your signal that your time is up. Or you can follow directions on the package to determine how long to remain in your bath.

Take a plunge. To get the total detoxi-fying effect, dip deep into the water so your shoulders are covered. Wrap your hair in a soft terrycloth towel, lean back, and relax.

Sip something cool. Refresh by sipping a glass of spring or mineral water with lemon (which possesses detoxifying agents) or a glass of herbal iced tea.

Be careful in there! If the bath makes you dizzy or lightheaded, get out immediately. Also, if you have high blood pressure, heart disease, or are being treated for any chronic ailment, check with your doctor before doing a seaweed bath.

PLAYING WITH MUD AND CLAY

Sea muds and clays are also common spa detoxifying agents. They have been used for centuries in many cultures to beautify, refresh, purify, and heal the face. In fact, clay from the Nile River is said to have been one of the secrets to Cleopatra's beauty. Today, medical science has validated the use of clay for healing, based on its ability to draw, bind, and hold toxins.

At spas, sea mud that comes from the ocean floor is the basis of a purifying, deep-penetrating facial. Impurities in the body will often show up as impurities in the facial skin, explains Schneider.

(continued on page 198)

Add Oils to Boost the Bath

ESSENTIAL OILS ARE NATURAL SUBSTANCES extracted from flowers, herbs, fruits, trees, and grasses through a special distilling process. Many of these oils have been found to contain healing properties. Some are also known to affect the nervous system and can elicit either a calming or stimulating effect.

Essential oils are potent. A drop or two is often all that is needed to get the effect. (This is good, considering it takes about 100 pounds of plant material to produce 1 pound of oil.) Also, they should never be used directly on the skin or used alone. Keep all essential oils, even when diluted, away from mucous membranes (your mouth, nose, eyes, and vagina).

Keep in mind that not all essential oils are safe and that many types are best used only by trained aromatherapists. If aromatherapy and essential oils are new to you, refer to the list below when creating your own spa experience. Also, do not use essential oils if you are pregnant, have very sensitive skin, or are being treated for a health problem, unless you have the consent of your physician.

ESSENCES THAT SOOTHE

Basil. Helps ease muscle aches and pains. It is also used in skin toners.

Bergamot. Possesses antitoxin agents. Effective against acne and blemishes. *Caution:* Causes photosensitivity. Do not expose skin to the sun after using.

Cedarwood. Possesses antitoxin agents. Good for oily skin.

Chamomile. Helps skin conditions such as dermatitis, psoriasis, acne, and herpes.

Clary sage. Good for aging skin and varicose veins. Also known to have aphrodisiac qualities.

Cypress. Helps alleviate bruising, muscle cramps, and broken capillaries. Believed to help control cellulite.

Geranium. Helps ease breast tenderness and swelling.

Hyssop. Helps ease dermatitis, eczema, and acne. Helps reduce water retention.

Jasmine. A softener for dry, sensitive skin. Also believed to have aphrodisiac qualities.

Lavender. Helps soothe inflamed skin.

Mandarin. Good for scars and stretch marks. A great skin toner. *Caution:* Causes photosensitivity. Do not expose skin to the sun after using.

Marjoram. Has extra-strength calming qualities.

Neroli. Good for scars, stretch marks, sensitive and aging skin. Believed to have aphrodisiac qualities.

Patchouli. Helps soothe skin irritations. Good for aging skin and varicose veins.

Peppermint. Soothes muscle aches and pains. Helps constrict capillaries.

Rose. Good for aging skin. Believed to have aphrodisiac qualities.

Sandalwood. Good for dry and aging skin. Believed to have aphrodisiac qualities.

ESSENCES THAT ENERGIZE

Eucalyptus. Possesses antitoxin qualities. Helps heal blisters and other skin irritations.

Ginger. Helps fight congestion; improves circulation. *Caution:* Do not use on sensitive skin.

Grapefruit. Helps fight muscle fatigue and jet lag. Noted for its cleansing effect on the circulatory and lymphatic systems. Also good for oily skin. *Caution:* Causes photosensitivity. Do not expose skin to the sun after using.

Juniper. Known as a detoxifying agent. Also good for oily skin and blocked pores.

Lemon. Helps lighten skin pigmentation. *Caution:* Do not expose skin to the sun after using.

Lemongrass. Eases muscle soreness, bruising, and athlete's foot. Good for aging skin.

Pine. Helps fight eczema and psoriasis. *Caution:* Do not use on sensitive skin.

Rosemary. Eases sore muscles. Good for oily skin.

Chin blemishes are a perfect example. Smoking, poor nutrition, pollution, and certain medicines contribute to imbalances in the facial skin. Mud masks get below the surface and pull the impurities out.

Clay treatments are much more specialized. Because therapeutic clay is derived from mineral rocks and the Earth's crust, geographic location has much to do with the mineral content and other healing properties of the different clays.

Clays are commonly used for facial masks, body wraps, and baths, and as carriers for aromatherapy formulas. Clay works by generating heat that draws toxins out of the body. Clay absorbs oils, dirt, and bacteria from the skin's surface. It also pulls moisture and oil from the skin, so you don't want to use clay if you have dry or dehydrated skin.

Clays and muds are simple to use. Select a product that appeals to you and follow the directions on the package. Or, to make a detoxifying mask, all you need to do is take 2 tablespoons of powdered clay or mud and mix it with small amounts of mineral water or cider vinegar until it forms a paste. Presto! You're ready to go. Apply it generously to your face in small, circular motions. Make sure to avoid your eyes and hairline. Leave it on for 10 to 15 minutes. Remove the mud with warm water and a washcloth. To enhance the experience, you can also do the following:

Add some essence. Instead of using mineral water, use a floral water made from any of the essences recommended in "Add Oils to Boost the Bath" on page 196. Or add 2 or 3 drops of an aromatherapy oil.

Be still. Remember that this is spa time. Lie back, close your eyes, put on some soft music, and relax. You want your facial muscles to relax, so let the mask do its magic by being as still as possible. That means no talking or smiling!

Play misty for you. You do not want the mask to dry out before your 15 minutes are up. If you feel it beginning to crack, spray your face with a water mist, or a mist fragranced with a few drops of aromatherapy oil (but close your eyes first!). Keep your mister right by you so you can grab it without moving.

Steam first. Steaming before you apply a mask will help increase the effectiveness of the mask by opening the pores so dirt and impurities can escape. To steam properly and safely, do the following:

- Heat a pot of water on the stove until the water is simmering but not boiling.
- Pour the water into a ceramic bowl that is sitting on a nonslip surface.

Fill the bowl to no more than an inch from the top.

⊚ Drape a towel over your head to make a tent, close your eyes, and place your face 8 to 10 inches above the water. If the water gets too hot, lift the end of the towel to release some heat. Steam for 5 to 10 minutes.

Refresh. By the end of the mask, your pores will be tightened and your face will feel soft. Gently spray your face with the purified mist you have handy and let it dry.

Go for it all. Do a detoxifying mask and bath at the same time. Even though she runs a spa, this is something Schneider does for herself at home once or twice a week. "It's the best," she says.

A cuke makes it complete. About the only body part not accounted for at this point is the eyes. Put a slice of cucumber or a wet teabag on each eyelid to help pull out built-up fluid and reduce swelling. Some women prefer to wear a gel mask, which has the same effect plus offers the experience of bathing in a darkened room.

SALTS OF THE SEA AND OTHER PURIFIERS

Another secret super spa agent also comes from the sea: sea salt. Celtic Sea and Dead Sea salts are used in spas because they have a high mineral content and are slightly moist. Household Epsom salts have similar qualities. Therapeutic salts should not be confused with common table salt that has been stripped of its nutrients and, therefore, offers no healing qualities.

Salts have detoxifying qualities because they encourage perspiration. Like clays and muds, they leave your skin feeling silky, but they don't leave a ring around the tub!

Baking soda, also known as sodium bicarbonate, is highly alkaline and has been found to help leach from your system toxins caused by pollution, cigarettes, and alcohol. Baking soda is commonly combined with sea salts to make formulas for detox baths.

Making a detoxifying bath using sea salts is easy. Just combine the following:

1 cup of Dead Sea, Celtic Sea, or any marine sea salts (You can also combine different salts.)
1 cup Epsom salts
2 cups baking soda

Make a large batch of the salt solution and keep it in a jar with a tight lid. (You don't want moisture to get inside.) At bath time, add about ¼ cup of the salts to the bath as you are drawing the water.

To enhance the experience, try the following:

Turn up the heat. The hotter the bath, the better the results. Just make sure to get out of the tub immediately if you feel lightheaded. Also, if you have high blood pressure, heart disease, or are being treated for any chronic illness, get the okay from your doctor before trying this.

Add some essence. Salts do nothing to stimulate the senses, so add several drops of your favorite essential oil to the bath. For added pleasure, throw in a bunch of rose petals. It's the ultimate for your sense of smell.

Give it a boost. To enhance the detoxifying effect, add a tablespoon of powdered seaweed to the bath while you're drawing the water.

Another detoxifying treatment is what is known in some spas as an oxygen soak. In at-home parlance, it is called a peroxide bath. Mixing hydrogen peroxide in the bath creates a high concentration of oxygen that stimulates the circulatory and lymphatic systems. The water needs to be hot in order to create perspiration. To try this, add a cup of common drugstore-grade hydrogen peroxide to the bath water and soak, immersed to your shoulders, for 20 to 30 minutes. (Make sure you keep your hair up and out of the way, or you'll end up with unwanted streaks!)

FANCY FOOTWORKS

Sea salts are also great for soothing tired and aching feet and for softening the calluses formed by the abuses of everyday living. Put sea salts in a tub of tepid water with a few drops of rosemary, peppermint, and lavender essential oils to help stimulate circulation. To pamper your feet further:

Add some comfort. Do your footbath while sitting in the comfort of your favorite chair in your living room or den. Just make sure to set the foot tub on a rubber mat or towel to catch any water that may splash out.

Roll around. Put 8 to 10 equal-size marbles in the tub and roll your feet over them while you're soaking. The marbles will give you a minimassage. It feels great!

Do a scrub instead. Rather than a bath, make a scrub by mixing the salts and essential oils with enough olive oil to make a paste and vigorously rub it into your feet. Put your feet up, lean back, and relax for 15 minutes. Rinse your feet clean.

Have heat waiting. Before either the bath or the scrub, put a big, fluffy towel in the clothes dryer and time it to come

Stuff to Have on Hand

THE PURIFYING TREATMENTS in this chapter use the following household items. Keep them in your refrigerator or spa cupboard.

- Aloe vera gel
- Baking soda
- Cider vinegar
- Epsom salts
- Fresh flowers
- Herbal teas
- Lemons
- Mineral water
- Mist bottle
- Muslin
- Natural bristle brush
- Olive oil
- Powdered milk
- Rolled oats
- Sea salt
- Spring water
- Teabags or tea infusor

out as your treatment ends. Wrap your feet up in the warmth and relax for another 5 minutes or so.

Make it a couple thing. With your significant other, get on the couch covered in towels or linens and massage each other's feet at the same time. It's a great way to unwind right before bedtime, and it beats the stress of watching the news!

WHOLE-BODY TREATMENTS

The skin is not only the largest human organ, it is the only organ exposed directly to the harsh elements of the world. It takes a direct hit from all the pollution, dirt, and chemicals that we encounter on a daily basis. In addition to serving as an outlet for body toxins, it also has its own waste product to deal with—dead skin.

Sloughing away dead skin, also known as exfoliating, should be part of your daily detoxifying ritual. "An enthusiastic whole-body scrub is one of the best all-around body exfoliating spa treatments I know," says Valerie Gennari Cooksley, R.N., an aromatherapy practitioner and author of *Healing Home Spa*. A technique called dry skin brushing is simple and effective. It increases circulation and stimulates the lymphatic system to eliminate toxins and excess water.

To dry brush your skin, you should use a natural fiber brush, not plastic or nylon. Use the following technique several times a week in the morning before you step into the shower:

⚬ Using circular or figure-eight motions, brush your skin lightly, starting with your torso and working toward your heart.
⚬ Move to your legs, then your arms.
⚬ Give special attention to your thighs, buttocks, and the backs of your arms and legs.
⚬ Make sure to brush the palms of your hands and soles of your feet.
⚬ Do not dry brush your face. Use a dry washcloth, instead.
⚬ Be gentle. Remember, you are not scrubbing the floor!
⚬ Do not brush over any sore spots or open wounds.

On days when you have more time, give your body a salt scrub. This is an excellent whole-body treatment because the salts serve as both an exfoliant and a detoxifer. Getting a salt scrub in the luxury of a spa can cost $130. Salt scrub formulas can be purchased for $20 to $30 but are relatively inexpensive to make at home. Simply mix 1 ounce of ground sea salt with 10 to 12 drops of any stimulating essential oil to make a paste that you can spread easily over your body.

To get a salt scrub with more "feel," Cooksley recommends a scrub made with ingredients common to the kitchen. Mix together:

¼ cup Dead Sea salt
¼ cup ground oats
⅓ cup warmed virgin olive oil
10 drops essential oils of your choice

When using either scrub, rub small handfuls at a time over your entire body using small circular motions and following the recommendations above. Follow any whole-body scrub with a shower and an application of moisturizing cream.

GIVE YOURSELF A BODY WRAP

Detoxifying herbal body wraps are popular at spas and are the ultimate in decadence. They are an experience quite unlike any other. Wraps are especially good for drawing out nicotine and alcohol. They detoxify by increasing perspiration, encouraging circulation, and promoting drainage of the lymphatic system. You can mimic a spa-quality herbal wrap in your home, though be forewarned: It can get messy, especially the prep work and cleanup afterwards. But at a fraction of the cost, it can be worth it. Plus, the purifying benefits are beyond a dollar value.

Gathering the herbs is part of the fun—and the challenge. Detoxifying herbs that can be part of a wrap include:

- Dandelion roots and leaves
- Echinacea root
- Garlic cloves (if you dare!)
- Parsley leaves
- Alfalfa leaves
- Comfrey roots and leaves
- Dried cascara sagrada

You will need the following:

- Three large handfuls of detoxifying herbs
- A large super-clean bucket or utility tub
- Two very large, soft towels, such as beach towels
- A plastic sheet longer and wider than you are
- A clean tile or linoleum floor on which to lay out the plastic

Soothe Sun-Scorched Skin

TALK ABOUT CONTAMINANTS! Radiation from harmful ultraviolet rays and the resulting sunburn is about the worst thing that can happen to your skin. A milk bath can help make you more comfortable even though your skin looks as if it is on fire.

Milk soothes the skin and puts nourishment back at the same time. Simply add 2 cups of powdered milk to warm (not hot!) water as you are running the bath. To add to the healing effect, suspend two bags of chamomile tea from the faucet and let them steep into your bathwater.

Stay in the tub for 20 to 30 minutes. Afterwards, rub your burned skin with aloe vera gel.

Put the herbs in the bucket and fill it with hot water. Wait a few minutes, then submerge the towels in the water. Let everything steep for 5 to 10 minutes, but do not let the water cool. Remove the towels and squeeze them gently. (The idea is, you want to leave as much water in as possible but not have them dripping.) Remove your clothes and wrap the towels tightly around you. Remember, you must work quickly! The hotter the towels, the better the results. Lie down on the plastic and relax. Stay put for at least 15 minutes, then unwrap yourself slowly. To enhance the experience, you can also do the following:

Go alfresco. During warm—but not hot!—weather, do your herbal wrap outdoors. The exposure to nature and fresh air will heighten the mental aspect of the experience for you.

Soften the glow. Create a peaceful and comfy environment by placing the plastic on a stack of soft towels or soft cushions from an outdoor chaise lounge. Put a hot water bottle under the "bedding" to help extend the warmth.

Drink up. Body wraps are not intended to be a quick weight-loss device. Make sure to replace the fluid lost by drinking 8 to 10 glasses of mineral water over the next 24 hours. Also, skip refined sugars and foods and eat organic fruits and vegetables.

You can do a less-messy detoxifying body wrap by using essential oils. Mix 5 drops each of cypress, lemon, and juniper oils, plus 1 teaspoon of sea salt in a 12-ounce bottle of hot mineral water. Then simply spray the wet towels before applying.

KEEPING YOUR MAKEUP PURE

The irony of the spa experience is that many of the things we do to make ourselves look great and feel wonderful are actually contributing to the toxic abuse of our bodies. When it comes to chemically produced, commercial personal care products, cosmetics rank as the most toxic, says skin-care specialist Sunne Justice, chief pollinator and cosmetic expert for Burt's Bees, a small, entrepreneurial natural skin-care company based in North Carolina. Eye shadows, blushes, and mascara contain the highest percentage of chemically derived preservatives, she says.

Look at the labels of the products you are using. If the ingredients list looks like a jumble of letters with suffixes such as "ben," "ply," and "thyl," then you know

How to Make Aromatic Water

MISTING YOUR FACE with clean, fresh water during your spa treatment is nice, but misting your face with floral water is even nicer.

To make floral water, take 3 handfuls of petals from your favorite aromatic flower, put them in a large pot, and cover the petals completely with water. Heat the flowers and water over low heat and simmer until the water reduces by half. After the water cools, strain it into a clean, 12-ounce mist bottle. Gently squeeze water from the petals until the bottle is full.

If the water comes out tinted, it may stain your skin. Either use fewer flowers or choose another flower that doesn't discolor the water.

Caution: If you have hay fever or skin allergies (contact dermatitis), you should test whether you are allergic to a flower before using it. Rub some petals on a small area of skin and leave it overnight. If any irritation develops, don't use the flower in your bathwater or on your face.

the cosmetics you are using are not all-natural. Even water-based products like lotions, shampoos, conditioners, shower gels, and bubble baths contain chemicals. That's because water must be preserved in order to give the products a shelf life. (Remember, water is a favorite gathering place for mold and fungus.) For example, methyl peraben and propyl peraben are common preservatives in water-based skin-care products. "Ironically, these chemicals are drying," says Justice. Kind of defeats the purpose, doesn't it?

When it comes to chemical ingredients, Justice says petroleum derivatives are the most egregious. Anything that has "petro," "lum" or anything that sounds like petroleum-in-hiding is exactly that. Mineral oil, which is commonly found in cosmetics, is a petroleum derivative.

Skin keeps its softness and texture as a result of naturally occurring triglyc-

This Detergent Wears a Mask

HOW CHUMMY ARE YOU with sodium lauryl sulfate?

If you lather up your hair big-time in the shower, then it is pretty darn certain that sodium lauryl sulfate is an inhabitant in your household. Sodium lauryl sulfate is a foaming agent found in hundreds of over-the-counter shampoos, toothpastes, and cleansers. It is also a detergent—a strong detergent. It is so strong, in fact, that it is used to clean the dirtiest of floors.

The chemical is popular because it gives shampoos their foaming action. By comparison, natural shampoos produce almost no foam. It is also an inexpensive ingredient, which is why it is commonly used in products worldwide.

"Traces of it have been detected in the human body," says Patricia Schneider, director of the Arizona Biltmore Resort and Spa in Phoenix. "If it is one of the top three or four ingredients in your shampoo, you should switch to something else."

erides, wax esters, fatty acids, and vitamin E. As chemicals, pollution, and the sun sap the skin of these natural oils, they need to be replaced. Look for products that contain some of Mother Nature's best defenses. These include such things as avocado oil, clove oil, or any fruit or vegetable oil.

Going the all-natural route is the best way to minimize the toxic exposure your body gets as a result of making yourself look more beautiful in the morning. Short of that, you should read labels carefully, but most importantly, treat your skin to a daily routine that cleanses it of all makeup and environmental pollutions.

Cleanse twice a day. A morning-and-night cleansing routine is important, especially if you live in a big city where environmental pollution from things like car exhaust, diesel fumes, and chemical plants is high. Good cleansing is important even if you don't wear makeup. If you do wear makeup, it's a must!

Do not use soap and water to clean your face. Rather, use a mild, soap-free moisturizing cleanser that's right for your skin type. Ingredients that are particularly good for your skin include aloe vera, lanolin, olive oil, orange oil, sweet almond oil, vitamin C, and vitamin E.

Shed dead skin. Exfoliating tender facial skin requires a different tactic than the whole-body brushing routine described earlier. In addition to getting rid of dead skin, exfoliating helps get dirt and makeup out of your pores, preventing them from clogging and allowing them to accept nutrients. Exfoliate once a day, at night. Natural ingredients in exfoliants include such things as ground oats, ground almonds or spices, and natural plant oils such as almond, olive, and orange.

Give skin a daily tone. Applying a fresh, soothing toning lotion goes beyond making your skin feel refreshed; it decongests pores and equalizes the skin's pH. It also removes any traces of dirt still left on your face. Use a low-alcohol or a alcohol-free toner.

Moisturize, moisturize, moisturize. Got that? Moisturizers help feed the skin with important nutrients and help protect the skin from harsh elements. Depending on your skin type, you should moisturize day and night. Look for ingredients such as glycerin, vitamin C, borage oil, black currant oil, rice bran oil, and those that offer sun protection.

Chapter 10

Professional Purification Treatments: Options for a Thorough Cleanse

IF YOU WANT TO EXPERIENCE THE FULL GRANDEUR of a symphony, put away your CD player and buy tickets to a concert. If you want a great new hairstyle, put your scissors into a drawer and find a great stylist. And if you want to enjoy the full spectrum of beneficial effects you can get from body detoxification, locate a specialist and put yourself into his or her hands.

While juice fasting, herbal treatments, and exercising can be helpful, only trained professionals can safely apply many of the more potent body purification techniques. You may need to go to a clinic, office, or spa, and the cost may be higher than a do-it-yourself regime, but the effects you'll experience will be far more dramatic, and you can let the expert consider dosage requirements and any side effects.

In fact, the only real challenge you'll face will be in choosing from among the many great approaches available. Below are descriptions of some of the better-known techniques. These will help you decide which would be the best fit for your particular needs.

CHELATION THERAPY

Heavy metals are toxins that need to be removed for your optimum health. Chelation is a technique that removes these heavy metals, including nickel, lead, mercury, cadmium, and arsenic, from the bloodstream. "The word 'chelation' comes from the Greek root *chele,* meaning claw, like the claws of a lobster," according to Alan Magaziner, D.O., founder of the Magaziner Center for Wellness and Antiaging Medicine in Cherry Hill, New Jersey; president of the American College for Advancement in Medicine; and author of *The All Natural Cardio Cure.* "When you're given a substance to remove the metals from your body, it grabs onto them like a claw, binds with them, and pulls them out through the urine, sweat, or stool." These substances are called chelating agents. There are several of them, and each has an affinity for different metals.

Benefits of Chelation

For heavy-metal toxicity, chelation is the FDA-approved gold standard of treatment. If you went to a toxicologist, that's the treatment you'd receive. Chelation therapy is used, however, to treat many other illnesses as well, and

these uses are more controversial. But they do have a number of enthusiastic proponents.

"Some people with hypertension have higher than normal levels of lead and cadmium in their bodies," says Dr. Magaziner. "They are sometimes effectively treated with chelation therapy. Chronic fatigue syndrome, neurological disease, fibromyalgia, cardiomyopathies (disorders of the muscle tissue in the heart), hypertension, Parkinson's, and amyotrophic lateral sclerosis (ALS) all sometimes show a concentration of heavy metals.

"Another of the beneficial effects of chelation is that it reduces free radical damage," says Dr. Magaziner. Free radicals are harmful molecules that are formed in excess when we're exposed to toxins. "EDTA [ethylene-diamine-tetra-acetic acid] is one chelating agent we use that is in our food supply. It's in mayonnaise, for example. It's there because it prevents rancidity, which is the result of oxidation. On the other hand, smoking will negate the beneficial effects of chelation therapy, as will alcohol to some extent, and both create high levels of free radicals that damage the body."

Although some doctors use chelation to treat cardiovascular disease, its effectiveness for this condition is also still controversial. Clinical trials have either been too small or have not been designed well enough to come to firm conclusions. But Dr. Magaziner says we should soon have clearer answers. "There has been enough documentation that the National Institutes of Health in August of 2003 approved a 30-million-dollar, 5-year trial, so they're taking it seriously," he says.

How Is It Done?

"Chelation involves giving a patient an intravenous drip of vitamins, minerals, and a chelating agent," says Dr. Magaziner. "Nothing is taken out of the body, and blood is not run through a machine. The patient will lie on a recliner for anywhere from ½ hour to 3 hours, depending on what kind of chelating agent is used, and during that time they can read, talk, get up and walk, work on their laptop, do some needlepoint, just sleep, or have a conversation."

There are variants of chelation therapy that are administered orally and rectally, but Dr. Magaziner doesn't use these because he feels that their effectiveness is not well documented.

Because chelation can lower an individual's blood pressure or blood sugar level, some people may feel a little tired or dizzy after the first couple of visits. If this happens to you, immediately ask for some food during the chelation therapy, drink a glass of water, or take a little walk.

How Long Does It Take?

The number of treatments you receive will depend on which metal you're removing, but you may need as many as 30. Cost is typically around $100 per visit. If you can document that you have high levels of heavy metals in your blood, your insurance will pay for the treatment. But if you're there for a chronic disease such as fibromyalgia or chronic fatigue, even though chelation has been shown to improve those conditions, your insurance probably won't cover the treatment.

Who Does It?

Licensed medical doctors (M.D.s) and doctors of osteopathy (D.O.s) usually perform this procedure, but a couple of states are now allowing naturopathic doctors (N.D.s) to do it as well. According to Dr. Magaziner, "Any doctor doing this procedure should be in good standing with a group called the American College for Advancement in Medicine (ACEM), which administers oral and written exams to doctors who want to do chelation. Doctors may be designated to have basic proficiency or advanced proficiency. Obviously advanced is better."

Do-It-Yourself Chelation

CAN YOU ACTUALLY DO CHELATION AT HOME? Yes, but the effects will be very mild, according to Alan Magaziner, D.O., founder of the Magaziner Center for Wellness and Antiaging Medicine in Cherry Hill, New Jersey; president of the American College for Advancement in Medicine; and author of *The All Natural Cardio Cure*. "There are a lot of natural chelating agents, including garlic, cilantro, vitamin C, calcium, and magnesium," he says. "They're all mild chelating agents for metals, but they're only about 2 percent as effective as intravenous chelation." Adding garlic and cilantro to meals, however, is certainly a more pleasant way to do chelation, and vitamin C, calcium, and magnesium should be part of any general supplementation program.

COLONIC HYDROTHERAPY

Colonic hydrotherapy, also called high colonic, colonic irrigation, and colonic hydration, is a cornerstone of many professionally supervised detoxification programs. In fact, practitioners of alternative medicine will sometimes tell you that if you don't have one done, you'll miss half the benefits of body purification. Colonic hydrotherapy involves cleaning out the large bowel with water.

A colonic is like an enema, except that it is administered in a clinical setting using an apparatus that makes it possible to use more water and flush the colon more thoroughly. Symptoms that indicate that it may be time for colonic hydrotherapy include:

⑥ Bloating
⑥ Excessive burping
⑥ Flatulence
⑥ Poor digestion
⑥ Stomachache after meals

Many people, however, turn to colonic hydrotherapy simply to detoxify, even if they have no symptoms. Although almost anyone can benefit from colonic hydration, it's off-limits if you're pregnant.

Benefits of Colonic Hydrotherapy

After the very first colonic hydrotherapy session, "people notice immediately that bloat, distension, and the whole feeling of overfullness is gone or minimized. They also feel really energized," according to Trisha Rossi, N.D., founder of the Natural Alternative Center in New York City and former Northeast regional director of the American Colon Therapy Association (ACTA).

Better absorption is the long-term benefit, she says. "A sort of black plaque that accumulates on the inner walls of the colon can make absorbing nutrients difficult. In fact, we often see vitamins and medicinal capsules coming out whole, completely undigested. Nothing is being broken down. No wonder people complain their medicines and supplements aren't working."

Getting rid of parasites is another benefit. "We remove lots of different types of worms, although you can see only about ⅛ of them with the naked eye," says Dr. Rossi.

A high colonic can also clean out organs beyond the bowel.

As for side effects of colonic hydrotherapy, "sometimes people will feel a slight headache afterward, but nothing that lasts," says Dr. Rossi.

Eating Better for Bowel Health

YOU SIMPLY CAN'T DO COLONIC HYDRATION THERAPY without help from a professional, according to Trisha Rossi, N.D., founder of the Natural Alternative Center in New York City and former Northeast regional director of the American Colon Therapy Association (ACTA). You can, however, adjust your diet for better bowel health. "Don't overdo binding foods like pasta, bread, rice, and potatoes," she says. "They stick to us like glue. Anything alive and uncooked will be beneficial, and roughage will help. Eat lots of salads. Also drink raw vegetable juice. It's full of healthful enzymes."

How Is It Done?

"We recommend that hydrotherapy be done with a very professional treatment system that doesn't allow any sediments, impurities, or chlorine to enter the body," says Dr. Rossi. "We have a system that removes 106 of the EPA priority pollutants, including asbestos." The speculum, connected to a water feed tube and a waste tube, is inserted about 1 inch into the rectum. The tubing used in this process is disposable.

"Our ultimate goal is to recondition the shape of the colon to where someone would be able to go to the bathroom two or three times a day, which is normal," says Dr. Rossi. "One way we do that is to get rid of the hard, black, rubber-tire consistency that surrounds the walls of the colon. It's formed from years of additives, preservatives, processed foods, and junk foods."

How Long Does It Take?

The usual course is three treatments within 10 days of each other. "Any sooner, you're removing only fresh waste," says Dr. Rossi. "Any longer, and waste the body has failed to remove on its own is difficult to get out because it becomes too hardened."

The cost for colonic hydrotherapy may run anywhere from $35 to $75 per session.

Who Does It?

Colonic hydrotherapists do not have to be doctors, but they should be trained by a recognized association. Look for training and certification from ACTA or from the International Association of Colon Therapists (IACT). You can find referrals at www.i-act.org on the Web.

KNEIPP METHOD: EXTERNAL HYDRATION

The Kneipp method of purification uses water and herbs to cleanse and detoxify the skin and to improve circulation to the arms and legs. Sebastian Kneipp, a 19th-century naturopath, developed his method from spa culture, which dates back to the dawn of civilization. Kneipp combined five elements into what he called Kur (German for cure):

- Applying water to the body at contrasting hot and cold temperatures
- Balanced diet
- Movement and exercise (massage is considered to be a part of this element)
- Natural herbs, both applied directly to the skin with water and consumed in tea

⑥ Meditation, which integrates the first four elements through the mind/body connection

Benefits of the Kneipp Method

Proponents of this method of treatment tout a wide range of benefits. "Your whole circulatory system, respiratory system, lymph system, and digestive system improve, because you're stimulating them with herbs and water to contract and dilate," according to Jonathan De Vierville, Ph.D., owner and director of the Alamo Plaza Spa at Canyon Ranch in San Antonio. All of these are systems of detoxification in the body.

"You can use Kur for beauty, prevention, and wellness, but you can also use it for chronic disorders and major rehabilitation, especially for rheumatoid and skin disorders," says Dr. De Vierville. "You can also relieve pain and stress in your extremities. Applications of warm/cold contrast baths to the arms and hands can work wonders for people who suffer with carpel tunnel syndrome. A leg contrast bath would work well for people who are always on their feet."

How Is It Done?

"With the water treatments, we combine herbs such as lavender and rosemary to cleanse the skin with a hot herbal bath, which can be followed by a chilled bath, that is, an application of cool water after which the body itself reacts to warm itself up," explains Dr. De Vierville. "What you're trying to do is bring the heat out of the body. Most therapies bring heat into the body. We do that, but then we do a short effusion with cool water, over the legs, arms, back, or full body, and wait for the body's reaction to the chill.

"The warm water is applied by hand with a small brush. The added herbs can sedate, stimulate, or balance (harmonize). Rosemary, for example is a stimulant to the circulatory system. Hops or melissa would be more sedating."

After the initial cleansing, the person administering the treatment might apply even more heat using an herbal wrap or a warm bath, or by applying what is known as a hay sack. This is like a big teabag filled with herbal flowers that can be laid on various joints, such as the shoulder, or on specific areas of the stomach.

"After that, the therapist applies cooler water and allows the person's body to dry on its own," says Dr. De Vierville. "The next step is passive exercise, a massage, usually a traditional Swedish massage. We also do contrast baths for arms and legs. We warm the legs up to the knee in warm water, just above body tempera-

Kneipp Therapy in a Tub

"SPA CULTURE IN AMERICA encourages people to do spa treatments at home," says Jonathan De Vierville, Ph.D., owner and director of the Alamo Plaza Spa at Canyon Ranch in San Antonio. He recommends doing contrasting water treatments for arms and legs. "You can use tubs or large waste baskets. Showerheads don't do the job adequately. Stand with both feet in a large tub of warm water (100° to 105°F). The water should come up to your knees. Allow your legs to get good and warm. Then step into a tub of cooler water (65° to 70°F) until they cool down. Step out of the cool water and allow your legs to warm themselves up. Repeat this two or three times a day over several days or even a week. Allow ½ hour per session. Warm, chill, then walk around without drying." The herbs used at the spa include rosemary, but you can use any herbs you like, if you want to add them to the water, says Dr. De Vierville.

ture, then have them step into some cold water for a few seconds, so there's a constriction in the skin. Afterward you need a 20- to 30-minute rest or meditation of some kind."

How Long Does It Take?

Each session of hydrotherapy will take about ½ hour to complete, but you can't expect dramatic results right away. To get the full effect of the treatment, you have to do it several times over the course of 2 weeks.

Who Does It?

Hydrotherapy of this kind is usually done by a massage therapist, and that practitioner should have at least 2 years of training in physiotherapy. Massage therapists are often licensed by state, county, and local entities, so check to see if your state licenses therapists and whether the therapist you're considering has the proper credentials. Also ask if he or she belongs to the American Massage Therapy Association, which can be contacted through its Web site at www.amtamassage.org.

LYMPHATIC DRAINAGE MASSAGE

The lymphatic system is like a second circulatory system, distributing fluids and nutrients throughout your body. Lymph is the fluid collected in between cells. Sometimes the lymphatic system's drainage is inadequate and these fluids build up, causing problems such as swelling and discomfort. To make matters worse, the lymph can contain significant amounts of the toxic by-product of cellular metabolism.

"The way to combat this," says Mauro C. Romita, M.D., plastic surgeon and founder and executive director of AJUNE, The Center for Beauty Synergy in New York City, "is lymphatic drainage massage, which 'milks' the by-products of cellular metabolism (or toxins) through manipulation (pushing lymph into muscle where the muscle can then pick it up), physical therapy, and sequential compression."

Benefits of Lymphatic Drainage Massage

"Lymphatic drainage massage reduces cellular toxins that build up in tissue," says Dr. Romita. "It serves as the definitive treatment for lymphedema (accumulation of excess fluids resulting in inflammation); encourages postoperative healing, especially after liposuction; and improves the appearance of cellulite and tissue swelling due to varicose veins."

It may also be the treatment of choice for people experiencing swelling in their arms and legs as a result of cancer treatment. It's also helpful in reducing water retention during menstruation, flushing out toxins, and improving circulation.

How Is It Done?

This massage technique, created by Emil Vodder, Ph.D., in the 1930s, is similar to Swedish massage but is done with a lighter touch, as going too deep can actually close off drainage channels. The massage therapist will use rhythmic, nearly circular strokes to move lymphatic fluids back toward the nearest lymph node, starting from the area closest to the node and slowly working his or her way outward, while continuously pushing the fluid toward the node. This progressive movement away from the lymph node is called sequential massage. Afterward, you may have to wear compression stockings or bandages to keep your muscles clear of lymphatic fluid.

How Long Does It Take?

If you're having the treatment for cellulite, swelling, or water retention associated with menstruation or surgery, it'll take approximately 15 treatments to get noticeable results, says Dr. Romita. He recommends 2 treatments per week over the course of a month, followed by 1 treatment per month to maintain results. However, for those suffering from lymphedema, a medical condition affecting the lymphatic system, the treatment may be continuous. Each treatment lasts about 45 minutes.

The cost of a lymphatic drainage massage is usually in the $90 to $120 range, but your insurance may cover it if it's performed by a physical therapist following a physician's diagnosis.

Who Does It?

Physical therapists, trained clinicians, and massage therapists can perform lymphatic drainage. Physical therapists should receive training at an accredited institute, while clinicians and massage therapists should be trained in lymph drainage and experienced in using specific equipment, such as the pressotherapy and endermologie machines, which are specialized types of equipment

Draining Your Lymphatic System

WANT TO TRY LYMPHATIC DRAINAGE YOURSELF? If you're not suffering from a serious medical condition but are experiencing occasional swelling, here are some techniques you can try from Mauro C. Romita, M.D., plastic surgeon and founder and executive director of AJUNE, The Center for Beauty Synergy in New York City.

- Follow a low-salt diet
- Wear compression stockings or rent pressotherapy boots
- Elevate your lower extremities
- Self-massage your arms and legs
- Exercise your legs
- Refrain from sitting in a position with your knees flexed for a long period

sometimes used during this procedure. If the individual is experiencing swelling or complications as a result of lymphedema, cancer, or another medical condition, his or her physician would recommend that this procedure be done by a physical therapist.

PANCHAKARMA

Ayurveda, India's ancient tradition of medicine, includes a complete method for body detoxification called panchakarma. Panchakarma is a system that uses a number of different purification therapies to meet the cleansing needs of the person receiving treatment, explains V. Shekhar Annambhotla, who holds an Ayurvedic M.D. from India and is the founder and director of the Ojas Ayurveda and Yoga Institute in Macungie, Pennsylvania.

The therapies include herbal oil massage, herbal laxatives and enemas, body wraps, and herbal steam, all tailored to the individual's body type. The idea is to use these therapies to eliminate toxins from the body. Ayurvedic medicine views toxins as the root causes of disease.

Benefits of Panchakarma

Dr. Annambhotla offers a long list of special benefits that result from undergoing panchakarma treatment, including:

- Deep relaxation and a sense of well-being
- Elimination of fatigue
- Enhanced digestive power
- Faster elimination of waste products
- A feeling of lightness in the body
- Improved circulation
- Improved health and wellness
- Improved strength, endurance, energy, vitality, and mental clarity
- Minimized negative influences of stress
- Removal of toxins from body and mind
- Reversal of aging process
- Smooth skin
- Strengthened immune system

Panchakarma should not be administered to pregnant women or women who are having their period. Menstruation can become a significant issue if you've spent a lot of money to go to a week-long retreat, only to arrive and find it's the wrong time of the month, so it's best to plan carefully with your monthly cycles in mind.

How Is It Done?

In the United States, many practitioners have modified the more extreme traditional panchakarma techniques to make them kinder and gentler for Westerners. In India, for example, something like vomiting or bloodletting might be prescribed, but these more extreme kinds of therapies are less likely to be encountered in America. Among practitioners trained in panchakarma at the Maharishi Institute, for example, vomiting is not used, and if bloodletting is indicated, the individual will simply be advised to donate blood to the Red Cross.

"There are other ways to get the same results you get with these more aggressive techniques that are just as effective, if a little slower," says Nancy Lonsdorf, M.D., medical director at the Maharishi Vedic Health Center at the Raj in Vedic City, Iowa.

Because the therapies can vary among clinics that offer panchakarma, it would be a good idea to have a clear understanding of what to expect at a particular clinic before you take the plunge.

Dr. Lonsdorf says that for a typical panchakarma experience at the Raj, the cleansing process gets underway well before an individual arrives for treatment, because panchakarma has a preparation phase. "In India they go to the clinic and eat a special diet, but in our country, people do the first stage at home. First, we gather details about their health and habits, then put them on a diet of cooked vegetables, lentil soups, and light grains such as couscous, light basmati rice, and quinoa.

"They also ingest a liquefied, purified butter called ghee every morning, between six and seven o'clock, on an empty stomach. They start with a small amount, which increases over 4 days. When you eat it on an empty stomach at that time of day, it isn't processed the same way as it would be later. Instead of being burned for energy or stored, it gets deposited in the bloodstream and works its way through the tissues of the body, where it pulls out toxins by making them soluble. Those fat-soluble toxins then find their way to the bloodstream, the liver clears them into the bile, and finally they reach the intestine.

"At that point, we use a laxative to clean the bowel. We use the most traditional one, castor oil, because it starts moving the contents of the bowel from the very top of the small intestine. They take the castor oil in the morning, and by lunch they're having loose bowel movements. They'll usually eat liquid foods for the rest of the day."

Once clients arrive at the clinic, they receive a medical evaluation, which includes a look at lifestyle. They are then put on a vegetarian diet.

"They may not be feeling great at that point," says Dr. Lonsdorf. "When the body goes into purification mode, people don't feel like their usual, vigorous selves. If they came in with health problems, symptoms will sometimes get worse before they get better. But by the fourth or fifth day, people are feeling really good. They're feeling clearer mentally, lighter in the body, and they take on a healthy glow. They start thinking about doing things they haven't done in a long time, such as exercising or changing their diet—they

Panchakarma at Home

IT IS POSSIBLE TO DO A CERTAIN AMOUNT of panchakarma purification at home, according to V. Shekhar Annambhotla, who holds an Ayurvedic M.D. from India and is the founder and director of the Ojas Ayurveda and Yoga Institute in Macungie, Pennsylvania. Here's what he suggests.

You'll start with "oleation" to loosen impurities lodged deep in the cells and tissues. This process requires the consumption of ghee. Ghee (pronounced like the *gee* in "geek") is clarified butter, which can be purchased in many natural food stores and stores that carry Indian products. It's also possible to make your own. For directions, see page 55. Ghee can be heavy to digest and may cause slight nausea and dullness. Don't worry. You'll feel better after your system is flushed of the toxins through the laxative therapies later on.

Take ghee in liquid form on an empty stomach first thing in the morning, either with 1 cup of hot milk, soy milk, almond milk, or rice milk. Add a pinch of dry ginger powder and a pinch of cardamom powder.

During the ghee phase, eat no oil and maintain a low-fat or fat-free diet. Take one tablet of Trikatu (a combination of ginger, black pepper, and pippali available at health food stores and online) with each morning dose to keep the digestive fire strong, and one tablet before each meal of the day.

just mentally and physically have a lot more energy.

"Every day we rub herbalized oils onto their bodies from head to toe. It's not deep massage, but it's very complete, using the flats of the hands to rub the oil in classical Ayurveda style, with a massage technician on either side. After that they get either a relaxation treatment or a heat treatment to open up the circula-

Also during this phase, eat lightly and sip hot water throughout the day. Increase the dosage of ghee as follows:

Day 1:	2 teaspoons ghee
Day 2:	4 teaspoons ghee
Day 3:	6 teaspoons ghee
Day 4:	8 teaspoons ghee

On the evening of day 4, you'll take 1 teaspoon of castor oil at bedtime with hot milk, soy milk, almond milk, or rice milk, plus a pinch of dry ginger powder and a pinch of cardamom powder.

The purpose of this laxative is to cleanse the body of the impurities loosened by the oleation. If there is any loose stool, it should not last longer than 12 hours. One caution: Castor oil is a powerful purgative and laxative, so do not continue its use beyond this treatment. Anyone on heart medications should avoid this treatment entirely, due to the risk of electrolyte loss from diarrhea.

Your evening meal on day 4 should be very light, just warm vegetable soup. Before taking the laxative therapy, you might want to have a 15- to 20-minute hot tub bath to increase circulation and loosen the impurities in the body. You may need to get up during the night to evacuate, or it may not happen until morning. You can expect two to five evacuations, so you should plan to be at home throughout the morning. Eat a light meal after the laxative effect has worn off.

tory channels of the body, which increases circulation to the extremities. The relaxation treatment is called shiradara. In this technique, a person lies down while we pour warm oil back and forth over his or her forehead.

"In the heat treatment, herbalized steam is applied to the body or warm oil is poured all over the patient for an hour. For steam, people lie on a wooden table that has many holes in it, and steam comes up from pots below filled with boiling water and herbs. The head is breathing room-temperature air. It's important not to heat the head.

"For the oil treatment, the oil comes out of little hoses. There are other kinds of treatments, such as herbs wrapped in cloth and patted on the body, or rice, cooked with herbs and milk, wrapped in

Kick It Up a Notch

IF YOU REALLY WANT TO PUT YOUR BODY PURIFICATION INTO HIGH GEAR, you can add some Ayurvedic supplements to your at-home panchakarma program. According to V. Shekhar Annambhotla, who holds an Ayurvedic M.D. from India and is the founder and director of the Ojas Ayurveda and Yoga Institute in Macungie, Pennsylvania, here's what to use.

- Triphala, a remedy made of three types of medicinal fruits. It can help remove toxins from the GI tract as well as promote a strong environment in the entire digestive system. Take two capsules before bedtime with warm water or herbal tea.
- Turmeric Formula, which is a combination of turmeric, tippali, and kutki, three medicinal herbs commonly used in Ayurveda. It helps in digestion and also cleanses the blood and liver. Take two capsules with every meal.

You can purchase these supplements online or at stores that specialize in products from India. *One warning:* Dr. Annambhotla recommends that you check with an Ayurvedic physician before taking any Ayurvedic remedy.

cloth balls and then rubbed all over the body. The rice is especially good for fibromyalgia, muscle and joint problems, and pain in the body.

"At the end of each treatment day an enema is given. An herb-based enema is alternated with an oil-based enema day by day. Water alone tends to dry out the colon. We always give odd number days of treatment so the panchakarma can end with an oil-based enema. Ayurveda says that 80 percent of the value of panchakarma comes from the basti, which is the herbal enema."

How Long Does It Take?

Ideally, a course of treatment should last at least 5 days (not including 4 or 5 days of preparation done at home), although you can find programs that are longer or shorter. Traditionally, panchakarma is done once a year.

Panchakarma is among the more expensive detoxification treatments, running between $300 and $450 a day.

Who Does It?

In India, Ayurvedic physicians (vaidyas) generally administer these techniques. In the United States, they are often administered by massage therapists or others who have gone through specialized training. Indian universities offer a

5½-year course for a B.A.M.S. (Bachelor of Ayurvedic Medicine and Surgery) followed by 3 years for an M.D. in Ayurveda (Doctor of Medicine in Ayurveda). A number of Ayurvedic centers around North America provide panchakarma training programs. Ask about the practitioner's educational background.

SWEAT LODGE THERAPY

The body naturally uses sweating as a means of cleansing and detoxifying itself. Historians claim that cultures on five different continents have been consciously taking advantage of that process in various ways and that the practices go back a full 20,000 years. In North America, it took the form of the sweat lodge, which became pervasive among peoples from the Alaskan Inuit to the Mayans of Mexico.

The idea behind the sweat lodge is to cleanse the body, but perhaps even more so, to cleanse the spirit, according to Lewis Mehl-Madrona, M.D., coordinator for integrative psychiatry and system medicine, program in integrative medicine, at the Center for Biofield Science at the University of Arizona. Dr. Mehl-Madrona, who descends from Lakotas and Cherokees on his father's side, practices conventional medicine as a psychiatrist. He also incorporates traditional Native American healing techniques for those who ask for alternative treatments to complement their conventional care.

"The sweat lodge purifies the body, mind, and emotions," he says. "It's a journey of spiritual cleansing, although it's not actually considered a 'sacred ceremony.'"

Dr. Mehl-Madrona's sweat lodges are open to anyone. "We're completely ecumenical. Everyone is invited, regardless of age, sex, race, or religion. Some Native Americans believe outsiders shouldn't be allowed to participate in sweat lodges, but I disagree. We're all aware of the genocide against Native Americans, but now should be a time of reconciliation and healing. Besides," he adds wryly, "I'm only half Native American, so any sweat lodge I participate in will have at least half an outsider present."

Benefits of Sweat Lodge Therapy

Sweating can rid the body of heavy metals and other pollutants, as well as excess salt. It's particularly efficient at getting rid of nitrogen. "Fifteen minutes of sweat lodge expels as much urea nitrogen as the kidneys can expel in 24 hours," says Dr. Mehl-Madrona. Sweating can also make you look healthier and younger. "People's skin looks amazingly

better after a sweat lodge. I keep kidding my friends that I'm going to start a sweat lodge spa center for alternative face-lifts. People look lighter and feel lighter, and their skin is clearer."

Perhaps the most important benefit, however, is the purifying effect a sweat lodge has on the mind and emotions. "People feel spiritually more lightened," Dr. Mehl-Madrona explains. "There's a feeling we have when we say we're full of toxins. It's a heavy, sluggish feeling of being clogged up, where thoughts are kind of confused and foggy. When we go into the sweat lodge, we come out feeling the opposite way."

As with sauna therapy, people who have serious heart problems, are pregnant, or are on antidepressant medication shouldn't participate in sweat lodges. Likewise, sweat lodge therapy should be avoided by anyone who feels uncomfortable in dark, closed spaces.

How Is It Done?

Dr. Mehl-Madrona does Lakota-style lodges in the Black Elk family tradition, but he emphasizes that every family has its own way of doing things. "In the style that I do, we hold the ceremony in a wood-frame lodge, covered with blankets and tarps, although in the old days they used to use buffalo skins. Generally about 12 people attend. We enter the lodge and sit in a circle around a central pit. The ceremony is divided into four segments or 'rounds,' each of which begins with the door opening and fresh, hot stones being brought in. We pour water on the stones to create steam. The heat can be really intense at times.

"The first round is for physical, spiritual, and emotional purification. The second is for prayer. The third is to receive guidance. And the fourth is to offer thanksgiving. After the second round, water with herbs in it is brought in to drink for healing. After the third round, a pipe comes in to be smoked, which symbolizes prayers being answered. It's filled with a mixture of tobacco, bearberry bark, willow tree bark, and other sacred herbs.

"During the ceremony, someone is either singing or speaking continually. There is more singing than talking, and the prayers are always out loud, spoken in any language you wish to use. Everyone sings, but there's typically a designated singer (or singers) who knows the songs and picks them." When the fourth round ends, so does the sweat lodge.

How Long Does It Take?

It usually takes about 3 hours from the time you go in to the time you go out,

plus another hour or two to heat the stones. "Sometimes it can take longer because people can get really long-winded when they pray," says Dr. Mehl-Madrona. "Also, the singers can pick any songs of any length and in any combination, which can make the lodge last longer or shorter."

How often should you go? Dr. Mehl-Madrona either runs or attends someone else's sweat lodge once a week, every week. "That's pretty typical," he says.

Covering the costs of the sweat lodge is often handled in a communal way. "In Arizona, it costs a couple of hundred dollars to buy wood for each sweat lodge, so people make contributions," explains Dr. Mehl-Madrona. "There's no specific amount. If I know people are pretty well off, I sometimes bug them. But they're not going to get a bill in the mail. It's about being honorable."

Who Does It?

The person who holds a sweat lodge is called either the leader or the water dipper. He tells the singers it's time to sing, pours the water on the stones, and keeps the ceremony moving. "It has to be someone who's been spiritually trained in this, who's been steeped in the traditions," says Dr. Mehl-Madrona. "I would say that if there isn't such a person, then do a sauna. Don't dabble in these sacred ways."

How do you find a sweat lodge ceremony you can attend? Go to a powwow, or go to the local Indian Cultural Center and ask for referrals. "If you show interest and hang around long enough," says Dr. Mehl-Madrona, "somebody will invite you to one."

SAUNA THERAPY

A few months after the September 11th attack on the World Trade Center, David E. Root, M.D., M.P.H., of Sacramento, California, received a desperate call at his clinic from some folks in New York City. There were a lot of sick people, firemen and other rescue workers, suffering from the effects of poisons given off by the burning, collapsed buildings, who might greatly benefit from detoxification treatments—a specialty of Dr. Root's. That was the beginning of what came to be known as the New York Rescue Workers Detoxification Project.

"They got spectacular results," says James Dahlgren, M.D., professor on the clinical faculty of the University of California, Los Angeles, department of occupational and environmental medicine; director of the Toxicology Treat-

ment Center in Santa Monica, California; and member of the advisory board of the New York Rescue Workers Detoxification Project. "One guy's sweat actually turned blue from the chemicals he was excreting. It was dramatic. Of the 250 firemen treated so far, I'd say 95 percent are markedly better. Three-fourths of them have been able to stop all medicines; many of [those] had been on two or three inhalers, sleeping pills, and other drugs. The changes are dramatic."

The detoxification techniques that led to such remarkable improvements were first developed by L. Ron Hubbard, noted writer and humanitarian. Dr. Dahlgren and other scientists have since taken a more scientific approach to their use. They involve the use of some niacin (vitamin B_3), vegetable oil, exercise, and a whole lot of sweating in saunas. And you don't need to be a rescue worker to benefit from them. According to Dr. Dahlgren, we've all had enough exposure to toxic chemicals to have stored high levels in our bodies.

"Each decade we learn about a new group of chemicals that bio-persist, bio-accumulate," he says. "In the 1950s we heard about DDT, in the 1960s, PCBs, in the 1970s, dioxins and furans, and in the

1980s, we heard about polybrominated diphenyl ethers.

"These last were used as flame retardants in computers, polyurethane foam, and in thousands of other products. Everyone in the United States has fairly high levels in his or her body. These particular chemicals were banned in Europe decades ago, so now Americans have levels that are hundreds of times higher than those of Europeans.

"In the 1990s we started hearing about chemicals called perfluoroalkanes, which remain in the body for very long periods of time, some for 10 to 12 years. Then there are the fluorine compounds, which are used as surfactants in the manufacture of thousands of everyday products. These compounds don't break down. That's why they're so useful to industry. Unfortunately, they get into the body, and they don't break down there, either. They interrupt hormone function, cause cancer, and bring about a variety of other serious health problems. The way it manifests in people is that they don't feel good, they get sick all the time, and then they die young. It's really horrible."

Benefits of Sauna Therapy

People who come to see Dr. Dahlgren are often suffering from a whole host of symptoms, including fatigue, poor memory, lack of energy, greater susceptibility to infection, inability to concentrate, poor sleeping patterns, and generally feeling under par. Fortunately, sauna detoxification can change all that.

"The important point is that people feel better after this protocol," says Dr. Dahlgren, and laboratory results show that the improvement in his patients is real. "We've done objective measurements of neurological function and liver function after these treatments," says Dr. Dahlgren, "and a lot of these things get better, especially if they were abnormal to start with." In fact, when certain highly toxic chemicals called PCBs in the blood and fat of people are measured before and after sauna therapy, 63 to 75 percent reductions are not unusual. Other toxins are more difficult to measure, but they, too, show dramatic reductions, Dr. Dahlgren says.

In addition to all of its benefits, there doesn't seem to be any significant risk of side effects with sauna therapy, except perhaps for dehydration. "It's one of the safest things you can do, so long as a person isn't in a delicate state of health. Of course, if you have a weak heart or kidneys, it's not a good idea to stress those organs this way. The same thing is true if you're desperately sick and on multiple medications. And we don't want someone who's on tranquilizers or anti-depressants [to use sauna therapy] because the therapy will excrete those chemicals from the body and reverse their beneficial effects."

How Is It Done?

"We begin with an evaluation of health status," says Dr. Dahlgren. "We take a health history, and then do a physical, routine lab work, pulmonary function, electrocardiogram, and treadmill, and we do blood and urine tests to measure PCBs, DDT, and heavy metals. The patient starts the program by exercising for about a half hour on a bicycle or a treadmill to get his heart rate up, and then we give him a low dose of niacin, about 60 milligrams, and put him into a sauna bath.

"He may develop a little flush, because niacin causes the blood vessels in the skin to dilate. He'll stay in the sauna for 20 minutes of sweating, then come out for 10 to dry off, cool down, and take some fluids, supplementing with salt tablets, magnesium, and potassium as needed—basically taking an electrolyte solution to replenish what he lost during the sweating." (Electrolytes are important minerals that the body needs in

order to carry out many of its functions.)

"He'll go in and out of the sauna for anywhere from 3 to 5 hours, always 20 minutes in and 10 minutes out," says Dr. Dahlgren. "Along with sweating, all the fluids he's drinking will increase his urine flow. The niacin and exercise mobilize fat from the periphery, that is, they pull fat out of the adipose tissue and out of the liver and put it into the bloodstream." This is important because many toxins bind to fat.

"We've geared up all of the systems so there's a greater turnover, greater flow to the kidneys and skin, which tends to promote the excretion of unwanted elements from the body," explains Dr. Dahlgren. "Then, after he's finished the sauna baths, we give him vegetable oil—actually five pressed oils derived from nuts—which picks up chemicals that are being excreted by the liver and in bile and tend to be reabsorbed in the intestine. Many toxins in the body are reabsorbed this way. To interfere with that, we give this oil, which pulls the bile salts and the chemicals attached to the bile salts into the vegetable oil so it's excreted in the stool."

How Long Does It Take?

The treatment goes on 7 days a week over a period of 4 to 6 weeks. There are several ways to decide when to stop. The dosage of niacin is gradually increased over time to about 350 milligrams. When flushing from the niacin stops, the therapy has run its course. Another signal: The individual usually feels crummy for the first few days in therapy, but then starts to feel much better. When the person ceases to notice any further improvement, it may be time to stop. Ultimately, however, the supervising physician will make a judgment based on these and other factors.

In the state of California, an appeals

Can Saunas Keep You Sober?

SAUNA THERAPY CAN DO MORE THAN CLEAN POLLUTANTS from your fat cells. According to the folks at Narcanon Arrowhead in Canadien, Oklahoma, it has a special role to play in rehabilitating drug addicts. In fact, they report a 75 percent success rate in keeping people clean and sober by using this protocol in combination with a heavy dose of counseling, as compared to a 10 percent success rate with traditional approaches. They believe that metabolites of cocaine and heroin bind with fat cells and remain there for up to 3 years after a person quits using, and that any stressful situation can cause the fat to release those metabolites into the bloodstream, causing powerful cravings. Sauna therapy speeds up the process and cleans the fat within weeks. Of course, addicts who undergo this treatment also get some side benefits: "Sweat therapy can greatly improve your overall health; the appearance of your skin, hair, and eyes; and the clarity of your mind and emotions," says John Thomas Daily, C.C.D.C., director of drug education and certified drug withdrawal therapist at Narcanon Arrowhead. "You may even find yourself a little smarter. My IQ went up 12 points in 39 days, just by getting all that stuff out of my system." The benefits will cost you: Treatment at Narcanon comes with a hefty $22,000 price tag, but that covers a stay of any length, even 6 months or longer if you need it.

court has ordered that workers' compensation must pay for sauna detoxification if a worker has been injured by toxic exposure, but everywhere else in the country, you'll have to foot the bill. Health insurance generally will not cover it. Dr. Dahlgren's clinic charges $7,500 for the entire treatment, including initial evaluation and final evaluation to determine what changes have occurred.

Who Does It?

According to Dr. Dahlgren, sauna therapy is very safe, but he believes there are benefits to its taking place under medical supervision. "It's a medical treatment," he says. "It causes all kinds of complicated changes in the body, and a doctor will be more able to measure and gauge the benefits you're receiving. But it is a very safe procedure and can be done without a doctor's supervision."

One word of caution: If you try to do this therapy on your own in the sauna at your gym, you're unlikely to be successful. "The temperature of the saunas in health clubs and gyms is usually set too high," explains Dr. Dahlgren. "It's often up to 200°F. You can't stay in there long enough to get enough sweat out. At our clinic, we keep the temperature at 150°F."

ACUPUNCTURE-BASED THERAPIES: ACUPUNCTURE, ACUPRESSURE, SHIATSU, AND REFLEXOLOGY

This family of therapies bases its effectiveness on the traditional Oriental view that stimulating certain points on the surface of the body with either thin-gauge, painless needles or with the fingers, hands, and feet, can affect various organs and systems in the body. The points are located along "meridians," or energy channels that run through the body and along the surface of the skin, according to traditional Oriental medicine precepts.

The differences among the various approaches have mostly to do with the way they're applied. Acupuncture uses small needles, while acupressure uses the fingertips to stimulate various points. Reflexology does the same thing, but it concentrates on points located on the feet. Shiatsu adds massage techniques, such as stretching, rolling, and percussion to trigger point stimulation.

Acupuncture, in particular, can be helpful as a part of a general detoxification program. "Acupuncture has a natural diuretic effect, so it helps eliminate toxins through the urinary tract," says Laila Wah, O.M.D., DIPL. Ac., a Doctor of

Oriental Medicine trained in acupuncture, and founder of Healing Wisdom in Philadelphia. Dr. Wah practices all four therapies—acupuncture, acupressure, shiatsu, and reflexology—on her patients. Acupuncture, in fact, is such a powerful detoxification therapy that it is often used as part of an overall program of drug and alcohol rehabilitation.

Benefits of Acupuncture-Based Therapies

All acupuncture-based therapies strive to help the body reach a state of balance, and it is exactly that feeling of balance and well-being that you should come away with after a successful course of treatment. By improving the functioning of various detoxifying organs such as the liver, kidneys, and lungs, these therapies can also help clear the blood of poisons picked up from the environment.

Dr. Wah lists a host of conditions that can be helped: "Older patients come in with chronic conditions, such as arthritis, osteoporosis, and general aches and pains. Young people come in who have abused their bodies with drugs, alcohol, and sex, which often means their adrenals are blown, they have no energy, and they suffer from nervousness, anxiety, or depression. Another group of people I see have sports injuries. Then

there are those with psychological imbalances such as severe depression and anxiety. These techniques help all of these people. They can also help reduce the negative effects of chemotherapy."

Acupuncture, in particular, is used to help people quit smoking, as well as in the treatment of drug and alcohol problems.

How Is It Done?

The therapist begins by taking a medical history and doing a diagnosis. In making the diagnosis, the therapist considers not just the information that you've provided, but also things like how you look (with particular attention paid to the tongue), how you smell, and how your voice sounds.

After that you'll be asked to lie on a table, either face down or face up. If you're receiving acupuncture treatment, small needles will be placed at various locations on your body. If you're having one of the touch therapies, the therapist will begin either to press specific points on your body connected with various organs, or to knead and pound certain areas with his or her hands. With shiatsu, the therapist may also apply pressure by stepping with his or her bare feet on certain areas of your back.

"If someone comes in and needs detoxification to help purify the blood,"

Do-It-Yourself Shiatsu

A SHIATSU SESSION CAN BE REMARKABLY SOOTHING AND HEALING. You'll finish a session wishing you could do this for yourself. Alas, this is just not possible. There is, however, a milder related therapy that you can do yourself, according to Laila Wah, O.M.D., DIPL. Ac., a Doctor of Oriental Medicine trained in acupuncture and founder of Healing Wisdom in Philadelphia. She suggests a type of self-applied shiatsu called do-in. You perform do-in by kneading the muscles of your arms, legs, and abdomen the way you would knead bread, but always in a clockwise direction. You can also give yourself a reflexology treatment by pressing on the appropriate trigger points on your feet. You'll need to find a book with a chart to show you where they are. To learn more specifically how to do do-in, you can download a free instruction manual in Palm format from www.pilotzone.com/palm/preview/221045.html.

says Dr. Wah, "I work on clearing the back, because nerve endings affecting [the relevant] organs are lined up along the spine in the same way they are lined up in the body."

These techniques can be even more effective when used in combination with any other detoxification techniques you may be using, says Dr. Wah.

How Long Does It Take?

Sessions typically last anywhere from 30 to 60 minutes.

"For detoxification, people usually need to stay in their programs for 6 months or more," says Dr. Wah. "If you want to generally improve your health, then coming in for a tune-up once every few months is appropriate."

Although drug and alcohol treatment centers sometimes offer free programs that use these disciplines, for other kinds of detoxification, you'll have to see a private practitioner. Prices range from $35 to $125 a treatment, depending on what is being done.

Who Does It?

Acupuncture-based therapies are done by practitioners who train in the appropriate techniques. How do you find a good therapist? Start with a recommendation from a friend, or better yet, a referral from a physician. You could also try to find someone online. But do take some time to screen candidates before choosing one.

"It's always best to call and speak to a therapist personally," says Dr. Wah. "You can tell a lot about a person simply by listening to a person's voice and reflecting on how it makes you feel. But you should also ask how long a person has been practicing, and what kind of patients he or she takes care of."

Dr. Wah also recommends asking if the practitioner is licensed or certified, as many, but not all, states now require them to be. You can also get referrals from the National Certification Commission for Acupuncture and Oriental Medicine at www.nccaom.org. The American Organization of Bodywork Therapies of Asia (AOBTA) at www.aobta.org can help you find a shiatsu therapist.

HOLISITIC DENTISTRY

If you think going to a dentist is only about stopping a toothache or turning a crooked-toothed grin into a dazzling Hollywood smile, think again. The condition of your teeth and gums can affect your entire body, and "toxic teeth" can be a source of illness and poor health. Holistic dentists are particularly interested in helping you rid your mouth of any toxins that may be taking a toll on your general health. That includes removing amalgam fillings, which contain toxic mercury, and replacing them with nontoxic gold or composite fillings. Holistic dentists also try to be less invasive in their treatments than other dentists are.

"Dentistry is by nature an invasive science, but a lot of dentistry is optional and there are elective ways to go about it," says Lewis Gross, D.D.S., director of Holistic-Dentists.Com in New York City. "You may want to look for a less-invasive approach than doing your typical root canal, post, and crown. There are always choices."

Benefits of Holistic Dentistry

The health benefits of removing mercury amalgam fillings have been the subject of much controversy. The American Dental Association (ADA) has taken the position that while there does seem to be a direct correlation between the number of fillings a person has and the mercury level in his or her body, no documented proof exists (in the United States) that these levels are causing mischief with anyone's health.

Swedish scientists, who believe they do have proof, would beg to disagree. Based on their research, the World Health Organization named the following risks from mercury given off by amalgam fillings:

⊚ Impairment in kidney function
⊚ Impairment of the immune system
⊚ Neurological disorders
⊚ Problems in fetal development

So while no one may yet be able to give a definitive answer on the subject, holistic dentists would prefer to err on the side of caution. And whatever the health effects of mercury in our bodies, holistic dentistry has made the dental profession generally more aware of its effects on the environment, a benefit we all receive.

"ADA state offices are enacting much stricter protocols for dentists to use amalgam separators, which filter waste water before it goes into the general water system," explains Dr. Gross. "Until recently, they claimed that the mercury dentists were disposing of from their offices didn't pose any danger. Now they're accepting the fact that it's an environmental pollutant, and they're starting to change their opinion about how it should be removed—while still insisting there's no danger to the patient from these removals. They're in a bit of a difficult spot."

Mercury may not be your only worry when it comes to visiting the dentist. "People who are chemically sensitive should be concerned about all dental materials," says Dr. Gross, "as should those who are allergic to metals or who have a history of immune problems. Holistic dentists are going to be more concerned about the biocompatibility between you and the materials they use on your teeth."

Bottom line: You're far less likely to be exposed to things your body finds toxic when you're under the care of a holistic dentist.

You may also be less likely to undergo unpleasant, invasive procedures, such as root canals. "I believe that many root canals are unnecessary," says Dr. Gross. "They're done just because a tooth has a deep filling and the tooth is in pain. I believe a dentist should try to medicate the teeth first. They all know how to do that, so if you have a deep cavity or filling that hurts, rather than just jump into doing a root canal, you may be able to simply medicate the tooth and wait for the nerve to calm down."

If, on the other hand, you have a true abscess, a root canal may be necessary. "What happens is that often the patient will let it go for a very long time and the bacteria get organized in there. They're anaerobic, which means they live without oxygen, and they're virulent. Although they don't grow very quickly, they're tough, tough guys, and our bodies are not very good at eliminating them, so there is concern now that these bugs which can live in root canals and deep pockets in the gums may be a causal factor in heart disease."

How Is It Done?

If you're going to have amalgam fillings removed, you may be asked to take higher than normal doses of antioxidants both before and after your dental appointment, as mercury generates a lot of free radicals. These are harmful molecules that damage the body in many ways. Antioxidants mop them up. According to Dr. Gross, you should increase your intake of dark green vegetables such as parsley, and double your daily dose of vitamins E and C.

The beginning of a session with a holistic dentist will seem pretty much like a visit to any other dentist. But if you're having amalgams removed, you may notice some differences.

"When removing mercury fillings," says Dr. Gross, "we suggest that dentists follow the holistic protocol. They should use a rubber dam, which is a plastic barrier, sort of like a glove. It's essentially the barrier technique—a safe, simple procedure that every dentist is trained in. Because many dentists don't believe mercury is dangerous, however, and also because it's sort of a hassle to do it, many times they won't use a rubber dam. Any patient should feel free to ask his or her dentist to use one. High-speed drills vaporize amalgam, and without a rubber dam to protect you, the mercury will spread all over your mouth."

In the place of the amalgam, a holistic dentist will put in either a white composite filling or a gold filling.

Root canals present another toxicity danger, but not from metals or chemicals. In this case, after you've undergone this procedure, anaerobic bacteria (the kind that live where there is no oxygen) can remain in your tooth. Although the dentist has gone down the main chamber and cleaned it out, the roots of teeth are porous, providing hiding places for nasty, microscopic critters.

"There are thousands of little side tubules," explains Dr. Gross, "and the bacteria can live in them. You may not feel pain, but you know the tooth doesn't feel quite right. It's giving you a dull sensation, or it just doesn't feel like your other teeth. On an x-ray, we may pick up an infection running around the tooth, but it may not hurt that much.

"The problem is that this is a drain on your immune system. And since the tooth is dead, there is no blood supply, so the immune system can't reach the bacteria to kill them—it's like a dead zone. So your body is constantly throwing its immune forces into that tooth but can't reach it."

If the typical dentist sees an infection after a root canal, which often happens, he or she will sometimes recommend cutting the tip of the root off to remove the cyst, which is like a sack of bacteria created by the body to wall off the infection.

"When they cut the cyst off, it does not get rid of the bacteria living throughout the root of the tooth, so it's a short-term solution, and a very invasive and expensive one," says Dr. Gross. "At that point it's probably best to pull the tooth and do something called cavitation, which means cleaning out the socket, very thoroughly, usually by hand with a little spoon called a curette. That's also just normal, good dental technique, but many dentists don't do that—they pull the tooth and leave the ligament behind, or any of the other stuff that's in there after the extraction."

How Long Does It Take?

There is no prescribed course of treatment. Holistic dentists do everything that other dentists do, but they use some different protocols. Consequently some procedures can be done in one visit, while others might take longer.

Prices for holistic dental procedures are comparable to those done by non-holistic dentists, and insurance will cover almost anything you have done, including replacing amalgam fillings. (Make sure you check first, though, as insurance plans differ widely.)

Who Does It?

"Holistic dentistry is not a recognized specialty like orthodontics would be," says Dr. Gross. "Most holistic dentists have had extensive training through continuing education courses, but there is no certification given by any state. There is a Holistic Dentistry Society which most members would be a part of, so you can choose a dentist from a list at the holistic dental association." Such a list can be found at www.holisticdental.org.

THE PURIFICATION PLANS:
Your 3-Part Strategy
for Better Health

THIS SECTION DESCRIBES a three-part strategy that can move you toward your personal health goals.

For most of us, that means beginning with The 7-Day Purification Plan in chapter 11, a general purpose detoxification routine that introduces a variety of healing techniques. From there, paths will diverge into a variety of targeted plans and instant ideas in chapters 12 and 13. There you'll find strategies that are more specific to your individual health concerns. Chapter 14 closes the loop on detoxification by helping you to eliminate the sources of toxicity in your life for healthy, pure living.

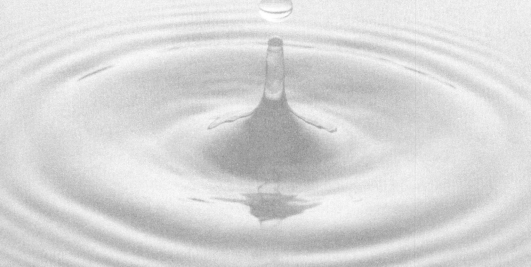

Chapter 11

The 7-Day Purification Plan: A Gentle Yet Powerful Body Cleansing Routine

GET READY TO GIVE YOUR MIND AND BODY a good spring-cleaning, regardless of the season. This simple yet powerfully effective program, developed exclusively for this book in conjunction with Peter Bennett, N.D., a naturopathic physician in Vancouver and coauthor of *7-Day Detox Miracle,* can help you:

◊ Eliminate the poisons that your body has absorbed from air, water, food, and household and personal-care products, as well as "autointoxicants" such as nicotine and white sugar
◊ Lose weight, gain energy, and increase mental clarity and well-being
◊ Relieve or even eliminate conditions caused or aggravated by environmental toxins, including headaches, fatigue, indigestion, constipation, and premenstrual syndrome (PMS)

In a perfect world, you'd devote a week or two each year to the full routine, preferably in the spring and fall, which naturopathic physicians consider key detoxification times. A spring cleansing helps rejuvenate your body after the excesses of the holidays, while cleansing in autumn prepares your body for

When Feeling Ill Is Good

SOME PEOPLE FOLLOWING A CLEANSING ROUTINE may experience a healing crisis, which occurs when toxins are released faster than they can be eliminated.

Don't be alarmed—these symptoms usually mean that your body is responding to the program. But this toxic "dump" can be uncomfortable, as the bowels, kidneys, lungs, sinuses, and skin may be operating in high gear. Symptoms might include headaches, diarrhea, skin rashes, or even vomiting. Other symptoms include bad breath, body aches, sweating, colds, flulike symptoms, and joint pain. (*Caution:* Watery diarrhea can be a danger signal that you could be depleting your body of important minerals. If this happens, you should stop the cleanse. Over the next few weeks, keep eating a healthy diet and take a multivitamin supplement daily. After a few weeks you can start the program again.)

To minimize a healing crisis, try the following:

- Add more protein to your diet (either two poached eggs or 4 ounces of fish or poultry)
- Drink at least 10 glasses of water a day
- Get some form of physical activity for at least 20 minutes a day
- Take cleansing baths
- Sweat by using exercise, baths, and diaphoretic teas, such as yarrow, catnip, chamomile, or blessed thistle during Days 3 through 5

If you do experience the symptoms of a healing crisis, you should begin to feel better by the third day of the program. However, if you have concerns or questions, stop the program and try again another time. You can also consult with your physician.

the rigors of winter, when it battles the viruses that cause colds and flu.

If your schedule won't allow you to devote a full week to the routine, however, simply adapt it to your busy schedule. For example, you can do a weekend "mini-cleanse" anytime you feel stressed or run-down. Feel free to pick and choose from among the meals, techniques, and treatments and create a customized program that meets your needs.

No matter how long you follow the program, get as much rest, sleep, and quiet time as you can while you're cleansing. If you follow the program for more than 3 days, you may experience a few less-than-pleasant symptoms (see "When Feeling Ill Is Good"). But rest assured: They're signs that your body is cleansing itself of toxins.

Follow this program only if you're a healthy, normal-weight or overweight adult. Don't attempt this or any cleansing regimen if you have a serious health condition (such as heart disease, diabetes, cancer, a kidney or digestive disorder, or an autoimmune disease such as lupus or fibromyalgia), are underweight, or if you are pregnant or nursing. Don't be discouraged from undertaking purification if you have any of these conditions. It may still be possible to detoxify, and you could well benefit greatly from doing so.

You just need to do so under medical supervision. Consult your physician for advice on what aspects of purification will be safe for you.

ABOUT THE ROUTINE

This program has five components that will work together to cleanse your mind as well as your body. Here's an overview.

1. Diet. For the next week, you'll enjoy three meals and two snacks a day, each composed largely of fresh fruits and vegetables, whole grains, and plant proteins. Unlike many detoxification diets, which allow only a few bland foods, this program features an appealing and varied vegetarian menu. You'll find a shopping list on page 246.

If you're overweight, you may lose a few pounds by the end of the week, which makes this program a fine way to jump-start a healthier diet. Remember, many toxins are stored in body fat, and when you lose excess body fat, you also reduce your body's toxic burden.

We'll also recommend herbal teas and supplements to help your body purify itself and build your immunity to toxins you can't avoid. For even more herbal options, refer to chapter 5, starting on page 81.

2. Physical activity. Each day, you'll get

(continued on page 244)

Everyday Cleansers

WHILE YOUR MENU AND ACTIVITIES WILL CHANGE EACH DAY, some things will stay the same. Do the following three cleansing techniques each day that you follow the program. You may continue to do the second and third cleansers after you complete the program, if you wish.

1. Take a multivitamin supplement and 1,000 milligrams of vitamin C every morning.
2. Perform alternate nostril breathing, a powerful way to stimulate your circulation and start the day off calm, mentally refreshed, and stress-free. You should do this immediately after waking up, before you've gotten out of bed.

   ⚬ Sit on the side of your bed, holding your spine straight. Gently exhale all the air from your lungs.
   ⚬ Press the thumb of your right hand against your right nostril, closing off the flow of air. Inhale slowly and deeply through your left nostril until your lungs are full.
   ⚬ While your lungs are still full, remove your thumb from your right nostril, press your left nostril closed with your ring finger, and exhale through your right nostril.
   ⚬ Inhale through the right nostril, slowly and deeply. When your lungs are full again, close your right nostril with your thumb, as before, and exhale through your left nostril.

   This completes one round. Begin with 10 rounds and work your way up to 30.

3. Perform the following end-of-the-day gratitude exercise before bed.

   This exercise was created by Steve Mensing, a counselor in private practice in Philadelphia and founder of Emoclear.com.

   Do a breathing exercise. Gently pinch your right nostril shut and breathe for 12 inhalations and exhalations, through your left nostril only.

Remember. Place your right palm on your heartbeat region and think back:

⊚ Recall any acts of love or kindness directed toward you in the previous 72 hours. These acts of love or kindness may have been performed by friends, family, or strangers.

⊚ Recall and feel how you felt at the time. Perhaps it was someone offering you a seat on public transportation, someone allowing you into the flow of traffic, a well-prepared meal, or errands someone ran so you wouldn't have to.

⊚ Notice your feelings and allow appreciation and gratitude to form.

⊚ Recall emotional issues that appeared within the last 72 hours. What valuable messages did they supply? What good things might they have done for you on some level? Notice them and allow your feelings of appreciation and gratitude to form.

⊚ Recall any of the acts of love and kindness or emotional issues that came up within the last few weeks, months, or years. Notice them and allow your feelings of appreciation and gratitude to form.

⊚ Recall the wonderful gadgets and tools in your home. These might be faxes, computers, TVs, food processors, juicers, refrigerators, cars, and other such items. Notice how these things add to the quality of your life and to your enjoyment. Review all of the great chain of people who produced and distributed these gadgets and tools. Then allow yourself to appreciate and feel gratitude toward all those people who brought these gadgets and tools into your home and made life more convenient and enjoyable.

In Sanskrit, the word *smriti* means, "what deserves to be remembered." Gratitude for the gifts you receive each day—and for life itself—is an important part of maintaining a sense of calm, peace, and balance. If you say nightly prayers, chances are you're expressing gratitude. If you are not, doing this brief exercise will allow you to express that gratitude. (You may do this exercise in addition to your nightly prayers, if you wish.)

at least 20 minutes—preferably 40—of gentle activity to stimulate blood circulation and lymphatic fluid. Don't panic; "detoxercise" doesn't require anything more strenuous than a brisk walk, and it can be enhanced through the suggestions on page 251 and on page 127 in chapter 6.

3. Spa treatments. Each day, you'll indulge in a treatment to purify or pamper your body, such as detoxification baths, facials, and other delights. You'll find a list of what you'll need, all of which is available in your kitchen or in health-food stores, on page 246.

4. Emotional cleansing. Every day this week, you'll learn a new "mind game." These games are designed to turn off the negative thoughts that lead to stress, anger, and depression and replace them with positive thinking, which will make you feel more optimistic and in control. The Mind Game exercises are cumulative, so once you learn them, make it a point to do one or two of them at least once a day.

5. Stress control. No detoxification program would be complete without addressing stress, which is just about the most toxic body state there is. We've included simple-yet-effective techniques that can help you learn to soothe yourself in healthy ways, rather than by smoking, abusing alcohol, or overeating. As you learn new stress-reduction techniques, continue to do the ones that seem to work best for you and make it a point to do one or two of them at least once a day.

As you embark on this program, give yourself a pat on the back. You're taking a giant step toward better physical health and a happier, more balanced lifestyle.

DAY 1

Menu

Your detoxifying tea: Drink up to 3 cups or 3 tincture dosages of any one of the following teas, hot or iced: dandelion leaf, buchu, or cleavers. These teas have a diuretic effect, helping the kidneys to eliminate toxins through the urine. *Caution:* Do not drink these teas if you are taking a medication that has a diuretic effect, such as spironolactone. These teas may increase the effect of these drugs and lead to possible cardiovascular side effects. See "Herbal Detox Recipes" on page 254 for preparation details and dosage information.

Breakfast: Breakfast Rice Pudding (see page 52)

Snack 1: Fruit Smoothie (see page 78) or

any of the cleansing beverages in chapter 4 (see page 78)

Lunch: Salad with Sunflower-Seed Dressing (see page 76), baked potato

Snack 2: Rice Protein Shake (see page 79) or any of the cleansing beverages in chapter 4 (see page 78)

Dinner: Eggplant Casserole with Herbed Tomato Sauce (see page 57)

Detoxercise

Take a brisk 20-minute walk, preferably in the morning. In the afternoon or evening, take a second 20-minute walk, or do one of the exercises on page 251 for 20 minutes. Do not work above your ability level, and stop and rest as often as you need to.

Spa Care

Hot Epsom Salts/Lavender-Oil Bath, Followed by Dry Skin Brushing. Epsom salts, or magnesium sulfate, help draw toxins out of the body, including some heavy metals (mercury, lead, and aluminum), car exhaust, solvents, and other toxins. Most people are deficient in magnesium, and many of the body's detoxification pathways are dependent on it. The lavender oil smells heavenly and promotes tranquility. Several studies have shown that lavender has profound stress-reducing benefits.

1 cup Epsom salts
2–3 drops of lavender oil

Fill your tub with the hottest water you can stand (to promote sweating) and add the Epsom salts and oil. Soak for up to 30 minutes. Afterward, take a cool shower to wash toxins from the surface of your skin.

Dry Skin Brushing: In this technique, you brush your whole body with a soft, natural bristle brush (available in health food stores) to stimulate the circulation of blood and lymphatic fluid.

The technique is simple: Using short, brisk strokes, brush each body part in the order below, and always brush toward your heart. Do not wet the brush, and do not allow anyone else to use it. (You wouldn't let someone else use your toothbrush, would you?)

- The fronts and backs of your arms, moving from your fingertips up into your armpits
- Each leg, front and back, starting at your feet and brushing upward
- The bottoms of your feet
- Your buttocks, abdomen, and lower back
- Your chest and upper back
- With a dry washcloth (not a brush): Your face, brushing with downward strokes

Your Shopping List of Detox Benefits

THIS SHOPPING LIST contains everything you'll need for the 7-day menu plan, as well as the spa treatments. (If you plan to follow only a few days of the routine, you won't need everything on this list.) The list also explains the detox benefits of each ingredient. Go ahead and splurge a little on items you have never tried or don't usually use, such as fresh herbs and exotic seasonings.

PRODUCE (organic if possible)

Basil. 1 bunch. Contains monoterpenoids, compounds with antibacterial properties.

Cilantro. 1 bunch. Contains volatile oils found in the leaves, which may have antimicrobial properties.

Mint. 1 bunch

Parsley. 1 bunch. Contains terpenoids, compounds that delay the onset of cancer and reduce the number of cancerous tumors.

Thyme. 1 bunch. Its volatile oil, thymol, has been found to increase the percentage of healthy fats in cell membranes and other cell structures.

Assorted fruits and berries for fruit salads and smoothies—pick your favorites. Fruits' fiber, vitamins, minerals, and plant compounds support liver detoxification.

Broccoli. 1 bunch. Contains isothiocyanates, compounds that stimulate cells to produce detoxification enzymes.

Carrots. 1 bunch. Rich in carotenoid antioxidants that disarm free radicals, which alter cells' DNA in a cancer-promoting fashion.

Celery. 1 bunch. Contains coumarins, compounds that help prevent free radicals from damaging cells, reducing the risk of cells becoming cancerous.

Eggplant. 1 small, 1 medium. Contains nasunin, an antioxidant shown to protect cell membranes from damage.

Garlic. 1 bulb. Rich in the trace mineral manganese, which helps formulate the antioxidant defense enzyme superoxide dismutase.

Green beans. 4 ounces. Good source of the trace mineral copper, needed to produce superoxide dismutase.

Lemons. 2 or 3 small

Mushrooms (optional). 2 medium or

small packages. Contain significant amounts of selenium, which plays an important role in the immune system.

Onions. 1 small bag. Contain quercetin, an antioxidant shown to protect colon cells from certain cancer-causing substances.

Pepper. 1 green, red, yellow, or orange. Rich source of the powerful antioxidants vitamin C and beta-carotene.

Potatoes. 1 small bag. Contains chlorogenic acid, a compound that blocks the action of cancer-causing nitrosamines found in cigarette smoke.

Raisins. 1 container (8 ounces)

Scallions. 1 bunch. Contain allium, a chemical that may lower cholesterol levels and blood pressure and reduce the risk of certain cancers.

Sweet potatoes or yams. 3 medium. Contain phytochelatins, chemicals shown to bind to harmful substances such as copper, cadmium, mercury, and lead.

Swiss chard. 1 bunch. Good source of vitamin C and isothiocyanates.

Tomatoes. 5 medium. Contain lycopene, a nutrient found to protect against a variety of cancers, including those of the stomach, colon, mouth, and esophagus.

Tomatoes, cherry. 1 cup

Zucchini. 5 small. Contain glutathione, a sulfur-containing amino acid that is an important part of the body's antioxidant defense system.

REFRIGERATED/FROZEN FOODS

Broccoli florets. Frozen, 5-ounce bag. Contain B vitamins and vitamin C, both of which help phase one detoxification.

Cheese, blue. 1 tablespoon (optional)

Cheese, Cheddar. Reduced-fat, 8 ounces

Cheese, cottage. Reduced-fat, 8-ounce container

Cheese, Gouda. Smoked, 3 ounces

Eggs. Organic if possible, 1 dozen. Rich in choline, a substance that assists with the removal of fat in the liver.

Milk. Fat-free or soy

Rice milk (optional; for protein shakes)

Shrimp. ½ pound. Excellent source of selenium, used to make glutathione peroxidase, needed for phase one detoxification in the liver.

Sour cream. Fat-free, 8-ounce container

Tofu. 1 package soft, 1 package firm. Good source of the trace mineral zinc, necessary for good immune function.

Yogurt. Fat-free plain, 24 ounces. Yogurt that contains live bacterial cultures helps fortify the immune system.

(continued)

Your Shopping List of Detox Benefits (cont.)

CANNED GOODS

Cannellini beans. Sodium-free, 15-ounce can

Garbanzo beans. Sodium-free, 15-ounce can. Excellent source of the micronutrient molybdenum, which helps the body's immune and energy systems function properly.

Kidney beans. Sodium-free, 8-ounce can. Contains phytic acid, shown to prevent colon cancer in animals.

Tomato puree. 8-ounce can (organic if possible)

Tomato sauce. One 15-ounce can and one 4-ounce can (organic if possible)

Tuna, albacore. 1 can

NUTS AND SEEDS

Almonds. 1 small bag. Good source of trace minerals manganese and copper.

Sunflower seeds. Raw, 1½ cups. Good source of selenium.

Walnuts. 1 small bag. Rich in the compound ellagic acid, which detoxifies potential cancer-causing substances.

GRAINS

Barley. 1 small box. Good source of soluble fiber, which reduces the amount of time cancer-causing substances spend in contact with cells in the colon.

Brown rice. 1 small box. Rich in manganese, selenium, and magnesium. Enzymes that manage detoxification in the cells need them to become active.

Oatmeal. 1 small container. Good source of selenium, a critical component of the body's antioxidant defense system.

OILS AND FATS

Tahini. One 16-ounce jar. 1 tablespoon provides 12 percent of the Daily Value for copper and thiamin, a B vitamin that helps convert food into energy.

Any one or more of the following:

Butter. Organic

Flaxseed oil. High in essential fatty acids, which support liver detoxification.

Olive oil

Sunflower seed oil. High in essential fatty acids.

HERBS, SPICES, AND FLAVORINGS

Apple-cider vinegar

Balsamic vinegar

Basil

Chile-garlic paste

Cinnamon. May help stop growth of bacteria and fungi, including candida yeast.

Cumin. May stimulate the secretion of pancreatic enzymes, necessary for proper digestion and assimilation of nutrients.

Curry

Dill. Contains volatile oils that may help neutralize such carcinogens as the benzopyrenes in cigarette smoke.

Fennel seeds

Ginger. Fresh or dried. Gingerols, its main active components, may inhibit the growth of cancer cells.

Honey

Hot-pepper sauce

Minced onion

Oregano. Contains thymol and rosmarinic acid, plant chemicals that have potent antioxidant properties.

Red pepper

Rice vinegar

Rosemary. Contains substances that stimulate the immune system, increase circulation, and improve digestion.

Sesame oil

Soy sauce. Reduced-sodium

Turmeric. Reverses liver damage caused by toxins; lowers levels of cancer-causing compounds in smokers.

Pure vanilla flavoring

Worcestershire sauce

MISCELLANEOUS

Baking soda

Buffing cream

Chamois skin buffer

Epsom salts

Nail polish formulated without dibutyl phthalate (DBP) (optional; for manicure and/or pedicure)

Nail-polish remover formulated without toluene and formaldehyde (optional; for manicure and/or pedicure)

Paraffin wax (optional; for foot treatment)

AT THE HEALTH FOOD STORE

Almond oil. ½ cup

Aloe vera gel. ¼ cup

Bentonite or green clay. 1 cup

Chamomile tea. ¼ cup

Essential oil of lavender, grapefruit, juniper, and rosemary. 1 small bottle of each

Kelp powder. 2 tablespoons

Lemon balm tea. 1 to 2 teaspoons

Natural-bristle dry skin brush

Passionflower tea. 1 teaspoon

Rice protein powder. 1 container (optional; for rice protein shake)

Sea salt. Approximately 3 cups

Tamari. 1 small jar

Mind Game

A Forgiveness Exercise. A survey conducted by the Institute for Social Research at the University of Michigan found that nearly three-quarters of respondents felt that God had forgiven them for their sins, but that only 52 percent had forgiven someone else. Forgiving those who have wronged you—or forgiving yourself—may help you purge emotional toxins such as sadness and anger, opening the way for purer emotions such as peace and joy. Try this exercise to help yourself feel forgiveness.

Sit in a quiet, comfortable place. Close your eyes and imagine that there is a circle of light around you.

Ask yourself a few questions. "Who have I not forgiven?" Wait for someone's face to appear in your mind's eye. It may be a parent's face, a sibling's, or a friend's; it may even be your own.

Invite this person into your circle. Visualize looking into his or her eyes and complete one or both of the following sentences:

What I learned from you is . . .

You taught me . . .

When you've finished, thank that person. If you wish, you may repeat the exercise, continuing to thank him or her until you feel at peace. Then say:

I forgive you.

I release you.

Go in peace.

Say goodbye. And with love, watch him or her leave your circle and disappear. Repeat this exercise as often as you need to with as many people as you need to.

Stress-Reduction Technique

Soak in a Sound Bath. To take a "sound bath," put some relaxing music on your stereo and lie in a comfortable position on a couch or on the floor near the speakers. (Some people lie down in front of or even between their speakers.) For a deeper experience, you can wear headphones to focus your attention and to avoid distraction.

As the music plays, allow it to wash over you, rinsing off the day's stress. Focus on your breathing, letting it deepen, slow, and become regular.

You can "bathe" to any music you find soothing, including light classical music such as Beethoven's *Spring Sonata for Violin, Opus 24*, Schubert's *Ave Maria*, or Gregorian chants. Other options include *Sounds of Light: The Pure Tones of Crystal Singing Bowls* by Crystal Voices and Deborah Van Dyke; *Golden Portal* by Xumantra; *Seapeace* by Georgia Kelly; and *Spectrum Suite, Inner Peace,* and *Comfort Zone* by Steven Halpern, Ph.D.

Detoxercise Options

MODERATE DAILY EXERCISE is a critical part of the detoxification process because it stimulates the circulation of blood and lymphatic fluid. This improves the body's ability to eliminate its cellular waste products as well as man-made chemicals and pollutants. Exercise also helps burn fat, which is where many of the body's toxins are stored, and it promotes deeper, more restful sleep.

The 7-Day Body Cleansing Program includes 40 minutes of gentle exercise each day. If you already have an exercise routine, you may follow it for the duration of the Body Cleansing Program. If you don't, you'll break your physical activity into two 20-minute sessions, morning and afternoon or early evening. In the morning, take a brisk 20-minute walk, outdoors if possible. (If you have a treadmill, you may use it during cold or inclement weather.) In the afternoon or early evening, take another 20-minute walk or do 20 minutes of one of the exercises below:

- Ballroom dancing
- Bicycling (outdoors or on a stationary bicycle)
- Jumping rope
- Step aerobics (class or video)
- Strength training
- Swimming
- Yoga

If you are overweight or have back, hip, or knee pain, you should perform a low-impact exercise, such as swimming or walking.

If you're in good shape, jumping rope is an excellent workout because it encourages the circulation of lymph. Do as many skips as you can, trying to add 10 skips each day. Rest or catch your breath as often as you need to.

If you are already a regular exerciser, make sure that you're working at a moderate level of intensity—enough to work up a good sweat, but not so much that you abuse your joints. Exercising too long or too hard can deplete the immune system.

If you'd rather listen to the sounds of nature—ocean waves or the calm rustlings and twitterings of a deep forest, for instance—that's fine, too. You can buy tapes of these sounds in many music stores. If you have a tape recorder and live near a babbling brook, a waterfall, the ocean, or the woods, take a walk and make your own tape.

DAY 2

Menu

Your detoxifying tea: Drink up to 4 cups of the same teas you enjoyed on Day 1. (See caution in Day 1 on page 244.)

Breakfast: Fresh Fruit Salad with Almonds (see page 68)

Snack 1: Fruit Smoothie (see page 78) or any of the cleansing beverages in chapter 4 (see page 78)

Lunch: Salad with Tomato-Dill Dressing (see page 77), Minestrone Soup (see page 71)

Snack 2: Rice Protein Shake (see page 79) or any of the cleansing beverages in chapter 4 (see page 78)

Dinner: Very Veggie Omelet (see page 62)

Detoxercise

Take a brisk 20-minute walk, preferably in the morning. In the afternoon or evening, take another 20-minute walk, or do one of the exercises on page 251. Do not work above your ability level, and stop and rest as often as you need to.

Spa Care

Sea Salt and Baking Soda Bath, Followed by Sea Salt Body Scrub. Along with sea salt, baking soda helps relax the body and may also eliminate trace toxins that your body has been exposed to in your workplace.

1 cup baking soda
1 cup sea salt
1 or 2 drops essential oil of your choice

Fill your tub with the hottest water you can stand (to promote sweating) and add the baking soda, sea salt, and oil. Soak for up to 30 minutes. Afterward, take a cool shower to wash toxins from the surface of your skin.

Enjoy this fragrant scrub after you've completed today's hydrotherapy treatment.

1 cup fine sea salt
½ cup almond oil
10 drops each grapefruit and juniper essential oils

Combine all the ingredients in a small bowl and blend thoroughly. Standing in the bathtub, spread the mixture onto your damp skin and massage into your skin with gentle circular motions. Shower off the mixture, using water as cold as you can stand.

Mind Game

Autogenic Training. Autogenics, which means "self-generation," was developed in the 1930s by Johannes Schultz, M.D., a neurologist and psychiatrist from Germany. Dr. Schultz, who compared the feelings generated by autogenics to taking a relaxing bath, wanted people to be able to generate deep relaxation in a practical way. Proponents of autogenic training believe that it stimulates blood-flow and deep relaxation. In essence, the idea is to get comfortable and give your body a series of instructions.

To begin, sit or lie in a comfortable position. Close your eyes and take a few deep breaths. As you exhale, repeat the following instructions to yourself:

> *"My hands and arms are warm and heavy." (5 times)*
> *"My feet and legs are warm and heavy." (5 times)*
> *"My abdomen is calm and comfortable." (5 times)*
> *"My breathing is deep and even." (10 times)*
> *"My heartbeat is regular." (10 times)*
> *"My forehead is cool." (5 times)*

> *"When I open my eyes, I will remain relaxed and refreshed." (3 times)*

Take a moment to move your hands, arms, legs, and feet around a bit. Rotate your head, open your eyes, and if you're lying down, sit up.

While doing this exercise, note what is happening to your body, but don't consciously try to analyze it. If your mind wanders, simply bring it back to your instructions.

Do the exercise for 2 minutes at least once a day.

Stress-Reduction Technique

Shavasana Yoga Pose. The Shavasana Pose is also known as the Corpse Pose, because you're simply lying on your back with your eyes closed. In reality, however, you'll emerge from this pose (which takes only 5 minutes) feeling more refreshed and alive. Do Shavasana twice a day all week—once after you perform your daily Detoxercise, and again right before bed.

Lie on your bed on your back, and spread your feet about 18 inches apart. Place your hands, palms up, about 6 inches from your sides. Ease yourself into the pose, making sure your body is symmetrical. Let your thighs, knees, and toes relax and turn gently outward.

(continued on page 256)

Herbal Detox Recipes

DOUGLAS SCHAR, DIP.PHYT., MCPP, MNIMH, a European-trained clinical herbalist based in Washington, D.C., recommends the following dosages for the herbs recommended in this cleansing routine. You'll find dosages for two forms: dried herbs and tinctures. You should be able to purchase most of these herbs in tea-bag form from a health food store and follow the dosage instructions on the label, says Schar. The doses provided assume that you are taking only one of these herbs at a time, so do not take all of these herbs at once using the faulty assumption that more is better. You'll find more information on herbal detox, including a discussion of choosing between tinctures and teas, in chapter 5 on page 81.

Note: Consult with your health care practitioner before adding herbal remedies to your health care regimen.

Blessed thistle *(Cnicus benedictus)*
Dosage: Three doses per day.

Tea Preparation: Boil ½ to 1½ teaspoons in 1 cup of water for 10 minutes. Strain and drink.

Tincture: Take ¼ to ½ teaspoon of tincture 1:1.

Buchu *(Barosma betulina)*
Dosage: Three doses per day.

Tea Preparation: Boil 1 teaspoon in 1 cup of water for 10 minutes. Strain and drink.

Tincture: Take ½ teaspoon of tincture 1:5.

Catnip *(Nepeta cataria)*
Dosage: Three doses per day.

Tea Preparation: Boil 1 to 2 teaspoons in 1 cup of water for 10 minutes. Strain and drink.

Tincture: Take ½ to 1 teaspoon of tincture 1:1.

Chamomile *(Matricaria recutita)*
Dosage: Three doses per day.

Tea Preparation: Boil 1 to 4 teaspoons in 1 cup of water for 10 minutes. Strain and drink.

Tincture: Take ¼ to 1 teaspoon of tincture 1:1.

Cleavers (Galium aparine)

Dosage: Three doses per day.

Tea Preparation: Boil 1 to 2 teaspoons in 1 cup of water for 10 minutes. Strain and drink.

Tincture: Take ½ to 1 teaspoon of tincture 1:1.

Dandelion leaf (Taraxacum officinalis)

Dosage: Three doses per day.

Tea Preparation: Boil 1 tablespoon dried dandelion leaf in 1 cup of water for 10 minutes. Strain and drink.

Tincture: Take 1 teaspoon of tincture 1:5 diluted in water, juice, or tea.

Lemon balm (Melissa officinalis)

Dosage: Three doses per day.

Tea Preparation: Boil 1 to 2 teaspoons in 1 cup of water for 10 minutes. Strain and drink.

Tincture: Take ½ to 1 teaspoon of tincture 1:1.

Passionflower (Passiflora incarnata)

Dosage: Three doses per day.

Tea Preparation: Boil 1 teaspoon in 1 cup of water for 10 minutes. Strain and drink.

Tincture: Take ½ teaspoon of tincture 1:5.

Uva ursi (Arctostaphyllos uva-ursi)

Dosage: Three doses per day.

Tea Preparation: Boil 1 teaspoon in 1 cup of water for 10 minutes. Strain and drink.

Tincture: Take 1 teaspoon of tincture 1:5.

Yarrow (Achillea millefolium)

Dosage: Three doses per day.

Tea Preparation: Boil 1 to 2 teaspoons in 1 cup of water for 10 minutes. Strain and drink.

Tincture: Take ½ to 1 teaspoon of tincture 1:1.

Close your eyes and breathe deeply and slowly from your abdomen. Feel your weight pulling you deeper into relaxation. Sink deeper with each exhalation, allowing your hands, feet, abdomen, throat, and eyes to get heavier and heavier. Repeat for 50 deep, relaxing, cleansing breaths.

DAY 3

Menu

Your detoxifying tea: Drink up to 3 cups of any one of the following teas: yarrow, catnip, chamomile, or blessed thistle. These herbs are diaphoretic, meaning that they increase elimination of toxins through sweating. See "Herbal Detox Recipes" on page 254 for preparation details and dosage information.

Breakfast: Fruit Melba Breakfast "Sundae" (see page 52)

Snack 1: Fresh Fruit Salad with Almonds (see page 68)

Lunch: Salad with Tahini Dressing (see page 76); rice or baked potato

Snack 2: Minestrone Soup (see page 71) or any of the cleansing beverages in chapter 4 (see page 78)

Dinner: Mexican Red Rice and Beans (see page 59; save the remaining serving for tomorrow's lunch)

Detoxercise

Take a brisk 20-minute walk, preferably in the morning. In the afternoon or evening, take another 20-minute walk, or do one of the exercises on page 251. Do not work above your ability level, and stop and rest as often as you need to.

Spa Care

A 30-Minute Facial.

Step 1: Cleanse Gently but Thoroughly

In a blender, combine ½ cup of oatmeal, ¾ cup of hot water, and 1 tablespoon of olive oil. Let the mixture sit until the oatmeal has absorbed much of the water.

In the meantime, apply a warm, damp washcloth to your face; the warmth will open your pores. Keep the washcloth on your face until it cools, then repeat the process. (Do not scrub your face with the cloth.)

Apply the cleanser, and gently rub it into your skin, making small circles with your fingertips. Rinse well with lukewarm water for at least 30 seconds. Pat your face dry with a clean, dry towel or washcloth.

Step 2: Apply an Herbal Compress

Mix 5 to 10 drops of lavender oil with 1 teaspoon of vinegar. Add this mixture to a quart of cool or lukewarm water. Place another clean washcloth in the warm water, wring it out, and apply the cloth to your face. Hold the washcloth to your face for 5 to 10 seconds, rinse the cloth, and repeat the process. Repeat three more times. Pat your face dry with a clean, dry towel or washcloth.

Step 3: Steam Away Impurities

Bring a large pot of water to a boil. Place 3 tablespoons of dried chamomile or rosemary in an old stocking or cheesecloth. Remove the boiling water from the burner and add the herbs. Let them steep for 10 minutes. Pour the hot water into a large bowl on a nonslip surface.

Lean over the bowl and drape a towel over your head so that the steam from the water hits your face. (Be careful! Keep your face at least 12 inches away from the top of the pot.) Steam for 10 minutes, being careful not to scald your skin. *Note:* If you have blemished or sensitive skin, steam for only 5 minutes.

Step 4: Slip Into a Seaweed Detoxifying Mask

Mix 2 tablespoons of kelp powder (available at health food stores) and ¼ cup of aloe vera gel in a small bowl. Add water until the mixture is thick and smooth. Apply to your face. Relax for 10 to 20 minutes. Rinse.

Step 5: Tone and Rebalance Your Skin

Mix 2 tablespoons of apple cider vinegar in 1 cup of water (preferably dis-

tilled water). Apply to your face with cotton balls, avoiding your eyes.

Step 6: Replenish Moisture

Apply a very thin coating of olive, sunflower, or flax oil to your skin. If you have oily or acne-prone skin, you can skip this step.

Mind Game

Anger Detoxification Game. This comical exercise is a lesson in deflating the power of anger. Try it today (even if you're not angry), and see if it doesn't help the next time your blood is boiling.

Thinking aloud, describe a situation in your life that makes you angry—really angry. It can be a situation from the past or present. As you speak, consciously try to make yourself as angry as you can—really whip yourself into a frenzy about it.

Stop! Think about whether this situation is worthy of such anger. Do you really need this kind of toxic emotion in your heart, threatening your physical and mental well-being?

Now, "talk" about the same problem, using only the words "blah, blah, blah." Think the anger words, but say only "blah." Chances are, you'll start to chuckle. Right now, you have just relieved yourself of a small part of the toxic burden anger places on you.

Stress-Reduction Technique

Calming Visualizations. In visualization, which is also called guided imagery, you create relaxing images to calm your mind and body. By controlling your breathing and visualizing a soothing image, you can enter a state of deep relaxation.

Read through the following visualization once or twice before you begin this exercise. It's not important that you follow the images to the letter, just that you understand the basic premise. Let your imagination soar and create the most soothing scenario for you.

Either sit or lie in a comfortable position and close your eyes. Now, see yourself sailing high in the sky in a large, translucent bubble. You are floating above an expanse of breathtakingly beautiful countryside. Peer out from your bubble and take in your surroundings. What do you see? A perfect little farmhouse next to a waving field of corn? A patch of pine trees surrounding a crystal-clear lake? Whatever you see, try to create as vivid a "mind picture" as you can.

Now, "land" your bubble. Step out and begin to walk. Soon, you come to a beautiful rushing waterfall. At the bottom of the waterfall, there is a deep pool of water. Step into the water. Stay there for a while and feel all of the stress in your body leave.

Allow yourself to relax. Spend some time in this tranquility. Feel the sun warming your head, enjoy the cool water, hear the soothing rush of water. When you are ready, step out of the water, walk back to your bubble, step in, and sail off again into the sky, calm and refreshed.

DAY 4

Menu

Your detoxifying tea: Drink up to 3 cups of the same teas you enjoyed on Day 3.

Breakfast: Berry Morning Crush (see page 51)

Snack 1: Raw vegetables with Garlic-Herb Dip (see page 70) or Fruit Smoothie (see page 78) or any of the cleansing beverages in chapter 4 (starting on page 78)

Lunch: Mexican Red Rice and Beans (see page 59)

Snack 2: Rice Protein Shake (see page 79) or any of the cleansing beverages in chapter 4 (see page 78)

Dinner: Moroccan Carrot Salad with Toasted Cumin (see page 72)

Detoxercise

Take a brisk 20-minute walk, preferably in the morning. In the afternoon or evening, take another 20-minute walk, or do one of the exercises on page 251. Do not work above your ability level, and stop and rest as often as you need to.

Spa Care

Hand Massage Followed by Manicure. While the ritziest spas worldwide offer hand massages, it's just as easy to give yourself one using a detoxifying essential oil, such as lavender or rosemary. And it's so simple that it's easy to overlook how soothing it can be.

Hand Massage

⚬ Place 5 drops of lavender essential oil into the palm of one hand. If using rosemary essential oil, combine 10 drops of the oil with 1 teaspoon of almond oil and place in the palm of one hand. Rub your palms together until you feel heat.

⚬ Squeeze the fleshy part of your right hand between your left thumb and forefinger, with your thumb on the top side, for 10 seconds.

⚬ Massage your entire right palm with your left thumb. Start from the outside of your palm, working in a circular motion to the inside. For deeper treatment, search out sore spots, press with the thumb, and hold for 10 seconds.

⚬ Massage your left hand in the same way.

Manicure

Note: Before you begin, sterilize your file with rubbing alcohol to avoid transferring bacteria from a previous manicure to your nails.

1. **Remove old nail polish.** Using an emery board, file your nails. To prevent splitting, draw your file back and forth or in one direction only underneath each nail at a 45-degree angle.

2. **Soak your cuticles** in lukewarm to warm soapy water for 5 minutes to soften them.

3. **Use an orange wood stick** (available in drugstores) to push back your cuticles. Be sure not to cut your cuticles, which can cause infection and damage your nails.

4. **Apply a small amount of buffing cream** to your nails and buff in one direction across each nail, using a natural chamois skin buffer. Rinse and dry your nails.

If you use polish:

5. **Apply a base coat,** which keeps your nails from discoloring and allows colored polish to go on more smoothly. In three careful strokes, starting at the base of each nail, apply up the middle of the nail, down the left side of the nail, and down the right side.

6. **Allow the base coat to dry** for at least 15 minutes. Then apply the first coat of color polish, using the same three-stroke method above. Wait 5 minutes, then apply a second coat.
7. **Apply a protective topcoat** and let it dry.

Note: To keep this spa treatment toxin-free, select nail polish removers formulated without the toxic chemicals toluene and formaldehyde. Also, avoid nail polish that contains the chemical dibutyl phthalate (DBP).

The following nail polishes are phthalate-free: L'Oreal Jet Set Nail Enamel, L'Oreal Jet Set Quick Dry Nail Enamel, Maybelline Shades of Your Nail Color, Naturistics 90 Second Dry! Super Fast Nail Color, Revlon Nail Enamel, and Revlon Super Top Speed.

Mind Game

Surrender to Tranquility. To purify yourself of toxic emotions, you need to learn to let them go. This simple but powerful exercise, which uses one blank sheet of standard-size paper, can help you do just that.

Think of a problem, big or small, that has been eating at you. Write it on the paper. Really focus on its negativity; state exactly how it's causing anxiety in your life and disturbing your tranquility. Feel free to write as much as you wish.

1. Now, fashion your paper into a paper airplane. Count to three, and as you reach three, sail your airplane—and your worry—into the air with a cheer or a whoop. If you don't know how to make a paper airplane, then place the paper in a deep bowl and light it on fire. As you watch it burn, cheer or whoop.
2. Close your eyes and give a soft sigh of satisfaction. Repeat the sigh three times, increasing the volume until your whole body gets into the act.

Stress-Reduction Technique

Circle Breathing. Circle breathing is a systematic way to relax and calm the mind and body. This exercise was created by Joan Borysenko, Ph.D., a scientist, psychologist, inspirational speaker, and author of *Inner Peace for Busy Women* and *Inner Peace for Busy People.*

Make the choice. Whenever you feel stressed, remember that you have a choice: to practice stress or to practice peace. Then take 5 to 10 "circle breaths." Try to perform this centering exercise at least five times today.

Begin your breaths. Inhale and stretch your arms over your head, then give a sigh of relief and lower your arms as you exhale.

Bring in the peace. Now imagine that you're inhaling a stream of peaceful energy into a spot just below your navel.

Move it on up. Inhale the warm stream into the base of your spine, then imagine it traveling up your back to the top of your head.

Complete the circle. Now exhale, and mentally follow your "out" breath down the front of your body to the point below your navel where you'll begin your next "in" breath. Your breath has now made a full circle up the back of your body, down the front, and back to the starting place below your navel.

Maintain a gentle focus. Continue this breathing pattern for 5 to 10 breaths.

DAY 5

Menu

Your detoxifying tea: Drink up to 3 cups of the following teas: lemon balm, chamomile, or passionflower. These teas have a sedative effect, helping to promote calmness and tranquility. See "Herbal Detox Recipes" on page 254 for preparation details and dosage information.

Breakfast: Very Veggie Omelet (see page 62)

Snack 1: Fruit Smoothie (see page 78) or any of the cleansing beverages in chapter 4 (see page 78)

Lunch: Barley Salad with Smoked Cheese (see page 65; save the remaining serving for tomorrow's lunch)

Snack 2: Rice Protein Shake (see page 79) or any of the cleansing beverages in chapter 4 (see page 78)

Dinner: Roasted Vegetable Salad with Balsamic and Basil Vinaigrette (see page 73)

Detoxercise

Take a brisk 20-minute walk, preferably in the morning. In the afternoon or evening, take a second 20-minute walk, or do one of the exercises on page 251 for 20 minutes. Do not work above your ability level, and stop and rest as often as you need to.

Spa Care

Soothing Scalp Massage, Followed by Yogurt Hair Mask. This simple treatment both melts away tension and improves the health and appearance of your hair by bringing fresh blood and nutrients to your hair follicles. Sitting in a comfortable chair, gently massage your scalp for 10 minutes, spreading your fingers wide and moving your fingertips in a circular motion across your entire scalp. Follow with the Yogurt Hair Mask, which is recommended for all hair types and which will restore life and sheen to damaged locks.

1 whole egg plus 1 egg yolk
8 ounces whole-milk plain yogurt

Put a clean towel in the dryer for 10 minutes. Beat together the egg and yogurt. Coat freshly shampooed hair with the mixture, and pile your hair on top of your head. Wrap your hair in the warm towel. Ease into a steamy bath and relax. After 20 minutes, drain the tub, remove the towel, and take a cool shower to rinse the mixture out of your hair. It's important to use cool water because water that's too hot will cook the egg and make it difficult to remove.

Mind Game

Think Yourself Tranquil. Virtually every second that you're conscious, you are listening to a silent interior dialogue with yourself. This internal chatter provides a running commentary about your life, feelings, and problems, as well as the world itself. It also has a powerful effect on your feelings, beliefs, and attitudes, and reinforces how you see yourself.

Affirmations are positive, powerful statements used to boost self-esteem and confidence. As you repeat the affirma-tions over and over, your subconscious mind comes to believe them and replaces that negative interior dialogue with a more positive one. Emil Coue, a French psychotherapist who practiced in the early 20th century, created perhaps the most famous affirmation: "Every day, in every way, I am getting better and better."

Affirmations are worded in a positive rather than negative way, and they are grounded in the present rather than the future.

Try to come up with five affirmations that will replace the negative inner dialogue in your head. Here are some examples to get you started.

My good thoughts and good actions pro-
duce good results.
I am blessed with right thoughts and
good actions.
I let go of the past.
I say yes to life.

Stress-Reduction Technique

Write Your Heart Out. Keeping a diary, or journaling, is a time-honored way to release your most private thoughts and feelings. While it might seem time-consuming, setting aside just 10 to 15 minutes to put your thoughts into words may help soothe your stress and its physical symptoms. As a bonus, writing about your feelings can help you increase your self-knowledge, nurture your spirituality, and tap into your unconscious mind.

Block out 10 to 15 minutes and just write whatever comes into your head. Do not write at the computer. Your feelings will flow more naturally when you use a pen or pencil and a pad of paper.

This exercise may inspire you to keep a personal journal. If you do, remember that there's no rule about how much or how often to write. Just one paragraph a day is fine, and you don't have to write a detailed report of your day. You might want to focus on one particular person, event, or problem and write about that.

DAY 6

Menu

Your detoxifying tea: Drink up to 3 cups of the same teas you enjoyed on Day 5.

Breakfast: Select any of the breakfasts from Days 1 through 5.

Snack 1: Fruit Smoothie (see page 78) or any of the cleansing beverages in chapter 4 (see page 78)

Lunch: Barley Salad with Smoked Cheese (see page 65)

Snack 2: Rice Protein Shake (see page 79) or any of the cleansing beverages in chapter 4 (see page 78)

Dinner: Indian-Spiced Potatoes and Spinach (see page 67; save one potato for tomorrow's lunch)

Detoxercise

Take a brisk 20-minute walk, preferably in the morning. In the afternoon or evening, take a second 20-minute walk, or do one of the exercises on page 251 for 20 minutes. Do not work above your ability level, and stop and rest as often as you need to.

Spa Care

Paraffin Foot Dip and Pedicure. Your feet work hard for you—now's their time to get the royal treatment. This three-step treatment will leave your feet looking and feeling soft and silky smooth.

Paraffin Foot Dip (optional)

Melt paraffin wax (available at any supermarket) in an old pot or saucepan that you will use just for this purpose. Massage 1 tablespoon of olive oil into each foot. When the wax is slightly cool to the touch, dip each foot into the wax four or five times. Wrap each foot in a plastic bag. Relax for about 15 minutes.

The paraffin will harden into a waxy

foot "mask." Remove the plastic bags, then peel off the wax. Your feet will be silky-smooth for about 2 weeks.

Pedicure

1. **Remove old polish.** Add a few drops of your favorite essential oil to warm water and soak your feet for 10 minutes. When you're done soaking, rinse your feet with cold water, dry them, and buff away calluses and dead skin with a pumice stone or foot file.

2. **Trim your nails** straight across using a straight-edged clipper. Using an emery board, file your nails. To prevent splitting, draw your file back and forth or in one direction only underneath each nail at a 45-degree angle.

3. **Soak your cuticles** in lukewarm to warm soapy water for 5 minutes to soften them.

4. **Use an orange wood stick** (available in drugstores) to push back your cuticles. Be sure not to cut your cuticles, which can cause infection and damage your nails.

If you apply polish:

5. **Twist a tissue** and weave it between your toes to keep them separate. Then apply polish, as in Steps 5 through 7 of the Manicure (see page 259). Let the polish dry for at least 30 minutes. For a more professional finish, dip a thin eye shadow or paintbrush into some polish remover and whisk it around the edge of the nail near the cuticle for a nice, clean edge.

If you don't use polish:

6. **Apply a liberal dollop** of a thick moisturizing cream. Then slip on a pair of big, fluffy socks to retain the moisture.

Mind Game

Giving Negative Thoughts a Makeover. If you believe in the power of positive thinking, then you'll probably benefit from this exercise in the power of rational thinking. Rational beliefs make sense—they're objective and based in reality. By contrast, irrational beliefs like "I am stupid and worthless," or "If I don't do what others want, they will be angry" fall apart when you stop to analyze them.

That's the goal of rational-emotive behavior therapy (REBT), which maintains that to a large extent we don't get upset by things or events, but by the view we take of them. When we give ourselves a "thought makeover"—that is, we replace irrational, self-defeating beliefs with rational ones—we are happier and more productive.

The following exercise can help sharpen

your ability to ferret out the irrational beliefs that may be causing you worry and stress and replace them with rational beliefs. You'll be amazed at how much stress relief is packed into this simple technique.

Pick your topic. On a piece of paper, write down a description of an event that provoked a specific negative emotion, such as fear or depression.

Describe your negative feeling. In one sentence, write down your number one anxious thought about this event.

Balance it out. In one sentence, write down a short, clear, and rational statement to counter the negative thought above.

Let's say that the anxiety-provoking event is that recently your boss called you into his office and told you that he was disappointed in your work on a certain project. Your number one anxious thought might be, "I'm afraid I'll get fired and never find another job." Your "thought makeover" might be, "I've always received good or excellent performance evaluations, and just last week my boss praised that report I turned in."

Stress-Reduction Technique

Lose Your Mind. Like our bodies, our minds are constantly going, going, going. We are either planning the future or lamenting the past. The solution? Being "mindful," which is to have a heightened awareness of the present. Mindfulness may not only diminish stress, anxiety, and depression, but may also transform a person's actual approach to life itself.

Mindfulness-based stress reduction (MBSR) is a meditation technique with proven benefits in the reduction of stress symptoms. Developed in 1979 by Jon Kabat-Zinn, Ph.D., and colleagues at the University of Massachusetts Stress Reduction Clinic, formal practice of MBSR involves true meditation. But informally, you can practice mindfulness in the most ordinary activities, even brushing your teeth or washing the dishes. The exercise below can help you experience mindfulness. To do this exercise, you'll need an orange.

Take a few deep breaths and relax your body. Now, tune everything out but this orange in your hand. Turn it this way and that, absorbing its orangeness. Examine its texture and shape, notice how it feels in your hand. Smell it. Don't make a judgment about this orange; simply see it. Let go of any ideas of how this exercise will help you; just be accepting and aware of each passing moment. Take a moment to appreciate where the orange came from. Notice the wonderful smell as you begin to peel it. Now eat the orange slowly, noting the taste and texture of every bite. Follow each bite with your attention as you slowly chew and swallow it. Now, take this nonjudgmental, accepting, observant attitude into your daily life.

DAY 7

Menu

Your detoxifying tea: Drink up to 3 cups of the same teas you enjoyed on Day 5.

Breakfast: Select any of the breakfasts from Days 1 through 5.

Snack 1: Fruit Smoothie (see page 78) or any of the cleansing beverages in chapter 4 (see page 78)

Lunch: Indian-Spiced Potatoes and Spinach (see page 67)

Snack 2: Rice Protein Shake (see page 79) or any of the cleansing beverages in chapter 4 (see page 78)

Dinner: Barley with Ginger and Broccoli (see page 54)

Detoxercise

Take a brisk 20-minute walk, preferably in the morning. In the afternoon or evening, take a second 20-minute walk, or do one of the exercises on page 251 for 20 minutes. Do not work above your ability level, and stop and rest as often as you need to.

Spa Care

The Scented Clay Body Wrap. A body wrap is a triple delight: It eliminates toxins, it calms your mind, and it revitalizes your skin. This treatment is thought to have originated in ancient Egypt, where the rich slathered their skin in scented mud, then wrapped up in soft cloth to beautify their skin and prevent illness. Today, virtually every high-priced spa offers wraps featuring detoxifying ingredients such as muds, seaweeds, and herbs.

A do-it-yourself body wrap requires only a few simple tools: an old cotton sheet to wrap yourself in, three towels, a pillow or cushion for your neck, and an inexpensive foil thermal blanket to keep you warm. Drink lots of water before and after your wrap to help flush out toxins.

2 cups water

¼ cup sea salt

1 cup bentonite or green clay (available at health food stores)

2 tablespoons olive oil

1 tablespoon essential oil

Begin by preparing the sheet. Heat a large pot of water on the stove until it's comfortably hot, but not boiling. Add the cotton sheet, stir until entirely saturated, wring it out, and place it in a plastic bag. Set it aside.

Then make the clay wrap. Boil the water in a large saucepan, add the sea salt, and stir until the salt is fully dissolved. Add the clay, olive oil, and essential oil, and stir again. Add more water if you need to so that the mixture has the consistency of a wet paste.

Now it's time to swaddle yourself in your soothing, scented cocoon. Head to the bathroom with the sheet (still warm in the plastic bag), three towels, pillow, and thermal blanket.

Take a warm shower to open your pores and fill the air with steam. Towel off slightly and wrap your hair in a towel. Place a dry towel on the bottom of the tub. Standing on an old towel, apply the clay mixture to your still-damp skin (excluding your face). Wrap yourself from ankles to chin in the warm, damp cotton sheet. Climb into the tub and lie on the towel, arranging the pillow to support your head and neck. Cover yourself with the thermal blanket.

Allow the clay to stay on your skin for 15 minutes or until the sheet cools. Unwrap and rinse in lukewarm water. When you're dry, follow with a dry skin brushing (see page 245).

Mind Game

Review of the Week's Techniques. Pick one or two of the Mind Games that you found to be most effective for you. Was it the Forgiveness Exercise? The Anger Detoxification Game? Disposing of your worries on the wings of a paper airplane? Practice these mind games again for a few minutes off and on throughout the day, with the goal of integrating them into your everyday life after you complete the program.

Stress-Reduction Technique

20-Minute Nature Walk. Bringing more nature into your life can reduce your stress and lift your spirits, according to proponents of biophilia, the term popularized by Harvard biologist Edward O. Wilson, Ph.D. According to Dr. Wilson, contact with the natural world may benefit health.

Exposure to nature has been shown to decrease heart rate, blood pressure, and other indicators of stress. Studies suggest that people who are exposed to nature, even through a hospital window, are likely to heal faster and require fewer pain relievers. In 2001, researchers at Johns Hopkins University used the sound of a gurgling brook and a mural of a mountain stream in a spring meadow to reduce the pain of patients enduring an uncomfortable lung procedure called a bronchoscopy.

This technique is short and sweet, but powerfully effective: Dress for the weather, then walk or drive to an area full of natural beauty, such as a park, a hiking trail, a lake, or a mountain path. As you walk, be aware of the sights, sounds, and even smells of the natural world around you. How many different birds, or bird calls, can you distinguish? Stoop and watch an anthill for a while. Marvel at the dozens of species of plants and wildflowers you see. Appreciate the beauty of the sun filtering through leaves, the muffled silence of snow, or the sound of rain. Chances are, you'll return home feeling more tranquil and grounded than when you left.

Chapter 12

Targeted Purification Plans: Detox Strategies for Specific Conditions

TOXICITY AFFECTS US IN LITERALLY HUNDREDS, IF NOT THOUSANDS, OF WAYS. Even though some detox remedies—the use of milk thistle to neutralize toxins and regenerate liver cells, for example—are used across the board to address a number of health concerns, many others are best used in a tailored approach to specific symptoms and conditions.

Are you tired and stressed all the time? You would probably benefit from a Swedish massage to drain your lymphatic system. Has your weight been creeping up? Eliminating a few key foods that trigger cravings could help tip the scale back in the right direction. Headaches sapping your strength? You may need to clear out harmful chemicals that inflame and irritate nerves and blood vessels in the brain.

In the following pages you'll find detailed detox strategies for some of the most common health threats—conditions that, year by year, can damage your health and perniciously erode your energy, motivation, and physical and emotional strength. It's always a good idea to work with a health care practitioner who combines detox procedures with mainstream medicine, but the plans have been designed with safety in mind. You can do them yourself at home, without spending a fortune on expensive procedures. Start now and feel the difference. You came into this world free of toxic chemicals. Why live with anything less?

If you have a particular condition that's been challenging you of late, turn directly to the pages that deal with it, and you'll find a range of practical tips and techniques that will help your body use the power of detoxification to help ameliorate—and in some cases even cure—the problem. You'll find strategies that employ herbal remedies and healing foods, helpful mental strategies, and other sage advice from the nation's top detoxification experts to speed you on your way to healing.

Remember, though, that curing a single condition wins a battle. If you want to win the war—returning your body to a state of vibrant health—you'll still need the essentials of purification detailed in the other sections of this book.

AGING
STAY YOUNGER LONGER

Every year, people are living just a little bit longer. This is partly due to our successes in battling childhood and adult diseases, but it's also because scientists are unlocking the secrets of aging itself.

Cells in your body divide a certain number of times, then die and are replaced by new cells. This process slows with age, however. Muscles get less flexible, bones weaken, immunity declines, and your organs essentially fatigue. Some of these changes are inevitable, but new research suggests that it may be possible to put the brakes on our own declines.

For example, laboratory animals kept in ideal conditions—given healthy foods and regular exercise in a toxin-free environment—can double their normal life spans. There's good evidence that people have the same potential, if they take the right steps.

Some researchers estimate that the average human life span could easy extend to 120 years if we did what we could to purge our bodies of environmental toxins as well as internal wastes. Here's what needs to be done.

Your Purification Plan

Strategy One: Eliminate Pollutants from Your Body

More than 1 billion pounds of pesticides are spread on produce each year. Our foods are spiked with thousands of additives and preservatives. Even "safe" drinking water contains up to 1,300 different chemicals. Over a lifetime, the liver, intestine, and other organs have to work overtime to eliminate these pollutants from the body, and all that extra effort accelerates the aging process.

A healthful diet and regular exercise are essential steps in any detoxification plan, says Emily Kane, N.D., L.Ac., a naturopathic physician and acupuncturist in Juneau, Alaska. At the same time, you need to cleanse your body of disease-causing chemical wastes.

Protect your liver with milk thistle. Nearly every toxin that enters your body passes through your liver. If your liver can't keep up, toxins accumulate and increase your risk of cancer and many other diseases. Milk thistle contains a chemical compound, silymarin, that enhances the liver's production of glutathione, a chemical toxin neutralizer, by 35 percent. It also helps damaged liver cells regenerate. The recommended dose is 200 mg three times daily.

Load up on beans. They contain phytates, which bind to toxins in the intestine and eliminate them from the body, says Dr. Kane. Just about any kind of beans will do the trick. Experiment with new recipes and learn to incorporate a variety of beans into your diet. Ideally, you should be eating beans a few times a week.

Drink a lot of water. You need at least eight 8-ounce glasses daily. Water dilutes chemical concentrations in the blood and helps all of the organs of elimination, including the liver and intestines, work more efficiently, says Dr. Kane.

Keep the colon clean. Toxins accumulate in the stools, and if you don't have daily bowel movements, many of these toxins seep back into your bloodstream. A high-fiber diet is the most efficient way to keep stools moving. Eating plenty of fruits and vegetables—at least two to three servings a day—will help anyone live longer, says Dr. Kane.

"I also encourage modified fasts, having only raw foods and fresh vegetables, several times a year," she adds.

Give yourself plenty of downtime. Doctors estimate that at least 90 percent of all doctor visits are for stress-related disorders. Uncontrolled stress lowers immunity, increases blood pressure in some cases, and can make you look and feel older than your years, says Dan L. Martin, N.D., O.M.D., a naturopathic physician and doctor of Oriental Medicine in Texarkana, Arkansas.

We all control stress in different ways, but a few techniques are especially effective. Start with exercise. It lowers levels of adrenaline and other stress hormones while boosting "feel good" brain chemicals called endorphins. Get a massage once a month if you can. It can lower the output of stress hormones from the adrenal glands. Definitely give yourself time just to relax, not just once in a while, but every day. It's not just about feeling good. The more you relax, the more efficiently your liver and other organs detoxify your body.

Strategy Two: Block Damage to Cell Structure

Many age-related diseases, as well as the aging process itself, are caused in part by free radicals, unstable molecules that are produced in profusion when you're exposed to pollution and other toxins, and which attack cell membranes throughout your body. The only way to stop the destruction is to increase your dietary intake of free-radical "scavengers," antioxidant nutrients that bind to tissue-damaging molecules and block their harmful effects. There are literally thousands of antioxidants. They work in different ways in the body and are most effective when consumed in combination from dietary sources rather than single-nutrient supplements, says Dr. Kane. Here are the antioxidants that doctors recommend most.

Boost your immune power with vitamin E. It blocks free-radical damage in the fatty membranes that surround cells, and it appears to counteract some of the negative effects of air pollution, heavy metals, and other environmental toxins, says Gary Dreger, N.D., L.Ac., a naturopathic physician and acupuncturist at Natural Health Works in Oregon City, Oregon. Vitamin E also improves immunity and reduces the risk of age-related diseases, including heart disease and some cancers.

Even though it's almost always better to get nutrients from foods rather than supplements, vitamin E may be an exception. You need 150 IU of vitamin E daily to glean its antiaging effects. You're probably not getting that amount from diet alone. Plan on taking a daily supplement, and increase your intake of vitamin E–rich foods, such as nuts, seeds, and wheat germ.

Strengthen E with selenium. It's a mineral that works together with vitamin E to reduce cell irritation. It binds to harmful toxins such as mercury, arsenic, and cadmium and reduces their harmful effects in the body. At the same time, selenium is a powerful antioxidant that strengthens the ability of the immune system to seek out and destroy cancerous cells. "Selenium is a cofactor in at least 75 percent of the enzymatic reactions in the body, including cellular repair mechanisms," says Dr. Kane. Selenium can be toxic in amounts greater than 900 mcg, and most people should not take more than 200 mcg per day.

Color your world. The beta-carotene in deep green and bright orange fruits and vegetables belongs to a chemical family called carotenoids. They're extremely powerful antioxidants that reduce damage to cellular DNA—damage that sets the stage for cancer and other degenerative diseases, including eye diseases. For example, people who get plenty of carotenoids from a produce-rich diet can reduce their risks of cataracts and macular degeneration, the leading causes of vision loss in older adults, by at least one-third.

Neutralize nitrites. In addition to

Fewer Calories, Longer Life

SCIENTISTS HAVE KNOWN FOR A LONG TIME that when animals are given about one-third fewer calories than normal, their life expectancy jumps by about one-third. If the same were true in humans, cutting about 600 calories out of your daily diet would increase your life expectancy from the current 83 years (for women) to an average of 100 years.

Consider life in Okinawa, Japan, where a low-calorie diet is typical—and where people are 40 times more likely than people in other parts of the world to celebrate their 100th birthdays.

No one knows for sure why reducing calories increases longevity, although it may be linked to accompanying reductions in insulin levels. "Calorie restriction is the only proven way to extend life," says Emily Kane, N.D., L.Ac., a naturopathic physician and acupuncturist in Juneau, Alaska.

Keep in mind, though, that cutting calories to this extent basically means going hungry all the time. Few of us have the stamina, or desire, to live that way. But eating less is certainly healthier in the long run. If most of us would follow this simple rule, we'd live longer, be healthier, and feel younger.

being a strong antioxidant, vitamin C prevents the conversion of nitrites, chemicals in meats and many other foods, into carcinogenic nitrosamines. Vitamin C also reduces irritation from air pollution and secondhand cigarette smoke, says Dr. Dreger. Try to get at least 200 to 500 mg daily.

Protect your cells with L-cysteine. It's a sulfur-containing amino acid that neutralizes free radicals and helps the liver produce glutathione, one of the most potent antioxidants. A study at the University of Michigan, Ann Arbor, found that people who got the most glutathione had lower blood pressure and cholesterol than those who got the least. Food sources of L-cysteine include avocados, grapefruit, and tomatoes.

Stay young with Bs. Many older adults have difficulty absorbing B vitamins, which strengthen nerve coatings and improve memory. The Bs are essential nutrients in any detox plan because they help the body eliminate homocysteine, an amino acid–like compound that increases the risk of heart disease. To lower homocysteine and improve brain function, take 50 mg of B_6, 1,000 mcg of B_{12}, and 1 mg of folic acid, according to Peter Bennett, N.D., a naturopathic physician in Vancouver and coauthor of *7-Day Detox Miracle*.

ALLERGIES AND ASTHMA
BETTER BREATHING

Mainstream medicine has always looked at allergies and asthma largely as an assault from without. If you avoid pollen, dust mites, or external "triggers," the thinking goes, you can prevent congestion, runny nose, wheezing, and other symptoms.

It's true that exposure to allergens such as pollens can unleash a flood of histamine, leukotrienes, and other inflammatory compounds in the body. Asthma is a bit more complicated, but the results are similar: Exposure to allergens or even a breath of cold air can cause tiny airways in the lungs to get constricted and inflamed.

But the immune system must literally come into contact with foreign substances for allergies to develop. This tends to happen when the body's defenses, such as mucous membranes or the lining of the intestine, aren't as strong as they should be, which allows allergens to breach their barriers, explains Gary Dreger, N.D., L.Ac., a naturopathic physician and acupuncturist at Natural Health Works in Oregon City, Oregon.

So it's not enough merely to avoid potential allergens—a nearly impossible task if you live in the real world. Besides doing your best to avoid these problematic substances, you also need to restore the strength of your body's protective barriers so that foreign substances can't trigger the symptom cascade.

Your Purification Plan

Strategy One: Cleanse Your Body's Filters

Nearly all of us have an overload of foreign substances in our bodies—not just potential allergens, but environmental toxins as well. Here's what doctors advise you do to boost your body's natural defenses.

Clean out fast. Even if you eat a healthful diet most of the time, sluggish digestion, caused by an accumulation of toxins, for example, can slow the passage of stools and make it easier for toxins and potential allergens to enter the bloodstream. "You need to lower the burden on the immune system so that it copes with airborne irritants more appropriately," says Emily Kane, N.D., L.Ac., a naturopathic physician and acupuncturist in Juneau, Alaska.

A 2-day water or juice fast is one of the quickest and safest ways to remove toxins from the colon and promote better digestion, says Dr. Dreger. At the very least, eat a lot more fruits, vegetables, and legumes. These and other high-fiber foods cause stools, and the toxins they contain, to move more quickly through your system.

Watch out for additives. Many people with asthma and allergies are sensitive to food additives and preservatives, including sulfites, tartrazine, and sodium benzoate. "Your first step should always be to eat organic foods and drink purified water," says Dr. Dreger.

Exercise often. Regular exercise improves the ability of the lungs to take in oxygen and dispel carbon dioxide. It helps the lungs, liver, and kidneys excrete toxins more efficiently. It also makes you sweat, and perspiration carries tremendous loads of toxins out of the body through the skin.

Strategy Two: Control Histamines

Histamine, the chemical that causes allergy symptoms, can be managed with some easy yet effective changes to your diet and lifestyle.

Go easy on the red. Austrian researchers report that red wine often contains histamine. Pouring additional histamine into your system when you're already loaded with the stuff can cause bronchial tubes to constrict and make breathing harder.

Shake the salt. A diet high in sodium

may make bronchioles, tiny airways in the lungs, more sensitive to histamine. You don't have to give up salt entirely, but you'll definitely want to eat less. Read labels and buy low- or no-sodium foods, and be a little less liberal with the shaker.

Have a cup of tea. While you're at it, munch a few apples and add more onions to your soup. Tea, apples, and onions are among the best sources of quercetin, an antioxidant that inhibits the release of histamine and also tames free radicals, says Dr. Dreger.

Cut animal foods. Toxins accumulate in fatty foods, which is why a diet high in meats or dairy can trigger more asthma attacks than a vegetarian diet. Eating fat, and the toxins it contains, increases levels of inflammatory chemicals in the airways, says Dr. Kane. One study found that about two-thirds of participants who ate a vegetarian diet for a year had a significant reduction in symptoms.

Strategy Three: Reduce Allergens

The combination of environmental toxins and less-than-perfect diets can cause junctions between cells in the intestine walls to get "leaky" and allow undigested food particles to pass into the bloodstream. The immune system reacts to these particles, potentially making you

more vulnerable to allergies, says Dr. Kane. Here are some simple ways to protect yourself.

Cut out dietary culprits. Millions of Americans are sensitive to milk, wheat, eggs, and dozens of other foods. Dr. Dreger recommends keeping track of everything you eat for a month or two. When you have an allergy or asthma flare-up, check your notes to see which foods you ate prior to the symptoms occurring. Then eliminate those foods, one at a time, for 3 to 4 weeks to see if it makes a difference.

Rotate your diet. In other words, don't eat any one food more often than once every 3 or 4 days. "When you eat the same food day after day, you're more likely to get reactions," says Dr. Dreger. Giving yourself a few days' break from specific foods can reduce allergy flare-ups and also reduce the risk that you'll develop new allergies in the future.

Strategy Four: Wash Out Inflammation

Histamine and other chemicals produced by the immune system cause an inflammatory response in the respiratory system. This is what causes much of the sniffling and sneezing of hay fever, as well as difficulty breathing when asthma flares. To reduce inflammation:

Oh say, can you C? Take 500 to 1,000 mg of vitamin C daily. It blocks the effects of free radicals, tissue-damaging molecules that are produced when the airways are inflamed and irritated. Vitamin C also appears to prevent asthma attacks by making the airways less likely to go into spasm.

Try tomato therapy. Lycopene, an antioxidant in tomatoes, is related to beta-carotene and has been shown to reduce asthma symptoms. In one study, more than half of those who got extra lycopene experienced fewer asthma symptoms.

Up your antioxidant quotient. Antioxidants include vitamin E, selenium, and beta-carotene, says Dr. Dreger. If you eat a lot of produce, whole grains, and legumes, you'll almost automatically get enough to help keep allergies and asthma under control. The one exception is vitamin E, since it's hard to get enough through diet alone. Take a daily supplement that provides 150 IU.

Strategy Five: Clear Out Congestion

The newer antihistamines for easing congestion and other allergy symptoms cause fewer side effects than older generations of drugs, but sedation—not to mention the high cost—is still a problem for some people. A better approach, at least initially, is to try some natural steps to help mucus flow more easily and to cleanse your body of congestion-causing chemicals.

Avoid milk, and drink a lot of water. Even though dairy foods don't appear to cause an increase in mucus, they may trigger congestion if you have lactose intolerance, an inability to digest the lactose (a sugar) in milk and other dairy products. So go easy on milk, and drink plenty of water. It makes mucus thinner so that it drains out of the body rather than accumulating in the respiratory tract.

Foil excess phlegm. Breathing hot, moist air, such as while you're lounging in the bath, can help eliminate mucus from your airways and make breathing easier, says Dr. Dreger. Another option during allergy season is sinus irrigation. Mix ½ teaspoonful of salt in a cup of warm water. Cup some in your hand and sniff carefully up into your nostrils. (The idea is to cleanse your nasal passages, not breathe it in.) You might find it easier to use a neti pot (nasal wash cup). It's a simple device that allows you to safely pour salted water in one nostril and allow it to flow out the other. For directions on purchasing and using a neti pot, see "Say Hello to Neti" on page 157.

The Kitchen Congestion Connection

IT'S ALWAYS A GOOD IDEA TO EAT LESS MEAT and bump up your consumption of fresh fruits and vegetables. But if you suffer from hay fever, some of that produce may be a problem.

For reasons that still aren't clear, the immune systems of people with hay fever sometimes react to certain fruits and vegetables, especially bananas and melons. If you're allergic to ragweed, for example, eating a banana or a slice of watermelon could trigger additional stuffiness. If you're allergic to grass pollen, then apples or cherries could set off a torrent of congestion.

Some people with this type of multiple allergy, known as cross-reactivity, are sensitive to trouble foods all year long. In most cases, though, congestion flares in the spring when pollen counts, and the body's level of histamine, are already high.

All of these foods are perfectly healthy—unless you're sensitive to them. The only solution? Watch your reactions whenever you eat these foods, and ask your doctor if these or other foods might be contributing to the problem. Of course, you should avoid them if that seems to help.

ARTHRITIS
CALMING THE FIRES OF INFLAMMATION

Imagine a building on fire. The alarm sounds, fire crews douse the flames with special chemicals, and the fire is reduced to embers. But even while the owner of the building is congratulating the firefighters on a job well done, things start to go wrong. Doors that once opened easily are now stiff and creaky. Windows are jammed. The floors creak and moan. The rescue effort saved the building, but all of those chemicals attacked the building's hinges and joints.

A similar thing can happen if you have arthritis. The body's immune system pours powerful cells and chemicals on the site of a problem—your knees or hips, for example—but at the same time those chemicals damage the tissue they're meant to repair, explains Joel Fuhrman, M.D., a family practice physician specializing in nutritional medicine and author of *Eat to Live* and *Fasting and Eating for Health.*

There are more than 100 forms of arthritis, the most common being osteo-arthritis, a "wear-and-tear" disease that gradually damages joint cartilage, and rheumatoid arthritis, which occurs when the immune system mistakenly attacks the joints.

Since rheumatoid arthritis is triggered by a misbehaving immune system, and the immune system is affected by what you eat, it makes sense that changes in your diet can make a real difference. Both long-term diet strategies and short-term changes can prove helpful. But some people aren't quite prepared to go that far—and even if they are, they still might experience periodic flare-ups. This is especially true if you have os-teoarthritis, which is caused by mechan-ical problems in the joints rather than a whole-body immune response.

Your Purification Plan

Strategy One: Switch Off Immune Response Triggers

The most important strategy is to elimi-nate toxins from your body, toxins that can stimulate your immune system to launch its misguided attacks.

Cut back on meat protein. In a study at Norway's University of Oslo, people with arthritis who switched to a vegetarian diet for a year had less morning stiffness, their joints were less swollen and tender, and they had more hand strength than those who followed their usual diets.

When you eat animal protein, small bits of undigested peptides (the con-stituent parts of proteins) can slip through the intestine and into the blood. "The immune system reacts against them and causes inflammation," explains Dr. Fuhrman. In people who are sensitive to them, the fats in animal products can switch on the body's production of inflammation-causing chemicals called prostaglandins.

"I advise everyone to switch to a vegan diet," says Dr. Fuhrman. "The secret to detoxifying the body is to eat a diet that consists entirely of all-natural foods with very high nutritional content that are free of preservatives, salt, or sugar."

Take fish oil supplements. "In high doses—usually 9 to 12 grams a day—fish oil acts as an immune suppressant and can reduce joint inflammation," says Dr. Fuhrman.

Track and eliminate. Many people with arthritis are sensitive to specific foods, possibly because the foods contain allergens that stimulate the immune system and trigger inflammation and pain. Oranges, grapefruit, and other citrus foods are common arthritis triggers, as is wheat. Vegetables in the nightshade family, such as tomatoes and potatoes, can also cause problems, though with less frequency. In people who are sensitive to them, these foods act like toxins.

"It's very individual," says Dr. Fuhrman. "Some people have more pain when they eat green apples, but not red ones. Or they're sensitive to one kind of lettuce and not another."

Since these are all healthful foods (unless you're sensitive to them), you don't want to eliminate them unless they prove to be problematic for you. So it's helpful to write down everything you eat—meals, snacks, everything—for a few months. At the same time, jot down when you have arthritis flare-ups. Comparing the two lists will give you a good sense of what foods are most likely to cause problems. "You usually have to be off a food for 3 or 4 weeks before you'll notice an improvement in symptoms," Dr. Fuhrman says.

Strategy Two: Stop the Pain with Vitamins and Supplements

The trick to quelling arthritis pain is to lower levels of pain-causing prostaglandins and substance P, a chemical messenger than carries pain signals from the painful area to the brain, says Timothy Douglass, D.C., founder and owner of Douglass Chiropractic in Glen, New Hampshire. You'll also need to take steps to flush your joints of waste products from your body's normal metabolism.

Clear out wastes with vitamin C. Boston researchers report that people who get more than 200 mg of vitamin C daily are three times less likely to experience a worsening of arthritis symptoms than those who get less than 120 mg. Vitamin C scrubs the joints of free radicals, oxygen molecules that cause joint damage and inflammation. "Vitamin C is absolutely wonderful for any kind of joint pain," says Dr. Douglass.

Take a pineapple pill. Supplements that contain bromelain, a chemical compound extracted from pineapples, lower levels of immune antigen complex, compounds that can contribute to pain and swelling. Pineapple also breaks down fibrin, a compound linked to some forms of arthritis. "It doesn't work for everyone, but many of my patients say that it helps," says Dr. Douglass.

Scrub out substance P. The next time you have an arthritis flare-up, apply capsaicin cream, available over the counter, to the sore area. It cleanses nerves of substance P, a pain-causing chemical. In one study, people who applied capsaicin were able to reduce their pain by about one-third.

Strategy Three: Put Nature's Pharmacy to Work

Mother Nature must have anticipated that our joints would need a lot of help because She provided us with dozens of healing remedies that strip away pain-causing chemicals and waste products. When using herbs, simply follow the directions on the package. Some natural healers include the following in a regimen intended to lessen the effects of arthritis.

Top off with turmeric. It contains chemical compounds that reduce levels of prostaglandins and other inflammatory substances. You can enjoy turmeric as a spicy addition to many foods (think curries), or you can purchase it in the form of an herbal supplement.

Jump for ginger. An Indian study found that more than 75 percent of those who ate 1 to 3 teaspoons of ginger daily experienced significant relief from pain and swelling. You can enjoy ginger as a spice in many dishes, drink it as a tea (it comes in tea bags), or take it as an herbal supplement.

Follow the way of the willow. Made into a tea, willow bark delivers high levels of salicin, an aspirinlike chemical that lowers levels of inflammatory prostaglandins.

Take out the sting. Eaten as a vegetable, an average serving of cooked stinging nettle provides more than 3 mg of boron, a mineral that is recommended for both rheumatoid arthritis and osteoarthritis. You won't be able to find this delicious herb in the supermarket, though stinging nettle does grow wild in many parts of the country. If you have access to this plant and are able to clearly identify it, add it to your diet whenever you feel like indulging. (You'll need to wear gloves when picking it, as the tiny nettles that cover the plant really do sting. But cooking destroys the parts that sting.) All you have to do is simmer the nettle leaves in water for 5 to 10 minutes, or until tender.

Befriend the good bacteria. Available in health food stores, probiotic supplements contain live, beneficial bacteria that take up residence in the intestine and crowd out less-healthful bacteria. "Bacterial toxins can be related to rheumatoid arthritis, and you can reduce their levels with probiotics," says Dr. Fuhrman.

Strategy Four: Take the Fast Path to Speed Recovery

Since rheumatoid arthritis may be triggered by undigested foods that slip into the bloodstream, fasting for several days (or even 1 to 2 weeks, if you're under the supervision of a physician) gives the entire body a chance to recover. Here's a painless way to get started.

Gimme the juice. If you don't like the idea of total deprivation, it's fine to drink fruit juices, vegetable juices, or herbal teas during your fast. A modified fast can usually help ease arthritis pain while providing your body with nutrients. Obviously, you don't want to fast for extended periods on your own. To be safe, check with your doctor before you try fasting.

After a few days on your fast, start adding "new" foods back in one at a time. For example, you might end the fast with a leafy green salad. A day later, have a small serving of chicken or fish. After that, add some vegetables. If the pain suddenly comes back, you'll have a clue as to what might be causing or contributing to the trouble.

"I recommend fasting only if someone has been following a very healthful diet for a few months," Dr. Fuhrman adds. "If you go from a traditional American diet into a fast, you'll detox too violently." For more information on safe and healthy fasting, see chapter 7 on page 143.

Strategy Five: Eat Right and Lose Weight

Many of the strategies above can provide temporary relief, but for the long term, changing the way you eat and losing some weight could be the best ways to outsmart your arthritis pain for good. Between 60 and 80 percent of people with rheumatoid arthritis get dramatically better when they overhaul their diets and switch to a natural style of eating, says Dr. Fuhrman.

Drop excess pounds. There's a simple reason that people who are overweight tend to suffer more pain from osteoarthritis: They carry a heavier load when they walk, and the extra pressure on their joints invariably causes more pain, says Dr. Fuhrman.

You don't have to lose a lot of weight to notice a difference. Studies suggest that people who lose as little as 10 to 15 pounds often feel a dramatic reduction in soreness.

Fish for relief. Even though it's a good idea to cut back on fats when you're trying to lose weight, there is one type you'll want to include in an antiarthritis diet: The omega-3 fatty acids, found primarily in cold-water fish (such as mackerel, trout, and salmon). These fatty acids reduce levels of prostaglandins and leukotrienes, both of which contribute to inflammation. Two to three weekly servings is probably enough.

BINGES
RECOVERING FROM TOO MUCH FOOD OR DRINK

See if this sounds familiar. Saturday night: Good food, good drink, good company, and a few too many trips to the punch bowl. When you wake up the next morning, your body lets you know in no uncertain terms that you should have stayed home and organized your stamp collection.

Or how about this: You sometimes get this irresistible urge to eat—and not just a little. Entire packages of chips, cookies, or chocolate disappear in a single sitting. Afterwards, you feel lousy and probably guilty, yet a few days later you're at it again. You can't seem to stop yourself, and you probably suffer in silence because you don't want anyone to know what's going on.

Between 1 and 2 million Americans have a binge-eating disorder. Most women (it affects three women for every two men) who have it are overweight, and most have some degree of depres-

sion. Binge eating can be life-threatening in some cases, so you'll obviously want to get medical or psychological help.

Binges seem like they come out of nowhere, but actually they are often triggered by physical imbalances in brain and body chemistry—imbalances caused in part by substances that are toxic to your body and that can make you feel as though you're out of control. Even if you overdo it only occasionally, you'll want to recover as quickly as you can, while at the same time taking steps to reduce future cravings. Here are some cleansing steps to start getting the cravings under control and reduce their harm.

Your Purification Plan

Strategy One: Squelch Sugar

Banish sugar from your life. In one study, women given a sugar-free diet (one that also eliminated alcohol, caffeine, and processed white flour) stopped binging within 3 weeks and remained binge-free for more than 2½ years. "Sugar is almost like a drug in its addictiveness," says Cynthia P. Buxton, N.D., L.Ac., a naturopathic physician and acupuncturist in private practice in Seattle. Once you give up sugar, the cravings usually end in 1 to 3 weeks, she adds.

Give up coffee for a few weeks. Along with colas and other caffeinated beverages, coffee lowers blood glucose levels and can produce intense sugar cravings, says Dr. Buxton.

Mop up the excess. The level of glucose (sugar) in your blood rises sharply when you overdo it. "The pancreas releases insulin to bring glucose back down, but sometimes it overshoots," explains Jessica Nesseler-Cass, N.D., a naturopathic physician in private practice in Portland, Oregon. When that happens, your blood sugar levels plummet and you crave food to restore a kind of balance. The minerals chromium and magnesium can help because they stabilize blood sugar and keep cravings under control.

You can get plenty of these minerals in a balanced diet, but you may want to supplement with 200 mcg of chromium and 500 to 700 mg of magnesium daily. You can divide each supplement into two doses, Dr. Buxton says. Take one dose in the late morning and another in the afternoon (times when blood sugar starts to sag). You'll still need to restrict your intake of dietary sugar, but the minerals will help keep cravings under control in the meantime.

Strategy Two: Turn Off the Triggers

It's easier than you think to stop the habits that may be causing you to binge. Here are a few ways to put yourself back in control of your cravings.

Calm cravings with zinc. This mineral derails out-of-control cravings by activating a brain chemical that sends "stop eating" signals to the brain, says Dr. Buxton. Get at least 15 mg daily—the amount found in most multivitamin supplements.

Clear out depression's cobwebs. Since nearly everyone who suffers from food cravings has some degree of depression, you'll want to take steps to clear it out of your life.

◐ Start with 5-HTP. Your brain converts this supplement, sold in health food stores, into serotonin, a brain chemical that improves mood while at the same time putting the brakes on appetite, says Dr. Nesseler-Cass. Take 50 mg of 5-HTP three times daily for 6 weeks. If you don't notice a reduction in cravings and binge-eating episodes, increase the dose to 100 mg. If you're taking other antidepressants, check with your doctor before supplementing with 5-HTP. Also note that the key studies on craving and 5-HTP used an even higher dosage, up to 900 mg per day. If you'd like to try a higher dose, consult with your doctor.

⑥ Take St. John's wort. This over-the-counter supplement has been shown to be just as effective as prescription drugs for treating mild to moderate depression. It improves mood, stabilizes appetite, and makes it easier for the brain to send stop-eating signals when you're full. Take 300 mg two or three times daily. As with 5-HTP, don't combine it with antidepressants without checking with your doctor.

Drink plenty of water. Your body often confuses dehydration with hunger. Doctors estimate that millions of Americans routinely let their tanks run a little on the low side, and people who don't get enough water tend to eat more than they really need. The next time you have a craving, immediately drink two glasses of water, preferably with a squeeze of lemon. Wait a few minutes. You'll probably find that your craving is gone.

"If nothing else, drinking more water means that you'll drink fewer soft drinks, which are loaded with sugar," says Dr. Nesseler-Cass.

Strategy Three: Head-Off Hangovers

Alcohol is a bit of a mixed blessing. The evidence is clear that moderate drinking (up to one drink daily for women and two for men) protects against heart disease and can help lower blood pressure and the risk of stroke. Drinking too much, on the other hand, can devastate your personal life along with your health.

Even if you drink sensibly most of the time, it's easy to overdo it on occasion—and that's when you'll find yourself wishing your head were attached to someone else's body. The fact is that your body views alcohol as a toxin, every bit as much of a threat as pollutants in the air you breathe or a trace of pesticide ingested along with a peach. And your body's detoxification systems need to work in order to clean alcohol from your blood.

It's unlikely that scientists will discover a miracle hangover cure any time soon. They have discovered, however, that you'll feel a lot better when you cleanse your body of alcohol-related toxins and waste products. Here's where to start.

If you must drink, think "light." Darker, sweeter drinks, such as red wine and whiskey, contain more cogeners— (organic molecules such as methanol that increase the head-pounding effects) than lighter-colored drinks such as white wine or vodka.

Eliminate acetaldehyde accumulation. If you experience hangovers even after modest drinking, it's possible that one of your liver's detoxification pathways is more sluggish than it should be. This can lead to buildups of acetaldehyde, a toxic substance that causes morning-after discomfort. To cleanse the liver:

⊚ Take a B-complex supplement. The B vitamins help the liver cleanse itself more quickly, says Dr. Buxton. Follow dosage directions on the package.

⊚ Make a detox blend. Mix a little lemon juice and a teaspoonful of cayenne pepper (brace yourself!) in a tablespoon of olive oil, and take it once or twice when you're suffering the next-day blahs, suggests Dr. Nesseler-Cass. It helps purge toxins from the liver. Don't take any more than a few tablespoonfuls of olive oil, she adds. Too much can cause the gallbladder to go into spasms.

⊚ Sip dandelion tea. It is among the best liver remedies and helps with cellular repair after exposure to cell-damaging toxins. "Dandelion is a mild diuretic, so make sure you drink extra water when taking it," advises Dr. Nesseler-Cass. This herbal tea is available in convenient tea bags.

⊚ Take milk thistle. This supplement contains a chemical compound, silymarin, that stimulates liver cells and helps them rid the body of alcohol and alcohol-related waste products. "It's an excellent liver herb," Dr. Nesseler-Cass says. Again, follow dosage directions on the package.

Fill your tank with water. When you have a hangover, it's almost impossible to drink too much water, so take in as much

Tropical Stomach Soother

OVERINDULGING CAN LEAVE YOUR STOMACH FEELING LIKE IT'S GONE ALL TOPSY-TURVY. You can calm it down in a hurry with a few slices of papaya. This luscious tropical fruit contains papain and other protease enzymes, which are similar to the stomach's natural enzymes. Eating papaya makes it easier to digest proteins and will soothe an upset stomach. Better yet, make yourself a fruit smoothie that contains papaya.

as you can. Water dilutes toxins and waste products and also reverses dehydration, the main cause of alcohol-related discomfort, says Dr. Nesseler-Cass.

Fiber up. High-fiber foods are essential for digestive health and can also make a difference when you've had too much to drink. Fiber is like the body's natural sponge. It sops up alcohol and alcohol by-products in the intestine and carries them out of the body in the stool. You might have a bowl of oatmeal for breakfast, for example, when you first wake up.

BLOOD CLEANSING HEALTHY BLOOD FOR HEALTHY CELLS

Every organ in your body, every cell and artery and bit of tissue, is linked by blood. The heart sends blood coursing through your system, delivering oxygen and nutrients and carting away wastes. The downside, now that we live in an industrial, pollution-filled world, is that blood also carries toxins that can damage your health.

We all ingest chemicals from the environment. We take high-powered drugs. We eat sugar and refined foods. We inadvertently flood our systems with synthetic, disease-causing toxins that weaken the body's ability to keep itself clean.

This has all sorts of consequences. For example, do you suffer from allergies? It could be because your liver isn't efficiently cleansing your blood of histamine, a biochemical produced by your immune system. Do you have creaky, painful joints? Blame blood buildups of leukotrines and prostaglandins, just two of the inflammatory substances that tend to accumulate when your organs of elimination are sluggish and congested.

"The only way to cleanse the blood is to ensure that all of the organs of elimination—the lungs, skin, kidneys, colon, and liver—are working well," says Margaret Beeson, N.D., a naturopathic physician at Yellowstone Naturopathic Clinic in Billings, Montana. "Imagine a kitchen strainer that's filled with mud. You can pour in fresh water, but nothing will flow out unless all the holes are clear."

Here's a powerful set of strategies to detoxify the blood and ensure that it is able to transport materials for health rather than toxins that cause decay.

Your Purification Plan

Strategy One: Cleanse Your Liver

It's the largest gland in the body, one that performs more than 500 functions, including filtering blood and detoxifying potential carcinogens. The liver has a remarkable ability to regenerate itself, but it can't perform efficiently without periodic cleansing.

Drink dandelion root tea. It's a very mild herbal remedy that enhances the flow of blood to the liver and bile (a digestive fluid that the liver makes) and expedites the cleansing of blood, says Dr. Beeson. It's especially important to use dandelion if you're taking antidepressants, which tend to impede the liver's detoxification pathways. You can buy the tea at health food stores and simply follow the directions on the package. Drink several cups daily.

Start the day with fiber. Sprinkle a tablespoonful of psyllium seeds or oat bran on your morning cereal. Eat more fruits, vegetables, legumes, and whole grains. All of these foods are high in fiber, which binds to wastes in the intestine and carries them out of the body before they enter the bloodstream.

Drink plenty of water—at least eight 8-ounce glasses daily. It reduces the body's concentration of toxins and makes it easier for the liver, kidneys, and other elimination organs to clear them from the blood, says Dr. Beeson.

Strategy Two: Cleanse Your Lungs

Your lungs do more than extract oxygen from the air you breathe. They also remove toxic wastes, including carbon dioxide, that are produced by your body's normal metabolism and carried in your blood.

Exercise daily. It's as simple as that. Anything that increases your normal rate of respiration—walking for half an hour, doing yoga, lifting weights, even vacuuming the floor—enhances the ability of hairlike filters in your lungs to carry out waste products along with any buildup of mucus. Exercise also increases gas exchange—the replacement of carbon dioxide and other waste gases in your blood with energizing oxygen.

Strategy Three: Cleanse Your Skin

This tough, supple membrane excretes as many toxins as the kidneys do. At the same time, though, it absorbs toxins from the environment. The only way you can hope to clear toxins from your blood is to ensure that your skin works at peak efficiency.

Dry brush daily. Use a soft brush to rub every inch of your skin, always brushing toward the center of your body. This pushes toxins out of the lymphatic system, the vast network of capillaries and storage sacs below the skin, so that they can be processed by the liver and kidneys, says Dr. Beeson. The best time to do this is right before you take a shower.

Scrub with salt. Health food stores sell

a variety of salt scrubs, stimulating salts that increase metabolism and speed the elimination of toxins when you rub them on your body. The salts also act like dry brushing and increase lymph drainage.

Soak in Epsom salts. Lounging in a warm bath opens blood vessels and helps the entire circulatory system purge toxins more efficiently. Adding Epsom salts (magnesium sulfate) to the bath is particularly helpful because it pulls toxins out of the skin, Dr. Beeson explains. You can find Epsom salts at many drugstores, and you'll find directions for how much to use right on the package. (It makes a good foot bath, as well.)

Follow hot with cold. One of the best ways to encourage the detoxification of your skin and lymphatic system is to follow a hot bath or shower with a cool rinse, and repeat the process three times. "Alternating hot and cold water creates a pumping action that sends fresh blood to the capillary bed and eliminates waste products," says Dr. Beeson.

Strategy Four: Cleanse Your Kidneys

These two powerful, fist-size organs filter blood and remove urea, salts, excess minerals, and other potentially toxic wastes from your blood. Their burden is tremendous: Every drop of your blood passes through your kidneys about 20 times an hour. If you don't take an active role in cleansing your kidneys, they get congested with wastes, work more slowly, and allow more impurities to stay in your bloodstream. Here's what you need to do to keep them clean.

Reach for the water pitcher. Once again, you need to drink at least 2 quarts of water a day, or more if you're bigger than average, live in a hot climate, or get a lot of exercise. Water dilutes minerals and other wastes and makes it easier for the kidneys to flush them out of the body in the urine.

Switch to dandelion leaf tea. You'll remember that we recommended dandelion root tea for detoxifying the liver. Teas made from the leaves act in an entirely different way. They have a diuretic effect, which means that they accelerate the removal of urine (and all the excess chemicals that it contains) from the body, says Dr. Beeson. At the same time, dandelion leaf is an excellent source of potassium. That's important because most prescription diuretics remove potassium from the body. When you drink dandelion leaf tea, you get the same kind of diuretic action without depleting your body of this essential mineral. You'll find the herbal tea at health food stores. Just follow the directions on the package.

Cleanse the Blood of Cholesterol

MOST PEOPLE CAN LOWER BLOOD LEVELS of cholesterol by eating less fat and more fruits and vegetables. And virtually everyone can lower their cholesterol by taking one of the statin drugs. In some cases, though, traditional approaches don't work, which is a serious problem because uncontrolled cholesterol greatly increases the risk of stroke and heart disease.

Now there's an alternative: cleansing the blood with a technique called cholesterol apheresis. Similar to kidney dialysis, it filters out cholesterol and can lower the risk of cardiovascular events by 50 to 70 percent, researchers at the University of Michigan Health System report.

People have the treatment every 2 or 3 weeks. Blood is removed from one arm, put into a machine that filters out cholesterol, and then returned to the bloodstream. Because people get their own blood back, there's little risk of infection or other complications.

Note that this high-tech treatment is reserved for people who can't get their cholesterol down by any other method and who are at risk of having a heart attack or stroke. If you fall into this category, ask your doctor whether this treatment is right for you.

Strategy Five: Cleanse Your Colon

You can't have clean blood unless your colon is regularly cleaned as well. This 6-foot tube, which can hold more than 30 gallons of fluid, is where most of the toxins in your body wind up. Many of these toxins are eliminated in the stools, but some are reabsorbed back into the bloodstream. Cleaning your colon regularly will help ensure that toxins leave your body when stools do.

Fast regularly. It's the most effective tool for detoxifying the colon, along with the blood, liver, kidneys, and virtually everything else in your body. "It reduces the body's toxic burden and can help relieve arthritis, eczema, and many other common conditions," says Dr. Beeson.

We talk about fasting in detail in chapter 7 on page 143. In a nutshell, plan on fasting for 3 days at least once a month. A water fast is acceptable, but it can be hard on your body unless you're already in good health. For most people, a juice fast, in which you drink vegetable or fruit juices throughout the day, is better because you'll get the cleansing effects without depleting your body of essential nutrients, says Dr. Beeson. Vegetable juices are optimal because they provide an abundance of fiber and phytonutrients, chemical compounds in foods that neutralize toxic molecules in the body.

Consider a colonic. Self-care enemas and professionally administered colonics are not uniformly recommended by health professionals. Many believe that they are, at best, unnecessary. Others, including Gaia Mather, N.D., believe these techniques are an important part of fasting. Dr. Mather, who offers colonics in a clinical setting and teaches about both colonics and enemas at National College of Naturopathic Medicine in Portland, Oregon, believes they are essential, especially if bowel movements are sluggish. What's more, if you are fasting, Dr. Mather warns that you can reabsorb some of the toxic material that you've just thrown off and lose some of

the benefits you've gained by fasting. For her advice on self-administered enemas during a fast, see "Flushing the Toxic Colon" on page 155.

Cancer Prevention
Keep Your Cells Healthy

Inside your body are some 50 trillion cells, the building blocks of bones, nerves, and everything else that makes you you. As time goes by, every one of these cells will grow, mature, and then divide, forming two new, identical cells to take its place.

At least, that's what's supposed to happen. Should a cell become damaged during the division process—as a result of chance or, more likely, exposure to harmful, toxic substances in the body—it can spin out of control. For example, a cell that should divide once a week could conceivably double, triple, or even quadruple its numbers in a matter of days. Each one of the new cells will also be abnormal, and just as prolific. The result is cancer-cell growth and multiplication that can't be stopped.

Your body is equipped to eliminate or neutralize toxins in the colon, kidneys, liver, and other organs. But our modern world is so full of toxins that the body can't always cope, says Judy Neall, N.D., a naturopathic physician at Natural Choices Health Clinic in Beaverton, Oregon. Air pollution, industrial chemicals, pesticides, and even chemicals or hormones in the body can disrupt the cellular machinery and trigger cancer growth.

Ideally, we should live in a pollution-free world, eat untainted foods, and drink pure water. Since this isn't possible at present, the next best thing is to avoid pollutants whenever possible and to minimize pollutants in the body with the following detoxification plan.

Your Purification Plan

Strategy One: Control Your Hormones

Two of the hormones that play key roles in determining who we are—estrogen in women and testosterone in men—are also the ones that often lead to tumor growth. Women with high levels of estrogen may have a higher risk of developing breast cancer. Men with high levels of testosterone may be more likely to get prostate cancer. You obviously wouldn't want to eliminate these hormones, but it's essential to take steps to minimize their potentially harmful effects.

Say yes to soy. Tofu, tempeh, and other soy foods are rich in plant chemicals called isoflavones, which appear to lower levels of estrogen in the blood and reduce a woman's breast cancer risk. This may explain why women in Japan, who eat soy foods daily, have a much lower rate of breast cancer than American women do. A soy-rich diet is good for men, as well, possibly because these foods temper the effects of testosterone, the "fuel" that causes prostate cancers to grow.

It's not difficult to add more soy to your diet. There are so many delicious possibilities to choose from. Add tofu to your next stir-fry, steam some fresh soybeans, or nosh on soy nuts and snacks. Switch from cow milk to soy milk. Try grilling your steaks with soy sauce and a hint of garlic.

Trim your risk with fiber. The less a woman is exposed to her own reproductive hormones, the lower her risk for developing breast cancer. A fiber-rich diet of fruits, vegetables, whole grains, and legumes lowers levels of estrone, a type of estrogen associated with higher rates of cancer. Fiber also helps flush toxins from the colon. You might also consider adding a commercially available fiber supplement to your diet under the guidelines described on the package.

Lose weight, lower your risk. Much of the body's estrogen is produced by fatty tissues, and much of the body's overload of toxins is stored in fatty tissues. Women who maintain a healthful weight or who successfully lose weight by exercising regularly and eating well have lower levels of estrogen and are less likely to get breast cancer than women who are overweight.

Strategy Two: Eliminate Toxins

Pollution, pesticides, plastics—we live in a remarkably toxic environment, and your body's cells pay the price. The solution isn't to hide out in some super-clean bubble. You need to take advantage of proven body cleansers that seek out potential carcinogens and carry them out of the body.

Load up on citrus. Lemons, limes, and oranges contain a powerful chemical compound called limonene, which stimulates the ability of the immune system to destroy cancer cells before they have a chance to multiply. Citrus fruits also contain glucarase, a compound that neutralizes carcinogens and rushes them out of the body. Laboratory studies show that animals given orange juice had 22 percent fewer colon tumors than animals who didn't get the juice. You might consider making orange juice your breakfast beverage of choice.

Eat dandelion salad. Or drink dandelion tea. This common "yard herb" helps the liver eliminate and break down toxins before they have a chance to damage cells, says Dr. Neall. Even if you have an organic lawn, you should purchase both greens and tea at a natural foods store. You can drink dandelion tea as often as you wish. It helps the liver detoxify the body and is helpful for preventing many conditions in addition to cancer. Just follow the directions on the package.

Clobber carcinogens with crucifers. Broccoli, brussels sprouts, cabbage, and other crucifers are rich in sulforaphane, a chemical compound that increases the body's output of cancer-fighting enzymes. Crucifers are especially important for women because they convert estrogen into a form that's less likely to trigger cell changes that can lead to cancer.

For recipes featuring broccoli, see pages 54 and 61.

Detoxify with garlic. Eat a lot of it. It's one of the most potent cancer-fighting herbs, says Dr. Neall. Garlic contains organosulfurs, chemicals that boost the production of enzymes that detoxify potential carcinogens. Researchers at Memorial Sloan-Kettering Cancer Center in New York City found that substances in garlic also slow the growth of breast, skin, and colon cancers. Other chemicals in garlic help the body to excrete carcinogenic toxins.

A study of nearly 42,000 women found that those who ate more than one weekly serving of garlic—either one fresh clove or a shake of powder—were 35 percent less likely to get colon cancer than those who didn't eat garlic.

Cut the saturated fat. It's among the main cancer risks. A high-fat diet increases levels of cell-damaging molecules, increases production of testosterone and estrogen, and steps up the body's production of bile acid, which may be transformed into cancer-causing compounds, says Dr. Neall.

The National Cancer Institute calls for limiting fat intake to no more than 30 percent of total calories, and less is even better. A study of women in 21 countries found that those who ate high-fat diets had more than five times the risk of breast cancer than women who got only 15 percent of their calories from fat. A diet low in saturated fat can also reduce your risk for colon and prostate cancers, as well as many others.

People who eat less fat invariably find themselves eating more plant foods. The fiber in these foods helps trap cancer-causing substances in the colon. Since the fiber itself isn't absorbed, it rushes these substances out of the body before they can trigger dangerous cell changes.

Strategy Three: Build Your Immune System

Detoxify with antioxidants. Every day your body's cells are damaged by free radicals, toxic oxygen molecules that strip away electrons and potentially set the stage for cancer-causing mutations. It's essential to load up on foods that contain the "big three" antioxidants— beta-carotene and vitamins C and E, says Dr. Neall. They reduce the harmful effects of free radicals and protect cells from life-threatening changes.

- Beta-carotene, found in sweet potatoes, spinach, and other richly colored vegetables, stimulates the release of natural killer cells, immune cells that hunt down and destroy cancer cells. The recommended dosage is 5,000 to 25,000 IU per day, according to Peter Bennett, N.D., a naturopathic physician in Vancouver and coauthor of *7-Day Detox Miracle.*

- Vitamin C, in addition to being one of the most powerful antioxidants, has been shown to prevent carcinogenic compounds from forming in the digestive tract. People who get the most vitamin C in their diets usually have the lowest risks of getting cancer. Dr. Bennett recommends a dosage of 500 to 3,000 mg per day. If you have any digestive problems with vitamin C, lower the dose until the symptoms go away.

⊚ Vitamin E also stimulates the immune system's fight against cancer cells and blocks the effects of free radicals in the body's fatty tissues. A study at State University of New York, Buffalo, found that women who got the most E in their diets were 80 percent less likely to get breast cancer than those getting the least. Since it's difficult to get enough vitamin E from food, consider taking 150 IUs in supplement form.

Detox Makeover

KELLEY SIMMONS IS A VEGETARIAN. She doesn't eat sweets, runs most days of the week, and takes yoga and spinning classes at her health club. She always took it for granted that she, like her parents, would live out her days free from serious illnesses. She was wrong.

In 1998, she was diagnosed with colon cancer. Kelley, who manages a computer store in Green Bay, Wisconsin, was lucky. Her doctors caught the cancer early, and 6 years after surgery she remains cancer-free. But she's not taking any chances.

"After I recovered, I began to read about all of the toxins that have been shown to cause cancer," she says. "I decided to do everything I could to get them out of my body."

After consulting with an herbalist, she started eating dandelion salads every day at lunch to get extra antioxidants. She tops the salads with alfalfa sprouts because they neutralize carcinogens and speed their elimination from the colon. "I never liked garlic very much, but I started eating at least two cloves a day because it breaks down carcinogens," she says.

Her doctors have told her that it's unlikely that the cancer will come back. Kelley believes them. "There aren't any guarantees in this life. All I can do is be smart and keep my diet, and my life, in balance."

COLDS
JUST SAY "NO" TO VIRUSES

Don't blame a virus the next time you're stuck in bed with a cold. It's true that there are more than 200 kinds of viruses that can slip into your nose or lungs and trigger symptoms. It's also true that exposure to even a few viruses can leave you hacking and aching and sneezing for a week or two. (They multiply with amazing speed.) But the virus itself is mainly a trigger.

The reason that you experience so much discomfort is that your body is churning out all sorts of chemicals to combat the infection—chemicals that make you feel a whole lot worse before you start to feel better.

Here's what usually happens when a virus infects a small patch of cells lining the nose. The immune system kicks out a host of histamine, kinins, and interleukins—chemicals known as inflammatory mediators that cause blood vessels to leak and dilate, stimulate pain nerve fibers, and turn on the mucus taps.

Within a day or two, you're wiping your eyes, sneezing until your nose hurts, and hitting the bottom of the tissue box. The virus will eventually get mopped up by your immune system, but you'll keep having symptoms unless you find some way to cleanse your body of all the chemicals and gunk that make you feel so lousy.

Your Purification Plan

Strategy One: Evict the Virus

Scientists have tried for years to find a cure for the common cold, and they're still trying. In the meantime, they've discovered that there are quite a few ways to purge your body of some of the viruses, along with symptom-causing substances spewed out by your immune system.

These techniques are worth doing when you consider that adults get an average of 3 colds a year and children get about 10. And here's some really good news: Some of the same foods and herbs that cleanse your body and reduce symptoms will also prevent these miserable infections from taking hold in the first place.

Get better with ganmaoling. Taken at the very first whisper of a cold, this Chinese herbal blend causes cold viruses to migrate out of the body through the nose, throat, or even the skin, says Alexcia Grimm Trujillo, D.O.M., a doctor of Oriental Medicine at East-West Acupuncture Clinic in Albuquerque, New Mexico. "You'll break into a very slight sweat, and the sweating pushes the pathogen out of the body," she explains.

The usual dose is three to six tablets taken three times daily. You can find this blend in health food stores and natural food stores that sell oriental medicines. If you can't find it near you, try an Internet search for companies that sell the product online. You can also look for Yin Qiao, a similar formula with the same dosage.

Reach for herbal remedies. Both goldenseal and echinacea have been shown to help relieve colds. Both are readily available in convenient capsules or tinctures (liquid drops that you can add to tea). To take these herbs, simply follow the directions on the package.

Sip ginger tea. It purges the body of excess kapha, an Ayurvedic term for a body condition that features "cool and moist" symptoms, such as sneezing and nasal congestion. Studies have shown that ginger contains chemical compounds called sesquiterpenes, which help suppress rhinoviruses, the most common family of cold viruses. Other compounds in ginger, gingerols and shogaols, reduce pain, fever, and coughing. As a bonus, ginger tea tastes a lot better than over-the-counter cold remedies.

To make ginger tea, add about ½ teaspoon each of ginger powder, cinnamon, and fennel seeds to a cup of hot water. Let the tea steep for about 10 minutes,

strain out the herbs, and drink it while it's hot. You can also buy tea bags that contain ginger and other spices at most health food stores. Drink several cups a day for the duration of the cold.

Load up on produce. It's probably the best way to rid your body of virus-causing toxins. Many fruits and vegetables contain glutathione, a chemical compound that stimulates the release of macrophages, your body's own immune cells that essentially mop up viruses for disposal. In addition, fruits and vegetables contain a variety of antioxidants, chemical compounds that knock out toxic cell-damaging molecules called free radicals, which are produced in abundance when you have a cold.

Which fruits and vegetables should you choose? Whichever ones appeal to you! All of them do you some good. If you need an excuse to tear into a couple of oranges, this is it.

Feed a cold. This traditional advice appears to be right after all. Dutch scientists report that eating causes an increase in gamma interferon, an immune chemical that stimulates the body's ability to destroy and clear itself of cold viruses.

Strategy Two: Clear Out Congestion

Since the mucus that forms in your throat and nose is a trap for toxins, you'll want to try some of these tips that also help you breathe easier and sleep more comfortably.

Press away congestion. Firmly pressing the web of skin between your thumb and index finger for about a minute will help break up congestion and remove mucus from your body. You can use the same acupressure technique on the upper ridges of your eye sockets close to the bridge of your nose, or just to the sides of your nostrils along your smile line. "Pressing there will open the sinuses almost instantly," Dr. Grimm Trujillo says.

Mop up with vitamin C. Vitamin C does double-duty. It significantly lowers levels of histamine—an immune chemical that floods your body when you have a cold and is responsible for stuffiness and congestion—while simultaneously knocking down levels of free radicals, says Dr. Grimm Trujillo. A scientific review of 21 studies concluded that taking 1,000 mg of vitamin C daily can reduce the duration of colds by 23 percent.

Breathe better with juice. Fresh pineapple juice is loaded with vitamin C and also helps the body break down mucus and expel it from the body. Drink 4 to 6 ounces of juice (diluted half-and-half with water) at least four times daily when you're battling a cold. If you own a juicer, now is a good time to break it out and drink a variety of fruit and vegetable juices. If you don't own a juicer, use your blender to whip up a smoothie that includes fresh pineapple chunks.

Get hydrated. While you're at it, drink as much water as you can hold, preferably about 2 quarts a day. Colds cause the body to lose tremendous amounts of fluids. Drinking lots of water will help reduce throat scratchiness and headache, while at the same time making mucus thinner and easier to eliminate from the body.

Add some cayenne to your soup. Along with other hot peppers, cayenne is rich in capsaicin, a fiery chemical that's similar to the active ingredients in over-the-counter cold and flu remedies. It will make your nose run almost immediately after you ingest it, a sign that your body is overcoming the head-stuffing congestion.

Steam away congestion. It's not a coincidence that people with colds usually spend quite a bit of time in the shower. Breathing that hot, moisture-laden air is among the best ways to liquefy mucus so that it drains from your nose and airways. Less congestion means less coughing, stuffiness, and chest pain.

Strategy Three: Invigorate Your Body

When you're battling a cold, your purifying plan should include techniques that have been shown to stoke your body's immune response.

Run hot and cold. Lounging in a warm bath stimulates immunity and eliminates toxins through perspiration. Following a warm bath with a quick rinse in cold water—a technique known as contrast hydrotherapy—is even better because it constricts blood vessels and reduces fever and inflammation.

Free yourself from stress. It doesn't matter whether you breathe deeply for a few minutes, do yoga for half an hour, or simply take a quick walk around the block, as long as you reduce anxiety and stress and get back into your comfort zone. Studies have shown that people with high stress also have high levels of interleukin-6, an immune chemical that makes you more vulnerable to cold symptoms.

Get out of bed. The very idea of exercise when you have a cold probably makes your sinuses hurt, but try to do it anyway. Moderate exercise causes infection-fighting white blood cells to leave the organs and enter the bloodstream, where they're better able to expel the cold-causing virus.

Strategy Four: Eliminate Irritants

It's important to take special care of your respiratory system when you are suffering from a cold.

Clear the air. Second-hand cigarette smoke or the clouds of carbon monoxide from a passing bus do more than irritate your throat when you have a cold. Air pollution also causes cells to dump inflammatory chemicals called cytokines into your body. These are the chemicals that make your eyes puffy, your nose run, and your eyes water. You can't avoid all air pollution, of course, but do what you can by insisting that people smoke outside, for example, or by staying indoors during high-traffic hours.

DIGESTION
DETOX YOUR DIGESTIVE TRACT

Even though detoxification therapy to clean out the digestive tract has been practiced for thousands of years, most mainstream doctors view it as unproven at best, and fraudulent at worst. Yet the need to detoxify the intestine and digestive organs could well be greater today than it's ever been.

By the time you reach adulthood, you've probably consumed close to 200 pounds of lead, mercury, and other dangerous metals. Across the country, drinking water contains dozens of known carcinogens. Studies have shown that the

Detox Makeover

MOST ADULTS GET AT LEAST THREE COLDS A YEAR. Molly Hopkins, a 60-year-old landscape designer in Albuquerque, New Mexico, hasn't had a cold in years. When she feels one starting, she takes quick action to make sure it doesn't progress to full-blown misery.

"I'm really tuned in to my body, so I recognize the signs right away," she says. "I take a goldenseal and echinacea tincture every hour for the first few hours. I also eat a huge amount of vegetables, along with chicken soup and Chinese mushrooms."

That's the first part of her cold-purification plan. She also avoids meat as well as dairy foods that cause an increase in congestion in some people. She drinks water by the pitcherful. And, on the advice of her doctor, she wraps a hot pack around her throat to promote lymph-node drainage.

"I hate colds more than just about anything, and so far I've been pretty lucky," she says. "Knock on wood!"

cellular tissue of the average adult contains 177 different types of chlorine substances, many of them carcinogenic.

Our ancestors ate whole foods grown organically and free of pesticides. They got an abundance of fiber in their diets, and none of the foods they ate were treated with preservatives. None of this is true today. In addition to external contaminants, our bodies also produce toxins in response to infections, drug use, and digestive disorders, explains

Anil Minocha, M.D., professor of medicine and director of the division of digestive diseases at the University of Mississippi Medical Center, Jackson, and author of *Natural Stomach Care*.

When you get overloaded with toxins, they begin to leak out of your digestive system and into your blood. From there they migrate to cells throughout your body, and there they stay until your body's natural cleansing processes get rid of them. In the meantime, they can damage cells, cause depression and fatigue, and possibly shorten your life.

Your Purification Plan

Strategy One: Try Dr. Minocha's 6 Tips for Fasting

Nearly everyone will feel better, and be healthier, if they undergo regular detoxification. Fasting is probably the best approach because it gives the digestive organs a chance to rest and recuperate, while at the same time it purges toxins from the intestine, liver, and other parts of your body. "It's like spring-cleaning," says Dr. Minocha. "You'll be surprised how much better you feel."

Obviously, you should fast only if you're in good health, and be sure to discuss your plans with a health professional before jumping in. You can potentially go without solid food for weeks, but 3 days is about right for most people. There are many different kinds of fasts, but a water fast is the simplest and often the most effective, according to Dr. Minocha. (For a more extensive discussion of the different kinds of fasts and how they're used, see chapter 7 on page 143.) Here's Dr. Minocha's recommended approach.

1. On the day you start your fast, drink two glasses of water as soon as you wake up, and two more glasses a few hours later. Follow this with a glass of water at mid-morning, lunch, late afternoon, early and late evening, and before you go to bed. Don't eat any solid food at all.

2. Give yourself time to urinate. With all of the water you're drinking, you'll need to urinate a lot, so make sure you don't get stuck on the freeway or in an area without a public restroom at an inopportune time. Urination is good because it flushes huge amounts of toxins from the body, so you want to make sure you can go whenever you need to.

3. Sip clear soups if you have to. Ideally, you won't ingest anything except water during your fast, but if your stomach won't leave you alone, have some bouillon or miso soup. If you're really desperate, have a few bites of a banana or applesauce.

4. Get plenty of rest, but at the same time, work some gentle exercises, such as walking or light stretching, into your day. Exercise increases metabolism and speeds the elimination of toxins in sweat and urine.

5. Take a multivitamin supplement once daily, along with 1,000 mg of vitamin C three times daily for the duration of the fast. You'll need the extra nutrients to stay healthy and energized.

6. On the third or fourth day, break the

fast by gradually reintroducing solid foods into your system. You might want to start out by eating a little yogurt, soft fruit, or vegetables. Later in the day have a little protein in the form of beans, chicken, or lean beef. Keep adding foods slowly back into your diet over a period of several days.

Most people who fast experience sensations of inner peace and energy, says Dr. Minocha. You may decide you want to have a quick, 1-day purification fast every few weeks or once a month. Some people schedule a longer fast every year—on their birthdays, for example, or on another date that's easy to remember.

Strategy Two: Eat Pure, Be Pure

There are many ways to detoxify the digestive tract. Some health care professionals swear by colonics, although there's certainly no consensus on that score. (See "Flushing the Toxic Colon" on page 155 for more information on colonics.) Others recommend saunas or steam baths, while still others depend on exercise or a dry brush massage—techniques that facilitate the excretion of toxins through the skin and open up your natural detox channels. But perhaps the most effective approach is to include in your diet easily digestible foods that have very specific (and different) toxin-fighting properties.

Recover from infections with B and C. If you've recently had a cold or a bacterial infection, take extra helpings of foods rich in B vitamins, such as whole grain bread, and foods with vitamin C, such as citrus, peppers, and cabbage. Each of these nutrients helps cleanse the body of toxins generated by harmful microorganisms, says Dr. Minocha.

Scrub out additives with sulfur. It's almost impossible to avoid food additives and preservatives—chemicals that can drain your energy and weaken your health. So it's a good idea to eat plenty of foods rich in sulfur, such as garlic, red peppers, egg yolks, and cruciferous vegetables. They help eliminate food chemicals, along with environmental pollutants, from the body.

Purify your gut with chlorophyll. Found in green foods like cabbage, lettuce, and parsley, chlorophyll cleanses the intestine, oxygenates the blood, and speeds internal healing.

Give beneficial "bugs" a home. Yogurt is among the healthiest foods you can eat. In addition to its generous payload of calcium and other nutrients, it contains probiotics, beneficial bacteria that take up residence in your intestine and help displace harmful organisms.

Strategy Three: Supplement Your Detox Diet

A healthful diet can do only so much to keep your system toxin-free. Fortunately, there are a number of over-the-counter supplements that break down toxins and help eliminate them from your body. Dr. Minocha recommends using only one or two at a time. "We know that each one is effective, but there isn't any research that has looked at their use in combination," he says. The supplements below are available at health food stores. Follow the directions on the label.

Psyllium husk powder. It absorbs water in the intestine and helps stools pass through more quickly. This is important because stools are loaded with potential carcinogens and other toxins. The more quickly they move through your body, the less likely it is that the toxins they contain will leak through your intestinal wall and into your bloodstream.

Milk thistle. Studies show that this herb helps neutralize a number of toxins, including carbon tetrachloride and alcohol, both of which can cause serious liver damage. The active compound in milk thistle, silymarin, helps damaged liver cells regenerate, and it also helps the liver eliminate toxins more efficiently.

Bentonite clay. It comes from volcanic ash and is very efficient at absorbing bacteria and contaminants and removing them from your body through the stool. (We're referring only to purified clay, of course.)

Flaxseed. It acts as a gentle laxative and helps eliminate toxins from the body. It's also an antioxidant that helps neutralize the effects of free radicals, which are harmful, oxygen-based molecules that have been linked to dozens of serious diseases, including cancer.

FATIGUE
BOOST YOUR ENERGY

Fatigue is such a "normal" part of our lives that it's easy to forget that it isn't normal at all. In fact, it's one of the most common health problems, accounting for up to 15 million doctor visits a year. It can sap your motivation, damage your relationships, and take the fun out of life.

You need to see a doctor if your energy levels have taken a sudden nosedive. There's a good chance, however, that all of the standard tests will show that you're perfectly healthy, even though you know in your tired bones that something's not quite right.

That "something" could turn out to be toxicity. When your body is working overtime due to accumulations of heavy metals, pesticides, or other toxins, you're going to have less energy to live your life. "By pushing so hard we exhaust the organs in the body; they just get tired," says Peter Bennett, N.D., a naturopathic physician from Vancouver and coauthor of *7-Day Detox Miracle.*

There are any number of herbs and supplements that can help restore physical and mental energy, but they're much more effective when you first cleanse your body of the toxins that are dragging you down.

Your Purification Plan

Strategy One: Reduce Your Toxic Load

Toxicity occurs when your body accumulates more toxins and wastes than it can eliminate. Conversely, every cell and organ in your body works more efficiently when you help it eliminate toxins. Here's what you need to do.

Start with a 2-day liquid fast. "Fasting is critical because it shifts the body into a filtering mode," says Dr. Bennett. For 2 days, don't eat any food at all. Drink at least eight full glasses of water each day, more if you're still thirsty. A water-only fast allows the liver, intestine, and other organs to focus on eliminating toxins rather than coping with digestion. If you

want, drink lemon water instead of plain water. Squeeze half an organically grown lemon into a quart of water, drop in the peel, and leave it there.

After the 2-day fast, eat plenty of fresh fruits, vegetables, and brown rice, and nothing else for 5 days. These easily digested foods will allow the intestine and liver to continue cleansing themselves.

Improve circulation with hydrotherapy. This technique stimulates the pumping action of blood vessels and helps flush out toxins, while at the same time bringing energizing oxygen to cells throughout your body, says Dr. Bennett.

Hydrotherapy can be as simple as letting hot water cascade over your back for about 5 minutes in the shower, followed by a 30-second, cold water splash. Repeat the cycle three times, then curl up in bed under the covers for about half an hour. You'll probably feel a surge of energy right away, and the energy will persist as more and more toxins leave your system.

Cleanse the intestine. When you switch to easy-to-digest plant foods after the initial liquid fast, you'll naturally get a lot of fiber in your diet. Fiber accelerates the passage of stools and also binds to bile, a digestive fluid, in the intestine. This is important because bile contains toxins that can be reabsorbed into the bloodstream and drag your energy down. The idea is to get bile moving out with the stools instead of hanging around waiting to be reabsorbed.

Get a lot of vitamin C. Plan on taking 1,000 mg three times daily. It speeds the transit of stools and toxins out of the intestine, and it also detoxifies the toxins so you're less likely to experience a "healing crisis" (a sudden increase in fatigue or other symptoms) during and after your fast.

Strategy Two: Stimulate Your Body's Best Filter

The liver is the body's recycling plant for toxins, the place where harmful substances are transformed and broken down into harmless by-products. Because of our modern diet and lifestyle, the liver often gets overburdened and congested, which can lead to profound fatigue. There are several ways to stimulate the liver.

Eat fish several times a week. Fish oils are essential for Phase 1 detoxification, the stage in which liver enzymes break down toxins. The problem with fish, of course, is that it often contains mercury. "Salmon seems to be the cleanest fish," says Dr. Bennett. Wild salmon has fewer toxins than farmed salmon. Or you can take 2 g daily of pharmaceutical-grade fish oil, which is mercury-free.

Eat more fruits and vegetables. They replenish your body's stores of glutathione, an amino acid that's essential for Phase 2 detox, which includes the breakdown of carcinogens as well as PCBs and other industrial chemicals.

Eat high-quality proteins. You get these from lean, organic meats, low-fat dairy products, and eggs. They act on the liver's sulfation pathways. Sulfation is the process that breaks down steroid hormones, industrial chemicals, and bacterial toxins. Vegetable sources of sulfur include onions, celery, kale, and soybeans, says Dr. Bennett.

For a recipe featuring eggs, see page 62.

Get a handle on stress. It acts almost like an energy vacuum because it triggers the release of a flood of "fight or flight" hormones such as cortisol. These hormones make the body work overtime and block the liver's ability to detoxify chemical compounds.

Alternate-nostril breathing is a quick, efficient way to reduce mental and emotional stress. While sitting in a comfortable position, exhale all the air from your lungs, close your right nostril with your thumb, and inhale slowly and deeply through your left nostril. Then close your left nostril and exhale slowly and deeply through your right nostril.

Repeat the same steps, only this time inhale through your right nostril and exhale through your left. Repeat the whole sequence 10 to 30 times.

Strategy Three: Eat for Energy

You've probably noticed that some foods make you sleepy and droopy, while others give you energy to burn. Studies have shown that the foods we eat have a direct effect on our hormones and other body chemicals that can elevate mood. At the same time, eating the "wrong" foods can have the opposite effect and leave you tired and drained.

After you've cleansed your body of toxins, here's what you need to do to keep your energy levels high.

Relief from Chronic Fatigue

SCIENTISTS HAVE ALL BUT EXHAUSTED THEMSELVES trying to figure out chronic fatigue syndrome (CFS), a mystifying and debilitating illness that causes extreme fatigue and other symptoms. There isn't a cure for CFS, but some purifying plans do seem to help.

Get sugar out of your diet. It stimulates the growth of yeasts and other organisms that may be linked to chronic fatigue.

Try an elimination diet. People who are sensitive to the gluten in wheat or the casein in dairy foods may have immune reactions that cause fatigue along with joint pain, headaches, and other symptoms. Eliminate these foods, one at a time, for at least a month to see if there's any improvement.

Try an herbal blend. The antiviral herbs echinacea, goldenseal, licorice, ginger, and lemon balm, combined in equal amounts to make a tea, may clean up infections that contribute to chronic fatigue. You can purchase the dried herbs in many natural food stores. Mix the herbs, then steep a teaspoonful in a cup of hot water for about 10 minutes. Strain and drink it two to three times daily.

Avoid processed foods. Even though food preservatives and additives are considered "safe" by mainstream experts, over a lifetime they dump a tremendous amount of chemicals into your body. These chemicals stress your liver and other elimination organs and can leave you feeling worn down.

Switch to decaf. Forget the quick lift that you get from coffee and other caffeinated beverages—it's almost always followed by an energy crash, says Diane Spindler, Ph.D., N.D., a board certified naturopath and owner of Mountain Holistic Health in Indian Hills, Colorado. Caffeine is a diuretic that can dehydrate you. Dehydration increases the concentration of toxins that put extra strain on the liver and can put your metabolism in low gear.

Take a pass on simple carbs. Whole grains, legumes, fruits, and vegetables are among the best foods you can eat because the complex carbohydrates they contain enter your body at a steady, energy-giving pace, says Dr. Spindler. Simple carbohydrates, on the other hand, send blood-sugar levels soaring. When you eat sugary cereals, sweet snacks, white bread, pasta, and other concentrated sources of simple carbohydrates that convert to sugar in your body, the body responds with a flood of insulin. Insulin quickly removes the sugars from the blood, and that's when your energy drops into the basement.

FERTILITY
INCREASE YOUR CHANCES OF CONCEPTION

Having a baby is one of life's most fulfilling experiences. Unfortunately, getting pregnant can be a long, difficult process for about 15 percent of couples who want to conceive. If you and your partner have been trying to get pregnant for more than a year, it's likely that something is interfering with your reproductive abilities, and that something could be linked to toxins.

Women often blame themselves when they can't get pregnant. Yet in about 40 percent of cases, poor sperm quality or quantity is a key factor. In both men and women, exposure to pesticides, industrial chemicals, and other toxins has been linked to drops in fertility.

An Environmental Protection Agency (EPA) study reported that women who were regularly exposed to pesticides were up to three times more likely to become infertile than women without the chemical exposure. And in the last few decades, sperm counts worldwide have plummeted.

"Couples need to remove from their bodies any toxins that alter their natural or chemical balances," says Janet Starr Hull, Ph.D., a nutritionist in the Dallas area and author of *10 Steps to Detoxification*. The estrogen-like effects of many environmental toxins, or xenoestrogens, can increase a woman's chances of getting endometriosis, a leading cause of infertility. In men, xenoestrogens can lower levels of testosterone and impair sperm health.

Your Purification Plan

Strategy One: Reduce Your Exposure

You can't entirely avoid environmental chemicals, of course, but you can eliminate all or most of them from your body. "When you clear out the toxins, the ability to conceive can significantly improve," says Dr. Hull.

Avoid plastics whenever you can. One way to cut your risk of harmful exposure is to avoid using plastic water bottles, plastic food containers, and plastic to heat foods in the microwave. Many plastics contain estrogen-like chemical compounds that leach into the body. Over time this can increase endometriosis in women and change the testosterone balance in men, says Heidi Weinhold, N.D., a naturopathic physician at The Enhancement Center in McMurray, Pennsylvania.

Strategy Two: Boost Your Body's Natural Cleaners

The more vitality you can bring to your skin and liver, the more your body will be able to rid itself of toxins you can't avoid. Here are some easy ways to accomplish that.

Work up a sweat. The skin is one of the main organs of elimination. When you perspire from exercise or when you lounge in a dry- or moist-heat sauna, toxins are released from fatty tissues and eliminated in perspiration.

Enjoy a very gentle massage. Once every few days, have your partner stroke your skin with a feather-light touch, moving from the outer parts of your body inward toward your heart. Then do the same for your partner. A "soft" massage stimulates the lymph glands just beneath the skin and helps accelerate the excretion of toxins that can interfere with fertility.

Drink marshmallow root tea. It improves the ability of the liver to process and eliminate wastes, says Dr. Hull. "Have a cup or two a day when you're trying to get pregnant," she advises. It essentially makes toxins less sticky and easier to purge from the bloodstream.

This herbal tea is available at health food stores. Follow the directions on the package.

Strategy Three: Control Yeast

Many women are infected with subclinical levels of yeast, which can make it harder to conceive. These approaches can help restore optimal balance.

Supplement with caprylic acid. It's a fatty acid extracted from plant fats, such as coconut and palm oils. It's very effective at eliminating yeast and restoring a woman's natural hormone balance, says Dr. Hull. Caprylic acid is available in health food stores. Take the amount recommended on the label.

Eat alkaline foods. Yeast thrives in acidic environments. To make your body more alkaline and yeast-resistant, eat only organic foods, especially rice, beans, whole grains, and produce, Dr. Hull advises.

Strategy Four: Improve Your Odds with Nutrition

Dozens of physical problems can interfere with conception, but for some couples, just changing what's on the menu can put them back on the baby track. Studies have shown, for example, that a man's sperm may go to sleep on the job if he doesn't get a few key nutrients. A woman's body may be more receptive to pregnancy if she eats wholesome, organic foods. Both men and women can enhance their ability to eliminate toxins if they make a few simple dietary changes.

Load up on vitamin C. Men and women need this nutrient more than ever because it helps eliminate toxins in the sweat and urine, says Dr. Hull. In addition, the sperm in men who get adequate vitamin C tend to pick up speed and maintain their forward momentum. Finally, vitamin C is a powerful antioxidant that helps neutralize fertility-impairing molecules called free radicals. Take 250 to 1,000 mg of vitamin C daily, Dr. Hull advises.

Get extra selenium and zinc. Like vitamin C, this trace mineral is a powerful antioxidant that mops free radicals from the body. "People who live in toxic environments, as just about all of us do, tend to be deficient in selenium," says Dr. Weinhold. "If you're having trouble conceiving, supplement your diet with about 400 mcg of selenium daily," she advises.

It's also helpful to take a multivitamin supplement that includes zinc, Dr. Weinhold says. "It increases sperm levels, which is especially important for men who have been exposed to environmental chemicals."

Fillings and Infertility

MERCURY IS PROBABLY THE MOST TOXIC of the naturally occurring heavy metals. Scientists now believe that mercury exposure is a common cause of health problems, including infertility. Dental amalgams, or fillings, are the main source of human exposure. In fact, you could be absorbing up to 100 mcg of mercury daily if you have a lot of fillings. You could also be overloaded with mercury if you eat a lot of seafood, especially fatty fish such as tuna, which can accumulate enormous amounts of heavy metals and other toxins.

Chinese researchers who studied 150 infertile couples found that more than a third of the men and 23 percent of the women had abnormally high mercury concentrations in their blood. Doctors who specialize in natural therapy sometimes use vitamin C to pull mercury out of the body. Other steps you can take to minimize toxicity:

- Don't chew gum if you have fillings. Mercury escapes up to 20 times faster during chewing.
- Try probiotics. Acidophilus supplements aid in detoxification by restoring intestinal bacteria that are damaged by mercury.
- Eat the right kind of fish. Small panfish, such as perch and stream trout, generally have lower levels of mercury and other contaminants than large fish do.
- Eat canned light tuna packed in water. It may have lower mercury levels than tuna steaks or canned albacore tuna.
- Consult a holistic dentist. Discuss the possibility of removing amalgam fillings, which contain toxic mercury, and replacing them with nontoxic gold or composite fillings.

Get the fat out of your diet. It's one of the most important things you can do when you're trying to get pregnant. High levels of dietary fat can change your natural hormone balance, Dr. Weinhold says. Fat increases levels of free radicals and inflammation. It also tends to raise levels of cholesterol, which clings to arteries and restricts bloodflow to the reproductive organs. Nutrition experts recommend that you get no more than 30 percent of your calories from fat.

Shop from the produce aisle. A plant-based diet floods the body with phytochemicals, plant compounds that block the harmful effects of toxic free radicals, says Dr. Weinhold. Women who improve their diets and eat more plant foods and less meat tend to have lower levels of toxins and a lower incidence of endometriosis, she adds.

Flush toxins from the colon. The liver, kidney, and other elimination organs are very efficient at removing toxins from your body. If you aren't having regular bowel movements, however, toxins that should be eliminated in the stools can be reabsorbed back into the blood. "A high-fiber diet will help clean out the colon," Dr. Weinhold says. Good sources of fiber include beans, most produce, and oatmeal.

Imbibe little or not at all. A few glasses of wine might put you in the mood for love, but they won't do a thing for your chances of having a baby. Harvard researchers found that women who had more than one drink a day were 60 percent more likely to be infertile than women who abstained. Wine and other liquors can cause problems for men as well. Even small amounts of alcohol lower testosterone and make sperm less hardy.

Cut the caffeine. A study of more than 1,400 women found that women who got about 300 mg of caffeine daily (about the amount in five cups of coffee) were 2½ times more likely to have trouble conceiving than women who drank less. Scientists speculate that caffeine may alter a woman's hormone balance and interfere with her ability to ovulate.

HEADACHES AND MIGRAINES
PAIN BEGONE

So many people get headaches that you'd have to look hard to find someone who doesn't get them. At least 50 million American adults see their doctors for headaches each year, and no one can even guess how many people simply take care of the pain themselves.

Headaches may be common, but

there's nothing normal about them. You can bet that something in your body is triggering the pain, causing a chemical cascade that irritates nerves, blood vessels, muscles, or a combination of all three.

"Impurities in the body can block the channels of circulation and prevent nutrients from effectively nourishing nerve tissue," explains Mercedes Williams, N.D., a naturopathic physician at Alternatives in Health in Scottsdale, Arizona. "This can also prevent waste products from being efficiently eliminated, allowing the buildup of toxins throughout your system."

About 90 percent of headaches are the so-called tension-type. Doctors used to think they were caused by muscle tension, but new evidence suggests that chemicals in the brain irritate nerves and blood vessels. Migraines are less common, but much more severe. They're probably triggered by the release of neuropeptides, substances that cause blood vessels to get dilated and inflamed.

Your Purification Plan: Headaches

Strategy One: Clean Out Triggers

Since there are probably hundreds, if not thousands, of potential pain triggers,

your first step has to be to get them out of your life. Here's what you need to do.

Identify and eliminate key offenders. It's not as easy as it sounds. Some people get headaches when they eat chocolate, eggs, or mustard. Others are sensitive to red wine, fermented foods, or artificial sweeteners. Others react to sugar, dairy, nuts, or pickles. "Eliminating some or most of these foods for a few weeks is a good way to test if they're a trigger for you," says Dr. Williams.

If you keep having pain, you'll have to look a little more closely at your diet. Write down everything you eat for a few months, and see if you can link headaches to specific foods or ingredients. As soon as you have a suspect, give it up and see if things improve.

Clear your home environment. Why bombard yourself with chemicals unnecessarily? "Make your home a safe haven by using air and water purifiers, along with nontoxic paints and cleaning agents," recommends Dr. Williams.

Keep your blood sugar stable. The sudden spikes and subsequent drops in blood sugar that occur when you follow the traditional, three-squares-a-day eating plan are a common cause of headaches, says Dr. Williams. "Eating small, frequent, nutritious meals will keep blood sugar more stable," she explains.

Strategy Two: Sweep Toxins from Your Body

You also need to purge your body of chemical buildups that make you much more susceptible to headaches in the first place.

You can avoid some toxins by eating organic foods and avoiding products loaded with chemical dyes, preservatives, and additives. But we live in a toxic world, and you can't possibly avoid every potential headache trigger. What you can do, however, is help your liver and other organs excrete toxins more efficiently. "You have to support your body's natural detoxification pathways," says Dr. Williams.

Learn to love the lowly dandelion. Drink several cups of dandelion tea each day to increase bloodflow to your liver and help it remove toxins. Other liver-protecting supplements include milk thistle and artichoke leaf. To use any of these herbs, follow the directions on the package.

Eat plenty of fiber. All of those fresh fruits, whole grains, legumes, and vegetables that form the backbone of an organic diet also help your intestines eliminate toxins more quickly, says Dr. Williams.

Brush yourself. Use a soft brush to dry rub every inch of your skin, always brushing toward the center of your body. This helps pump toxins out of your lymphatic system so that they can be processed by your liver and kidneys, says Margaret Beeson, N.D., a naturopathic physician at Yellowstone Naturopathic Clinic in Billings, Montana.

Warm up. Lounging in a warm environment opens blood vessels and helps your circulatory system get rid of toxins, says Dr. Beeson. If you don't have access to a sauna, spend an occasional half-hour in a hot bath spiked with 2 cups of Epsom salts. Just stir in the salts until they dissolve, climb into the tub, and relax. The salts (magnesium sulfate) help pull toxins out through the skin.

Get professional care. Buildups of heavy metals in the body are a common cause of headaches, says Dr. Williams. "Have a knowledgeable practitioner test for mercury or other environmental toxicities," she suggests. If these toxins are present, the medical professional you've consulted can give you information on how to get rid of them.

You also might want to see a chiropractor, who can check your spine for misalignment. "Back and neck pain may be related to headaches," she explains.

Strategy Three: Reduce Muscle Tension

For most of us, this means eliminating the stress from our lives; stress that causes muscles to bunch and tighten increases blood pressure and causes levels of pain-causing stress hormones to rise. Here are a few simple ways to relax.

Go yoga. This ancient practice is now one of the hottest trends in healthy living. It's a great way to reduce emotional and physical stress, and you don't have to be a human pretzel to do it. Just about every health club offers yoga classes for every level of experience and physical fitness. Even if you can't attend a class, you can benefit from some of yoga's principles by giving yourself time to breathe deeply for 10 to 15 minutes a day. Even doing simple stretches will help you feel mentally and physically refreshed, while also flushing chemicals and metabolic wastes from your body before they cause head-pounding pain.

Oil your temples. Mix a few drops of lavender essential oil in a tablespoon of a "carrier" oil (such as olive or almond oil) and rub it on your temples. Lavender relaxes muscles and helps reduce headache-causing stress, says Dr. Williams. Studies have shown, in fact,

that applying lavender can stop headaches that are already in progress.

Your Purification Plan: Migraines

Migraines affect less than 10 percent of people with headaches, but they cause a disproportionate amount of misery. It's not just that migraines are so painful. They can also cause nausea, intense sensitivity to light, and depression—and they rarely disappear entirely with conventional treatments.

Work with your doctor if you suffer from migraines, Dr. Williams says. In addition, here are a few supplements that can make a real difference. For each one, follow the manufacturer's instructions for proper dosage.

Strategy One: Find the Right Supplement Combination

Try feverfew. Studies have shown that this head-protecting herb, available in health food stores, can be used to treat as well as prevent migraines. It blocks the body's production of prostaglandins and other neurochemicals that cause inflammation and pain in blood vessels in the brain.

Feverfew has to be taken regularly to be effective, Dr. Williams says, so don't try it only when you have a migraine.

Pump energy into your cells. It's thought that abnormal functioning of mitochondria, the microscopic "engines" that keep your cells running, may contribute to migraines. An over-the-counter supplement, coenzyme Q10, seems to help mitochondria work more efficiently, says Dr. Williams.

Bet on butterbur. Petadolex, a patented form of the herb, appears to block the effects of inflammatory chemicals while helping brain blood vessels relax. In one study, people who took butterbur extract had an almost 50 percent reduction in the frequency of migraines after just 1 month. Another study showed even better results: People saw their migraine frequency drop by 62 percent, and the headaches that did occur were less severe and lasted a shorter time, says Dr. Williams.

Heart Disease
Clean Your Vessels, Protect Your Heart

More than half a million Americans die from heart disease every year. What makes this statistic especially sad is that

Do You Need a Drug Detox?

IF YOU GET MORE THAN A FEW HEADACHES A WEEK and also take over-the-counter or prescription drugs to control them, there's a good chance that your "treatment" is part of your problem. People who routinely use drugs for headaches often get "rebound headaches." The waxing and waning of drug levels in their bodies can trigger pain-causing changes in blood vessels or nerves in the brain.

Doctors in headache clinics routinely detoxify patients off painkillers, doing it gradually over a period of days, until they're entirely flushed out. In some cases, eliminating headache drugs also eliminates the headaches. (This should always be done under medical supervision to prevent sudden flare-ups of symptoms.)

heart disease is almost always preventable. You can probably recite your doctor's usual advice by heart: quit smoking, eat less fat, lose weight, and so on.

What you might not know is that most cases of heart disease are linked to substances naturally produced by the body. Consider cholesterol: It's essential in normal amounts to strengthen cell membranes and manufacture key hormones. But it turns deadly when you have too much. Other body chemicals can also rise to unhealthful, toxic levels and threaten your heart, your arteries, and your life.

Then there are external toxins, such as pesticides, preservatives in foods, and cigarette smoke. When you light up a smoke, for example, your lungs fill with chemicals that spread throughout your bloodstream, damage artery walls, and promote accumulations of plaque (fatty deposits that interfere with normal bloodflow and increase your risk of blood-stopping clots). Smokers have two to four times the risk of nonsmokers of dying suddenly from a heart attack. On a more positive note, smokers who quit and rid their bodies of the harmful substances eventually have the same lower risk as nonsmokers.

Here's some even better news. Nearly all of the major risk factors for heart dis-ease can be reduced and often eliminated by following an action plan to scour your arteries and keep your body waste-free.

Your Purification Plan

Strategy One: Tame Toxic Molecules

You can't live without oxygen, but that doesn't mean it's always good for you. Your body faces nearly constant assaults from free radicals, unstable oxygen molecules that damage tissues throughout your body, including in the arteries that carry blood to your heart.

Your body produces chemicals—antioxidants—that stop some free-radical damage. You don't produce enough of these chemicals to stay entirely healthy, however. That's why your body needs antioxidant-rich foods that contain healthful substances that essentially mop up free radicals and minimize their toxic effects, says Judy Neall, N.D., a naturo-pathic physician at Natural Choices Health Clinic in Beaverton, Oregon.

In addition to a low-fat diet rich in healthful grains and produce, here's what you need to do most.

Clean up with onions. They're among the best sources of flavonoids, a family of plant chemicals that are potent antioxidants. As a heart-healthy bonus, they act like a Teflon coating and make platelets (celllike structures found in your blood that are responsible for clumping) less likely to form blood-blocking clots.

In addition to onions, other flavonoid-rich foods include apples, celery, berries, tea, and red wine. A study in the Netherlands found that men who got the most flavonoids in their diets were half as likely to get heart disease as those who ate the least.

For a recipe featuring onions, see page 58.

Avoid highly processed foods. Basically, this means eliminating or drastically curtailing your consumption of most foods that come in a package or box, along with preserved foods such as bacon and sausage. Most processed and preserved foods contain chemicals that turn into free radicals in the body, Dr. Neall explains. What do you do instead? Try grilling or roasting some lean meat, chicken, or fish, and enjoying it with a great big salad. What could be simpler?

Scour your arteries with vitamin E. This is probably the most important antioxidant for heart health because it prevents free radicals from damaging the harmful, LDL form of cholesterol. Damaged LDL is more likely to cling to arteries, reduce bloodflow, and set the stage for a future heart attack.

Vitamin E is found mainly in cooking oils and nuts. You may want to get extra amounts by taking a daily supplement that provides 150 IU.

Recycle E with C. Like vitamin E, vitamin C is a powerful antioxidant—one that also recharges vitamin E and keeps it active in the body. Studies show that people who eat foods that are high in vitamin C, such as citrus and other fruits, have lower rates of heart disease. Sounds like another good reason to make orange juice your breakfast beverage of choice.

Bet on beta-carotene. It's a red-yellow plant pigment that turns into vitamin A in your body. At the same time, it mops up free radicals that can eventually damage your heart. The best food sources are dark green, leafy vegetables, such as spinach, and deep orange fruits and vegetables, such as sweet potatoes. Raw baby spinach, along with sliced tomato and onion, makes a great salad.

Strategy Two: Cut Down the "New Risks"

Many people with heart disease have obvious risk factors. They smoke, they don't exercise, or they eat high-fat foods. But heart disease also strikes men and women who appear to do everything right. The reason, scientists have recently learned, is that millions of Americans—anywhere from 25 to 50 percent of those with cardiovascular diseases—have chemicals in their bodies that greatly increase their risks. You can't eliminate these chemicals completely, but there are ways to knock them down to safer levels. Here's what doctors advise.

Fortify with fiber. The "roughage" in plant foods, especially the soluble form of fiber found in beans, fruits, and grains, removes cholesterol from the body and lowers levels of C-reactive protein, a liver protein that's been linked to inflammation in the arteries. "By promoting bowel function, it reduces the potential to reabsorb inflammatory chemicals from the intestine," says Dr. Neall.

You need about 25 grams of fiber daily to protect your heart. Super sources include chickpeas, kidney beans, dried fruits, and oatmeal.

For a recipe featuring beans, see page 58.

Fight back with folate. Folate is a B vitamin that lowers levels of homocysteine, an amino acid that can increase your risk of cardiovascular disease. In fact, people with elevated homocysteine may be four times more likely to have heart problems than those with normal levels.

Your doctor can check homocysteine levels with a simple blood test. If you have too much, make an extra effort to get plenty of folate and B vitamins in your diet. The best sources are green, leafy vegetables and fortified grains such as rice. You can also take a multivitamin supplement that provides 400 mcg of folic acid daily.

Quit smoking to lower fibrinogen. It's a blood protein that increases your tendency to form clots in your arteries. People who quit smoking often reduce fibrinogen to normal levels. Until you quit (and even after), ask your doctor if you should take an aspirin every other day. It reduces the tendency of blood to form heart-threatening clots in the arteries.

Strategy Three: Muster Your Defenses

Heart disease doesn't happen all at once. It's a decades-long process caused by incremental assaults on the arteries. It's essential to cleanse your body of substances that put unnecessary stress on your system—stresses that, over time, can cause permanent damage. Here's where to start.

Restrict sodium to lower blood pressure. Hypertension (high blood pressure) is a complicated disease with dozens of effective treatment options, but everyone should make an effort to get no more than 2,000 mg of sodium daily. Less than 1,500 mg is even better. (One teaspoon of table salt contains approximately 2,000 mg of sodium.) Reducing salt causes the body to accumulate less fluid, which in turn means less strain on the heart and arteries.

Douse inflammation with fish. People who eat several weekly servings of fish have a lower risk of heart attack, in part because the omega-3 fatty acids in fish lower levels of inflammatory chemicals in the body. "The fish has to be from a healthful source, such as wild salmon," says Dr. Neall. "Farmed fish tends to be higher in toxins."

If you're not a fish lover, it's fine to take a couple tablespoons or four capsules of fish oil daily, she says.

Burn belly fat. Being overweight is among the leading risk factors for heart disease, and the risk is even higher when you carry the fat around your abdomen. If you have a potbelly or spare tire, do everything you can to get back in shape. Losing as little as 10 pounds can significantly lower blood pressure and protect your heart. It's easy to do by taking smaller serving sizes, going for long walks, and working out regularly.

Don't overdo iron. Millions of Americans take iron supplements because they're concerned about anemia, but studies have shown that the risk of heart disease in women over age 60 is drastically increased by taking in extra iron. Bottom line: You might need extra iron (if you bleed heavily during menstruation, for example), but supplemental amounts can rise to toxic levels in the body. Don't take iron supplements without checking with your doctor first.

IMMUNITY
BUILDING YOUR RESISTANCE

One innocent "ah-choo" from a coworker sends a cloud of viruses into the air. Swarms of bacteria and fungi enter the body through the nose, eyes, mouth, or a break in the skin. Dust and environmental pollutants enter our lungs with almost every breath. When you consider all of the disease-causing organisms and toxins that we're exposed to over a lifetime, it's a wonder that so many of us live to celebrate old age.

Yet we do, and the credit goes to our immune system. It maintains a vigorous defense against infection, pollution, and even diseases such as cancer. Yet by the time you reach your fifties, immune cells no longer function at full capacity.

The immune system requires a healthful diet, as well as regular exercise and adequate sleep, to repair itself and maintain optimal defenses. But these things aren't enough by themselves. You also have to cleanse your body of toxins, both natural and synthetic, that weaken your immune defenses and can vastly increase your chances of getting sick.

In addition to cleansing your main organs of elimination—by drinking dandelion tea to purify your liver, for example, or undergoing a brief juice or water fast to empty your intestines—you'll want to increase your intake of core nutrients, the ones designed by Nature to knock out microbes and keep immunity strong.

Your Purification Plan

Strategy One: Start with Antioxidants

Every second, immune cells are hit by a barrage of free radicals, harmful oxygen molecules that careen through your body stealing electrons from other cells and damaging your immune system at the same time. The only way to stop the process is to take in plenty of key antioxidants, nutrients that offer up their own electrons and protect immune cells from crippling damage, explains Diane Spindler, Ph.D., N.D., a board certified naturopath and owner of Mountain Holistic Health in Indian Hills, Colorado.

Drink several cups of tea daily. Researchers at the Institute for Cancer Prevention in Valhalla, New York, report that green and black tea contain 8 to 10 times more antioxidant polyphenols than fruits or vegetables. Drinking tea can reduce cell damage caused by toxins, while at the same time helping the immune system purge free radicals from your system.

Reach for the beta-carotene. The amount of beta-carotene in two large carrots is enough to stimulate your body to produce more natural killer cells and lymphocytes, immune cells that sweep up and destroy disease-causing microbes. Beta-carotene also dampens the carcinogenic effects of some toxins in your body. Good sources of beta-carotene also include spinach, sweet potatoes, and winter squash.

For a recipe featuring spinach, see page 67.

Seek out citrus. It's among the best sources of vitamin C, an immune-enhancing nutrient that is one of the most powerful antioxidants ever discovered, says Dr. Spindler. Vitamin C also may increase levels of glutathione, a compound that strengthens immunity. In addition, it helps the body produce interferon, a protein that mops up viruses before they have a chance to make you sick.

Get E in nuts and seeds. Vitamin E helps neutralize free radicals and enhances the activity of key immune cells. Nuts, sunflower seeds, and cooking oils are the best sources of vitamin E. If you're not getting the recommended 150 IU of vitamin E daily from diet alone, you'll want to take a daily supplement.

Think zinc. It's among the most important minerals for immunity as well as the elimination of toxins. Many of the detoxifying enzymes in your body require zinc to work efficiently. When zinc is combined with copper and manganese in a healthful diet, it helps block the effects of free radicals triggered by exposure to smog, ozone, and other pollutants. You'll find all three minerals in the typical multivitamin supplement.

Strategy Two: Protect Yourself with Probiotics

Your intestine contains roughly 3 pounds of bacteria. This thriving colony usually maintains a balance between beneficial and harmful species. The balance shifts, however, when your body is bombarded with toxins—from drugs, pesticides, and alcohol, to name just a few. When harmful bacteria proliferate, they secrete their own toxins that can impair digestion. At the same time, your immune system gets so busy fighting intestinal bacteria that it loses strength for more important battles.

"Probiotics can be extremely helpful," says Peter Bennett, N.D., a naturopathic physician in Vancouver and coauthor of *7-Day Detox Miracle*. They restore a healthful pH in the gut and boost the activity of immune cells. They also detoxify environmental chemicals along with excessive levels of hormones or metabolic by-products.

Eat more yogurt. This tasty dairy product, which should be made with live cultures, and other cultured foods, such as kefir and natural sauerkraut, contain some beneficial bacteria.

Consider a supplement. Even if you eat yogurt daily, you need a more concentrated source to get the full benefits from helpful bacteria. Look for a probiotic supplement that contains a mixture of species. The supplement should be kept refrigerated, both in the store and at home, to keep the organisms alive, says Dr. Spindler. Each day, plan on taking one or two capsules that provide about 10 billion organisms, she advises. This is especially important when you fast.

Strategy Three: Detoxify Your Life

We can't escape the modern world. Toxic chemicals have become a fact of life. The immune system has an impressive ability to regenerate, but that won't happen unless you keep your whole body healthy, says Dr. Spindler. Detoxifying foods and herbs, along with traditional purifying practices such as saunas, are a good starting place. After that, you need to eliminate from your body and mind many of the stressors that drag immunity down.

Reduce the fat. You need to get rid of not only the fat in your diet, but also the extra weight around your middle. Both have been shown to weaken immunity and make you more susceptible to infections as well as cancer.

People who are obese (more than 20 percent over their ideal weights) are more likely to have impaired immunity and get sick more often than those who are at healthy weights, according to a joint study from Appalachian State and Loma Linda Universities.

Dietary fats, especially saturated and hydrogenated fats, may interfere with the ability of your immune system to target harmful germs or early-stage cancerous cells. Saturated fat is any fat that is solid at room temperature. It includes things like butter and the fat in meats. Hydrogentated fats include things like margarine and vegetable shortening.

The same advice that doctors give for preventing heart disease—limiting fat intake to less than 30 percent of total calories—will work for optimizing immunity as well.

Exercise often. You can't have a healthy immune system unless you do. Exercise bumps up your oxygen intake, flushes out carbon dioxide and other toxic gases, and helps your lymphatic system pump accumulated toxins to your liver and kidneys for disposal.

Give yourself some mental space. If you're always stressed and in hyper-gear, your immune system is paying the price. Prolonged stress elevates levels of cortisol, a hormone that, in excessive amounts, is literally toxic. It depletes immune cells from your blood and also lowers levels of beneficial prostaglandins, substances that help your immune system work efficiently.

Everyone manages stress in different ways. Maybe you go for a long walk after a hard day at the office. Maybe you listen to music, watch silly movies, or spend a decompressing hour in the kitchen. The important thing is not how you manage stress, but that you recognize when it's getting to be a problem in your life and

Extras for Immunity

A HEALTHFUL DIET WILL GO A LONG WAY toward detoxifying your body and strengthening your immunity, but you'll also want to take advantage of the following supplements to improve your body's defenses and stop harmful germs before they cause infection. All of these are readily available in natural food stores. Follow the dosage instructions on the packages.

Echinacea counters the effects of enzymes that allow harmful germs to penetrate cell walls. It also increases the activity of natural killer cells.

Licorice root contains two chemical compounds, glycyrrhizin and glycyrrhetinic acid, that increase the body's production of interferon, an immune substance that combats viruses.

IP-6 (inositol hexaphosphate), found in supplements as well as soy foods and grains, increases natural killer cell activity.

Vitamin A enhances the production of lymphocytes and antibodies, and also increases the activity of natural killer cells.

that you act quickly to get it under control, says Dr. Spindler.

MENOPAUSE
TAMING THE TRANSITION

You wouldn't know it from talking to some doctors, but menopause is a natural biological process, not a disease that requires treatment. Even the common discomforts of menopause, such as hot flashes and mood changes, are usually more of an inconvenience than a serious problem, and they can almost always be reduced with simple cleansing procedures.

The conventional medical wisdom is that the discomforts of menopause are due to plunging levels of estrogen. But estrogen doesn't drop appreciably until after a woman's last period. During the transition phase into menopause, the time when symptoms are most apparent, women are more likely to suffer from "estrogen dominance"—they have too much estrogen relative to the hormone progesterone.

During a woman's reproductive years, estrogen is the dominant hormone for the first 2 weeks of her cycle. After that, it's balanced by progesterone. As she approaches menopause and her ovulation cycle gets irregular, estrogen is less "opposed" by progesterone. This is what causes things like decreased libido, headaches, mood swings, and other menopausal symptoms.

Other factors that can cause estrogen dominance include a low-fiber diet, excess stress, impaired liver function, or a buildup of environmental toxins.

Your Purification Plan

Strategy One: Sweep Out the Overload

Some women experience estrogen dominance for up to 15 years before the actual onset of menopause. That's why the first step in a menopausal cleansing plan is to sweep excess estrogen from the body. At the same time, it's essential to remove metabolic wastes or environmental toxins that can make symptoms worse, says Miranda Grace, N.D., a naturopathic physician and owner of Awakening Health in Austin, Texas.

Fill your water tank. Most women need to drink at least half their body weight, in ounces, of water daily. If you weigh 120 pounds, for example, you should be drinking at least 60 ounces, or eight full glasses—more if you're active or live in a hot climate. "You need a lot of water to open up the kidneys and liver and support the drainage of toxins out of your system," says Dr. Grace.

Supplement with B complex. Most women don't get enough B vitamins, a lack of which can cause fatigue and other menopausal discomforts, says Janet Starr Hull, Ph.D., a nutritionist in the Dallas area and author of *10 Steps to Detoxification.* "After menopause, a woman's estrogen essentially gets sticky and doesn't flow efficiently," she says. "The B vitamins escort old estrogen out of the body so a new supply is always circulating."

Pack in the fiber. Women in their pre- and post-menopausal years need to eat plenty of fruits, vegetables, and other high-fiber foods. Fiber increases bowel regularity and helps pull estrogen out of the intestine before it's reabsorbed into the body.

Take a coffee enema. Coffee contains palimate, a chemical that promotes the flow of bile and toxins to the liver for purification. Add 2 tablespoons of brewed coffee to a quart of enema water. "Take the enema whenever you're not feeling well," Dr. Grace advises. "Regular coffee often contains pesticides, so you should use organic coffee." For more information on how to use enemas safely and effectively, see "Flushing the Toxic Colon" on page 155.

Clear out estrogen with soy. Tofu, tempeh, and other soy foods contain natural plant compounds called phytoestrogens, which block the effects of natural estrogen and help reduce hot flashes and other menopausal symptoms. Simply add more soy foods to your regular diet.

For a recipe featuring soybeans, see page 74.

Strategy Two: Promote Lymphatic Drainage

A healthy lymphatic system is one of a woman's best friends before, during, and after menopause. Here are some ways to help invigorate your body's system.

Ease aches with castor oil. In the months or even years leading up to menopause, many women have painful uterine cramps along with headaches, fatigue, and a general lack of zest—all signs that the liver isn't working efficiently. "Soak cotton or wool in castor oil and cover your entire abdomen, all the way around to the back," says Dr. Grace. Leave it in place for about 30 minutes. "It supports lymphatic drainage and helps the liver detoxify." You can purchase castor oil at many health food stores.

Brush away toxins. Use a soft, natural bristle brush to gently massage your skin, stroking inward toward your heart. This technique, known as dry brushing, stimulates the flow of lymphatic fluid and accelerates the excretion of toxins from your body.

"You can get the same effect by gently massaging the skin with your fingertips," says Dr. Grace. "Use as little pressure as possible, as though a butterfly were just touching your skin."

Strategy Three: Clean Your Emotional Cupboards

Mainstream doctors tend to focus on the physical causes and manifestations of menopause, but emotional factors are equally important, says Dr. Grace. "Women experience huge emotional changes during menopause," she says. "They might find they have a really short trigger, or increases or decreases in sex drive, or dramatic mood swings."

Clearing your body of toxins and restoring a healthier hormone balance will help, but you'll still need to clear out accumulated stresses and negativity. "Toxic emotional situations and even toxic relationships interfere with normal drainage and can cause the body to accumulate excess estrogen and brain chemicals that make you feel tired and depressed," says Dr. Grace. "You have to cleanse your mind as well as your body."

Take flaxseed lignans. The thin hull that wraps around flaxseed is a concentrated source of secoisolariciresinol diglucoside, a chemical compound that helps calm turbulent menopausal emotions and also gives relief from hot flashes, says Dr. Grace. You can buy flaxseed lignans at health food stores. Follow the directions on the label.

Breathe away stress. In today's hectic world, women naturally fall into a pattern of rapid, shallow breathing, which leads to energy-sapping buildups of fatiguing carbon dioxide and a shortage of invigorating oxygen, along with a rise in cortisol and other stress hormones.

"Deep, healthy breathing exercises the organs and helps improve the elimination of toxins," says Dr. Grace. "It also dispels stress hormones that can lead to anxiety and insomnia."

The next time you feel your stress level rising, take a deep breath, hold it in for about 5 seconds, then slowly empty your lungs. Repeat the cycle five or six times, and do it every day. "You want to be aware of your breathing," says Dr. Grace. Create little reminders to make sure you do it correctly. For example, take 10 slow, conscious breaths whenever you open the refrigerator door or when you're stopped at a red light, she suggests. "You'll feel the difference right away," she says.

Listen to your heart. A woman's menopausal years are often a time of change—changes in relationships, changes in careers, and changes in family dynamics. "Our previous experiences lay down deep tracks in the brain, and our minds tend to fall into the same tracks and patterns, even when they're not in our best interests," says Dr. Grace. "Real change comes from the heart. The only way to escape toxic thoughts and patterns is to look inward and ask for guidance about what you should be doing with your life."

MENTAL ALERTNESS SHARPEN YOUR MIND AND MEMORY

Doctors talk a lot about "normal" age-related memory loss. It's true that once you hit your forties, you'll probably start having so-called senior moments: forgetting dates, appointments, or the name of the novel you just read. Occasional memory lapses or a loss of mental agility may be common, but there's no reason you have to accept them as part of your life.

If you find that mental slowdowns are interfering with your ability to function normally, you'll obviously want to see

Detox Makeover

THE OCCASIONAL CRYING JAGS WEREN'T SO BAD. She put up with the daily hot flashes that made her face feel oven-hot. But the insomnia—that was a real killer. From about the time she turned 45 until she was almost 50, Maria B. rarely got a full night's sleep. It got to the point that her eyes were so heavy during the day that she was almost afraid to drive.

"My doctor wanted to start me on HRT (hormone replacement therapy), but I was afraid of the health risks," says Maria, now 52, a realtor in Sacramento. "I went to see a naturopath, and boy, what a difference it made!"

She started a 1-month cleansing plan after tests revealed that she was loaded with heavy metals and other toxins. She took milk thistle and other herbs to stimulate her liver. She switched to a vegetarian diet. She drank water by the gallon and sipped cranberry and cucumber tonics to cleanse her kidneys.

"I started sleeping better about a week after starting the treatments," Maria recalls. "At the end of the month I was getting 6 or 7 hours' sleep a night—better than I'd done in years. My energy is way up, too."

Even though "the change" is long behind her, Maria stuck with the program. "I don't even want meat anymore," she says. "I've just started yoga, and I meditate most days. I wish I'd started all this when I was younger. I feel great."

your doctor. Chances are, there won't be anything medically wrong, but that doesn't mean you're entirely healthy, either. Accumulations of pesticides and food and water contaminants can seriously impair your ability to think clearly.

Your body may have buildups of free radicals, toxic oxygen molecules that damage neurons. It's also possible that your mind is filled with emotional and mental disturbances that interfere with your body's ability to cleanse itself, which can leave you feeling tired and fuzzy-headed.

"Many of these changes are not only preventable, they're also reversible. It's never too late to turn things around," says Mercedes Williams, N.D., a naturopathic physician at Alternatives in Health in Scottsdale, Arizona.

Your Purification Plan

Strategy One: Clean Out Chemical Wastes

The human body wasn't designed to withstand endless assaults from pesticides, air pollution, or food and water contaminants. Even if you eat a healthful diet, years of toxic overload can cause your body to use only about half of the nutrients you take in, which in turn can leave you tired and fuzzy-headed.

No one should have to live with a lack of mental clarity. You can turn things around with a mind-clearing purification plan.

Cover your bases. There are literally dozens of conditions, including nutritional or hormonal deficiencies, that can cause mental slowing. Thyroid disease is a big one. Even though thyroid hormone isn't a toxin in the usual sense, high levels in the blood (hyperthyroidism) can cause toxic effects, including mental slowing, along with vision and hearing loss and persistent memory problems.

"Lycopus and lenorus are botanical medicines that work to down-regulate the thyroid in overactive conditions," says Dr. Williams. Since thyroid disease is potentially serious, however, work with your doctor to determine whether you have the problem and how to treat it if you do. Attempting to treat this condition yourself is never a good idea, she says.

Eliminate free radicals. These toxic oxygen molecules damage neurons as well as the tiny arteries that carry blood to your brain. Your body naturally produces some free radicals, but exposure to environmental toxins vastly increases their numbers, says Dr. Williams. The only way to block their effects is to get extra antioxidants, chemical compounds in foods and supplements. An 18-month study of 442 older adults found that those with the highest levels of antioxidants in their blood had better memory performance than those with lower levels.

Combine vitamins C and E. They're among the most powerful antioxidants, and they work best when used in combination. You can get plenty of vitamin C by eating at least five servings of produce daily. To get brain-protecting levels of vitamin E, however, you need to take a daily supplement that provides 150 IU.

Eat blueberries daily. Researchers at the USDA Human Nutrition Center found that blueberries have more antioxidant activity than any of the 40 fresh fruits and vegetables they studied. The pigment that makes blueberries blue, anthocyanin, blocks an enormous number of free radicals. Laboratory animals given blueberries experience less memory loss than animals given their usual diets.

For a recipe featuring blueberries, see page 51.

Take alpha lipoic acid. The body manufactures small amounts of this powerful antioxidant, but it's mainly found in foods (such as spinach, brewer's yeast, and meats) and supplements. Take 100 to 200 mg daily. Other important antioxidants include selenium (100 to 200 mcg daily) and grape seed extract (100 to 200 mg daily). Research shows that you'll get the most benefit when you combine different antioxidants, Dr. Williams says.

Exercise away stress hormones. People who are chronically stressed accumulate massive levels of cortisol and other stress-related chemicals. Over time, they can cause the parts of the brain associated with memory to literally shrink. Exercise reduces levels of stress hormones almost instantly, and it also gives brain cells the oxygen they need to function at peak capacity. At the same time, exercise stimulates the release of trophic factors, brain proteins that repair damaged neurons.

All kinds of aerobic exercise do the trick—bicycling, walking, swimming, even vacuuming the house or weeding the garden.

Fortify your liver. When your liver is overwhelmed by toxins, your energy and mental abilities pay the price. Several daily cups of dandelion tea increase bloodflow to your liver and help it remove toxins more efficiently. Other liver-protecting supplements include milk thistle, artichoke leaf, and celandine. You can purchase the tea and any of these supplements at a health food store. Then simply follow the directions on the label.

Fill your tank. Get in the habit of drinking at least eight full glasses of water daily. Water reduces your body's concentration of mind-slowing toxins and makes it easier for your liver, as well as your kidneys, skin, and lungs, to remove those toxins from your body.

Eat plenty of fiber. Here's another reason to fill your shopping cart with fresh fruits and vegetables, along with plenty of whole grains and legumes. The fiber in these foods helps your intestines move toxins along more quickly. At the same time, fiber lowers levels of LDL cholesterol and makes it less likely to cling to your arteries and reduce bloodflow to your brain.

Strategy Two: Clear Your Mind

You can't think clearly when you're overwhelmed with negative, toxic thoughts. That's why it's just as important to purify your mind as your body when you notice slowdowns in mental energy. The breathing and meditation exercises in chapter 8 on page 161 are essential for detoxifying your mind. So are the following simple steps.

Give anxiety the boot. Along with chronic stress, anxiety increases levels of cortisol, a "fight or flight" hormone that damages neurons and makes it harder to concentrate and absorb information. Relaxation techniques such as yoga and tai chi have been shown to reduce anxiety and also improve bloodflow throughout the body, including to the brain. "Taking time for yourself every day is one of the most beneficial ways to improve feelings of self-worth and decrease stress and anxiety," says Dr. Williams.

Don't live with depression. It's the second leading cause of memory loss. And because it's often accompanied by anxiety, it can lead to elevated levels of cortisol. Studies have shown that people who manage depression with antidepressants often have memory improvements within 6 weeks.

An alternative to drugs is the herb St. John's wort. It's just as effective as drugs are at treating mild to moderate depression. Take 300 mg three times daily. Hypnosis, visualization, deep breathing, and meditation are also very effective ways to get a handle on depression, Dr. Williams says.

Clear the distractions from your life. It's getting harder all the time to focus on the things that count because we're so overwhelmed with new information. Here are a few key ways to sidestep distractions and keep your mind focused.

Pay attention up front. Be aware of things you'll want to remember later, like where you left your car. Inattention is the

Drugs, Toxicity, and Memory

MANY OF THE PRESCRIPTION AND OVER-THE-COUNTER DRUGS we depend on can cause memory or mental agility to slip. This is especially common in older adults, who metabolize drugs slowly and can accumulate toxic levels in their blood.

As you might expect, the worst offenders tend to be sedatives and painkillers, but they aren't the only ones. Medicines for Parkinson's disease, high blood pressure, and allergies often cause mental slowdowns. Even antiulcer drugs are a problem for some people. It can be a challenge to get the benefits of medications without the risk of toxicity.

"Most conditions that are treated with prescription drugs respond effectively and safely to natural therapeutics," says Mercedes Williams, N.D., a naturopathic physician at Alternatives in Health in Scottsdale, Arizona. If you have to take drugs, the daily choices you make—eating organic foods; drinking pure, filtered water; exercising daily; and so on—can make all the difference in minimizing toxicity. "Lifestyle cannot be emphasized enough," Dr. Williams says.

If you need to take prescription drugs and suspect that they may be affecting your memory or mental alertness, let your doctor know. It may be possible to either lower the dose or find an alternative medication.

main cause of most memory problems.

Visualize what you want to remember. If you just met someone, for example, picture her name in your head. You can do the same thing with phone numbers and addresses.

Fill the air with floral scents. A number of studies show that floral scents can increase learning speed and the retention of new material by 17 percent, probably because they promote concentration and alertness. Don't rely on chemical air-fresheners, however. A few drops of essential oil placed in a diffuser will do the trick nicely. Ask about these products at places that sell aromatherapy supplies.

MUSCLE PAIN
SOOTHE SORE MUSCLES

Muscles move only two ways: They shorten and tighten during their exertion phase, such as when you're pulling a stubborn dandelion from the lawn, and they lengthen when you relax. You're not likely to get hurt during the relaxation phase, but tighten a muscle harder or longer than it's used to, and ouch! You might find yourself out of commission with soreness or a painful cramp.

These painful conditions are two completely different problems. Cramps occur when a muscle tightly contracts and then refuses to let go. They rarely last more than a few seconds, but they're excruciatingly painful. More importantly, cramps can strike at precisely the wrong time, such as when you're scuba diving or playing in the ocean.

Soreness is a different kind of pain. It usually occurs when you've overdone it—running 5 miles when your body is used to 3, for example, or spending long hours gardening on the first day of spring. This kind of pain, known as delayed-onset muscle soreness (DOMS),

usually begins a day or two after the activity and can last up to a week.

Your Purification Plan

Strategy One: Get Muscles Back in Motion

Delayed-onset muscle soreness is caused by microscopic tears in the tissues, and also by accumulations of pain-causing fluids and chemicals. The soreness usually goes away on its own, but it can make your life pretty uncomfortable in the meantime. You'll heal a lot faster if you follow a detoxification plan to pump out pain-causing substances and bring in fresh blood and nutrients, says Timothy Douglass, D.C., founder and owner of Douglass Chiropractic in Glen, New Hampshire.

Ice it fast. At the first hint of pain, stop what you're doing, wrap some ice cubes in a washcloth or towel, and apply cold to the area for about 20 minutes at a time throughout the first day. Cold causes blood vessels to constrict, which prevents pain-causing fluids and chemicals from flowing into the injured area and causing swelling.

Wrap the area. Using an elastic bandage, lightly wrap the area where you have the most pain. This technique, called compression, helps prevent additional (and painful) fluids from entering the area. The wrapping should be firm, but not so tight that it cuts off circulation. You should be able to just about wiggle your little finger under the edge. If you can't, the bandage is too tight and you should back it off a bit.

Raise it high. If possible, elevate the injured area higher than your heart. This will allow pain-causing fluids to drain out, while keeping more fluids from coming in and causing swelling, says Dr. Douglass.

Follow up with massage. We instinctively rub our muscles when they hurt, and research suggests that it works. Massaging the sore area pushes out lactic acid and hyaluronic acids, metabolic by-products that cause a lot of pain. Massage also increases serotonin, a brain chemical that eases pain, and lowers levels of stress hormones that cause it, says Dr. Douglass.

Don't massage the area if the pain is too intense, however. It's normal to feel minor discomfort when massaging a sore muscle. Anything worse than that means that you should keep applying ice and wait at least a few hours before trying massage again.

Drink a lot of water. Even if you don't normally top your tank with the recommended eight full glasses of water daily, make sure to drink a lot when your muscles are sore—and especially after a massage. Water will help dilute chemical compounds that make soreness worse, says Joel Fuhrman, M.D., a family practice physician specializing in nutritional medicine and author of *Eat to Live* and *Fasting and Eating for Health*.

Take vitamin E. Boston researchers found that men who took vitamin E and kept taking it for 3 months experienced less post-exercise soreness than those who didn't take it. Vitamin E helps mop up tissue-damaging by-products that form in muscles when you've pushed them long and hard. The recommended dose is 150 IU daily.

Run hot and cold. After the first 24 hours, treat the muscle to alternating hot and cold compresses. Soak a towel in hot water, wring it out, and drape it over the area for a few minutes. Follow that with a cool cloth, and repeat the cycle several times. The contrast in temperatures works like a pump to increase the flow of toxins and torn muscle fragments out of the area and to bring in fresh blood and nutrients.

"Do this only if you have a healthy cardiovascular system," Dr. Douglass warns. "It can be risky for those with heart disease or a history of other cardiovascular problems."

Drain the fluid. Once the worst of the muscle soreness is gone, gently move the injured area through its full range of motion. If the pain is in your wrist, for example, gently bend your wrist up, down, and from side to side. Keep moving it for about 2 minutes, but don't push yourself to the point of pain.

Moving the muscles pumps fluids and lactic acid out of the area, says Dr. Douglass.

Reduce toxins with MSM. While you're waiting for the soreness to fade, you can help things along by taking a supplement called MSM (methyl sulfonyl methane), a form of sulfur that makes

Banish Bruises

EVEN IF YOU HAVE THE GRACE AND BALANCE OF A GAZELLE, there will be times when your clumsy side will get you into trouble, such as when you smack your head against an open cabinet door. Your lack of grace will be visible for the world to see in the form of an ugly, blue-black bruise.

Bruises occur when tiny blood vessels under the skin, called capillaries, leak and bleed. They usually aren't serious, but they can hurt like the dickens and are ugly, to boot. To help them heal more quickly:

Load up on blueberries. They're loaded with vitamin C and bioflavonoids, chemical compounds that help blood vessels heal more quickly. As a bonus, the chemicals in blueberries make capillaries stronger and better able to resist future damage.

Pop some bromelain. In addition to its ability to quell muscle pain and cramps, bromelain is like a miracle cure for bruises. In one study, researchers gave bromelain to 74 boxers four times daily. All signs of bruising disappeared in 4 days. In a control group of 72 boxers who got only placebos, only 10 showed similar results. Bromelain supplements are available in drugstores and health food stores. Follow the directions on the package.

muscle cells more permeable and allows accumulated fluids in the injured area to flow more readily back into circulation. Follow the directions on the label, and keep taking MSM until the soreness is gone, says Dr. Douglass.

Take a B-complex supplement. "I often advise patients to take a B-complex vitamin to relieve muscle soreness," says Dr. Douglass. "It helps heal injured nerve fibers that cause the pain."

Heal faster with creatine. A supplement available in health food stores, creatine is thought to aid in repairing microscopic muscle tears following overuse injuries. Follow the directions on the label, and keep taking it until the pain is gone.

Strategy Two: Take Care of Cramps

Since muscle cramps rarely last very long, there isn't a lot you can do to treat them. What you can do, however, is make sure they don't come back. For starters, you might want to take a mineral combo—500 mg each of calcium and magnesium. Muscles need these nutrients to function properly. In addition, here are a few steps you'll want to take when a cramp lays you low.

Grab it hard. As soon as a cramp begins, use one or both hands to really dig your fingers into the muscle. This "breaks up" the painful contraction and also forces out lactic acid.

Relax in a salted bath. As soon as you can, set aside half an hour to relax in a warm bath spiked with a few cups of Epsom salts (magnesium sulfate). This natural form of magnesium dissolves in water and helps pull fluid out of the injured area and will help cramped muscles relax. "Epsom salts are inexpensive and work as well as anything else," says Dr. Douglass. "I use them a lot for patients with arthritis."

Supplement with bromelain. An enzyme extracted from pineapple, bromelain reduces levels of inflammatory chemicals and also flushes fluids from the injured area, says Dr. Douglass. Follow package directions.

OVERWEIGHT
PURGE THE POUNDS

It's not exactly breaking news that a lot of us are heavier than we'd like to be. About two-thirds of Americans at any given time are attempting to lose weight or keep the weight they've lost from coming back. Diet plans dominate the best-seller lists and television talk shows, and collectively we spend about $33 billion a year to banish those extra pounds.

Our lifestyles have to take their share

of the blame. We're surrounded by calories in one form or another, and our exercise habits could use some improving. But there's more to it than that. Over our lifetimes we eat, drink, and inhale thousands of chemical compounds, everything from pesticides and food preservatives to secondhand smoke, all of which can end up as extra weight on our bodies.

Your Purification Plan

Strategy One: Eliminate the Toxins That Trigger Weight Gain

One significant way to peel off the pounds and, more importantly, keep them from coming back, is to cleanse your body of the toxins that may be triggering the whole weight-gain cascade in the first place, according to Diane Spindler, Ph.D., N.D., a board certified naturopath and owner of Mountain Holistic Health in Indian Hills, Colorado. Here's the four-step approach that she recommends:

Step 1: Optimize colon health. "You have to make sure that wastes are moving through the colon efficiently," says Dr. Spindler. "Toxins accumulate in stools, and anything that doesn't move out of the body quickly is going to get reabsorbed into the bloodstream."

Most people need a simple colon cleanse—a combination of a high-fiber diet and fiber supplements. Putting more fiber in your system causes stools to move more quickly. In addition to eating more fruits, vegetables, whole grains, and legumes, Dr. Spindler recommends taking psyllium or fruit fiber supplements daily. Available at drugstores and health food stores, these supplements draw water into the colon and make bowel movements more regular as well as more comfortable. Just follow the directions on the package.

If you have a history of constipation or your diet has been a little low in fiber for the last few years, you might need colon hydrotherapy, a thorough cleansing done by a professional. Once your colon is purged of wastes, a high-fiber diet is probably all you'll need to keep your bowel—and toxins—moving. For information on colonics, see "Flushing the Toxic Colon" on page 155.

Step 2: Flush your kidneys. Throughout your detox plan, drink as much water as you can. You need at least eight 8-ounce glasses daily. More is better. Water flushes chemicals and toxins out through your kidneys in the form of urine. "Make sure it's purified water," says Dr. Spindler. "The last thing you want is to dump more chemicals into your body." You also might want to stop by the health food store to pick up teas or supplements that contain uva ursi, juniper berry, or dandelion. They help flush out toxins and strengthen the kidneys and bladder. Follow the directions on the package.

Step 3: Detoxify your liver and gallbladder. "The liver is like the body's oil filter," says Dr. Spindler. "If it's not functioning properly, you're going to absorb toxins that can lead to weight gain." Cleansing your gallbladder is equally important because it secretes fat-digesting enzymes. When it gets clogged with stones, more saturated fat enters the bloodstream, she explains. For all the supplements listed below, follow the directions on the packages.

◐ Take a liver detox formula. Many of the liver-cleansing products in health food stores contain a variety of active ingredients that help the liver eliminate heavy metals and other toxins.

◐ Get rid of heavy metals. Alpha lipoic acid is a sulfur-based product that helps the liver eliminate heavy metals. It's also a cofactor that helps promote energy in liver cells.

◐ Take milk thistle. This traditional herb for liver problems has been shown to help liver cells regenerate after exposure to cell-damaging toxins or infection from hepatitis and other diseases.

◐ Think red. Red beet root helps the gallbladder work more efficiently at digesting fats and promoting the absorption of fat-soluble vitamins. Simply add more beets to your diet. If cooking beets is not your cup of tea, however, you can buy a beet root supplement.

Step 4: Cleanse your lymphatic system. "It contains three to four times more fluid than the blood," says Dr. Spindler. "The lymph system pulls toxins out of cells and carries them to the liver and kidneys to be eliminated." Even if you haven't been exposed to unusual amounts of toxins, your lymphatic system can get sluggish when you've had an infection or eaten foods you are sensitive to. (Common food sensitivities include dairy and wheat products.) To remove lymphatic toxins:

◐ Drink red clover tea. "It cleans the lymphatic system and eliminates offending substances," says Dr. Spindler. Feel free to enjoy this tasty beverage a couple of times a day. It comes in convenient tea bags.

◐ Take vitamin C. You'll need between 1,000 and 2,000 mg daily. It essentially scrubs toxins from your body's cells, washing them out through the lymph system.

◉ Dry brush your skin. Use a soft brush to gently rub every inch of your skin, moving toward the center of your body. Most of the lymphatic system is just beneath the skin, Dr. Spindler explains. Dry brushing stimulates the flow of lymph and accelerates the elimination of toxins.

"Be sure to cleanse the colon and liver before detoxifying the lymphatic system," Dr. Spindler warns. If the colon isn't moving and the liver isn't in top shape when you purge the lymphatic system, toxins will "back up" and essentially clog the liver. "You could get some pretty nasty symptoms," she says.

Strategy Two: Eat to Keep Away the Pounds

You already know the basic rules for losing weight: eat smaller portions, reduce daily calories, exercise more, and so on. It's good advice, yet millions of people continue to gain weight, even when they try to stick to the program. Part of the reason, says Dr. Spindler, is that most of us continue to do things that almost guarantee that we'll gain weight.

Once you've detoxified your body, it's time to move to the next step of the weight-loss plan. Here's how.

Eat small meals more frequently. Americans love the traditional three-meals-a-day style of eating, but it's a terrible approach when you're trying to lose weight. "You want to eat small, frequent meals," Dr. Spindler says. "It keeps your furnace burning all day, rather than at selected times." A higher, steadier metabolism means more calories burned, even when you're doing nothing more vigorous than watching TV.

Cut the caffeine. It stimulates the adrenal glands to release "fight or flight" hormones, which in turn shut down digestion and stimulate surges in glucose (blood sugar). This process could save your life in a true emergency, but in modern life—say, when you're at your desk drinking coffee—about all it does is stimulate surges in insulin, which sponges sugar from the blood and stores it as fat.

Don't skip meals. Even though fasting can be an effective way to purge your body of toxins, skipping meals is not. "If you starve yourself, your body thinks it's facing a crisis and will begin to store fat," says Dr. Spindler. Studies have shown, in fact, that people who skip meals tend to gain more weight than those who eat smaller portions throughout the day. For dozens of recipes that assist in detoxification, see chapter 4 on page 50.

Expert Advice

IT'S BECOME COMMON MEDICAL KNOWLEDGE that toxins tend to collect in our fat tissue, which means that carrying a little too much weight means that we're also carrying a toxic load that we can reduce through weight loss. But Diane Spindler, Ph.D., N.D., a board certified naturopath and owner of Mountain Holistic Health in Indian Hills, Colorado, doesn't stop there. She's convinced that toxins in our bodies are actually the triggers of weight gain.

"Fat is one of the body's protective mechanisms against toxins," explains Dr. Spindler. "Fat absorbs toxins in order to prevent them from damaging the organs. So when you ingest toxins from the environment, you're going to manufacture fat as a way of protecting the cells."

She has found that toxins interfere with metabolism, energy, and the elimination of wastes, all things that can contribute to gaining weight. "Detoxification is one of the keys to healthy weight management," says Dr. Spindler.

"If you want to lose weight in a healthy way, detoxifying the intestinal tract is paramount. A healthy intestinal tract is dependent on the food we eat, water we drink, and supplements we take," says Dr. Spindler. She recommends a high-fiber diet as the best way to maximize the elimination of unwanted wastes.

"A simple and tasty way to add fiber to your diet is to replace simple carbohydrates, like bread and pasta, with complex carbohydrates, like legumes, fruits, nuts, and seeds," she says. Dr. Spindler also advises her clients to take fiber supplements if they are having trouble adding high-fiber foods to their diets.

POLLUTION
PROTECTION FROM
PERVASIVE TOXINS

Maybe you eat organic foods. Maybe you exercise often, avoid sugary snacks, and keep your physical and emotional life in balance. Are you truly healthy? Not unless you've discovered how to live without air and water. It's a sad irony that the two things we need most to survive are the same ones that bring the greatest threats to our health.

In 1 year alone, more than 1 billion pounds of chemicals are released into the ground and trickle down to the water that we drink. Lakes and rivers catch more than 188 million pounds of chemicals. The air you breathe? All you have to do is spend a few minutes sucking fumes near a busy intersection to understand just how toxic it gets. The world's industrial nations pump more than 2 billion pounds of emissions into the air each year.

It's no wonder that asthma, allergies, and other respiratory diseases are on the rise. Researchers have discovered heavy metals in the tissues of people who live thousands of miles from industrial centers. Millions of Americans feel tired, stressed, and sluggish, even though their doctors insist that they're perfectly healthy.

Air and water pollution aren't going to disappear. It's easy to feel helpless—but don't. You can minimize, if not completely eliminate, your body's accumulation of pollutants that can have lasting repercussions on your health.

Your Purification Plan

Strategy One: Purge the Poisons

A generation ago, people would have laughed at the idea of paying actual money for water when you could get it free from the tap. Today, millions of us drink only water that's been purified and filtered. It's a good starting place if you're trying to avoid chlorine or other chemical compounds, but it's not a perfect approach because some waterborne chemicals invariably slip into our diets. The only long-term solution is to cleanse these chemicals from your body before they reach toxic levels.

Clean up with chlorella. A type of green algae available in drinks and supplements at health food stores, chlorella contains more chlorophyll than any other plant-derived food. Some practitioners believe chlorophyll binds to heavy metals in the intestine and carries them out of the body. It's not certain that chlorophyll actually has this effect. However, it does contain antioxidants that reduce tissue-damaging inflammation that's caused by chemical exposure, says Gary Dreger, N.D., L.Ac., a naturopathic physician and acupuncturist at Natural Health Works in Oregon City, Oregon.

Eat for elimination. Over your lifetime, about 500 pounds of toxic materials pass through your nasal passages and lungs, but anywhere from 5,000 to 25,000 pounds will pass through your intestine, says Emily Kane, N.D., L.Ac., a naturopathic physician and acupuncturist in Juneau, Alaska. Some of these toxins invariably get reabsorbed into your blood. The only way to prevent this is to have regular bowel moments, and that means eating a diet rich in fruits, vegetables, legumes, and other high-fiber foods.

Work up a sweat. Once or twice a week (or daily, if you can), spend a few minutes in a steamy bathroom or in the sauna at your health club. Your body stores toxins in fatty tissues. Sweat therapy stimulates cellular receptors and promotes the excretion of toxins—everything from lead and cadmium to PCBs.

One study looked at firemen who experienced neurophysiological problems after chemical exposure. The men who completed 3 weeks of a sauna program had significant improvements in memory tests compared to those who didn't "sweat it out."

Strategy Two: Tune Up Your Liver

This is where most of your body's detoxification takes place, explains Dr. Dreger. The liver breaks down toxins into harmless forms and excretes them from your body. If your liver isn't working at optimal efficiency, pollutants from air and water stay "active" and can damage cells throughout your body. To keep your liver healthy:

Be a dandy. Drink dandelion tea or take dandelion supplements. Both are available at natural food stores. To take them, follow the package directions. Dandelion promotes the flow of blood and bile to the liver and expedites the cleansing process.

Get hydrated. Drink at least eight full glasses of purified water daily. It reduces toxin concentrations and makes it easier for your liver to process and break them down.

Take milk thistle supplements. Available at health food stores, they contain silymarin, a protective plant chemical that helps damaged liver cells regenerate. Again, just follow the directions on the package.

Take a break. Avoid alcohol, meat, wheat, and medications (if possible) for 2 weeks, and eat lots of beets and artichokes, both of which promote liver health, says Dr. Kane.

Fast once a month. The liver, kidneys, and other organs of elimination are very efficient at breaking down and eliminating toxins. But the toxic load from water and air is so heavy that your body can barely keep up with the daily assaults, let alone years of accumulations. Fasting gives your detoxifying mechanisms a chance to rest and eliminate the backlog.

You don't need to fast rigorously or for extended periods. You shouldn't, in fact, unless you're under medical supervision, because your body needs a steady intake of nutrients to fuel the detox machinery. Set aside 2 days and have nothing but water and vegetable juices. Or use a product such as Ultra Clear, a supplement drink available at health food stores that provides nutritional support during a fast, says Dr. Dreger.

Strategy Three: Cleanse Your Lungs

You can survive weeks without food and up to a week without water, but you can't survive more than a few minutes without oxygen. Unfortunately, the air we breathe is a toxin repository. Toxins that slip deep into the lungs travel through the blood and can potentially damage every cell in your body.

You can't completely avoid airborne toxins, but you can neutralize their harmful effects. Here's what you need to do.

Breathe steam. Luxuriating in a hot shower or wet sauna essentially bathes the lungs with moisture, which thins and loosens toxin-filled secretions. Steam therapy also improves the elimination of toxins through the skin.

Breathe deeply. Taking a few minutes every day to breathe deeply improves the ability of your lungs to eliminate toxins as well as waste gases, says Dr. Dreger. Spend some time each day pulling air as deeply into your lungs as it will go, then blowing every bit of it out. Strong, deep breaths also stimulate the lymphatic tissues surrounding your lungs and help them transport chemicals to your liver for disposal.

Move aerobically. This basically means doing some activity—any activity—fast enough that it increases your breathing rate. The faster you breathe, the more efficiently hairlike filters in your lungs carry out mucus and waste products.

Fight back with watercress. This pungent salad green contains a chemical compound, phenethyl isothiocyanate (PEITC), that appears to neutralize some of the cancer-causing chemicals in tobacco smoke. Laboratory studies show that animals given PEITC are 50 percent less likely to get lung cancer than those given their regular diets only.

Watercress won't wash away all of the toxins from smoke, of course. But adding it to your daily diet can block some of the harmful effects while you try to quit, as well as protect you from secondhand smoke.

Get extra antioxidants. Vitamin C, vita-min E, selenium, and beta-carotene, along with the thousands of protective phytonutrients in plants, are your body's shields against air pollution, says Dr. Dreger. Pollution causes tissues to unleash floods of free radicals, toxic molecules that damage tissues in the lungs and other parts of your body. Antioxidants block this process and can reduce damage caused by asthma or other lung diseases.

Good lung-protecting foods include spinach, kale, broccoli, and winter squash. These and other fruits and vegetables with deep, rich colors usually

Fish for Health

NEARLY ALL FISH CONTAIN TRACE AMOUNTS OF MERCURY, dioxins, or other contaminants. Large fish such as bass may accumulate 1 million times as many contaminants as the surrounding water. To get the health benefits of fish without the toxic risks:

Limit your fish intake. Eat no more than 12 ounces of fish weekly, especially if you're pregnant. Toxins in lakes and streams that accumulate in fish can harm a developing fetus.

Select wisely. Eat small pan fish, such as trout and perch. They have lower levels of contaminants than larger fish do.

Eat canned light tuna packed in water. It has less mercury than tuna steaks or canned albacore tuna.

contain the largest antioxidant payloads. For a recipe featuring kale, see page 66.

Supplement with glutathione. It's an antioxidant that's often deficient in chemically overloaded people, says Dr. Dreger. "Glutathione is very important for reducing inflammation and general detoxification," he says. In fact, studies have shown that people exposed to heavy metals have less tissue damage when they supplement with glutathione. Follow the directions on the label.

If supplements aren't for you, buy whey protein and add it to smoothies or cereal. It boosts glutathione levels in the body, says Dr. Dreger.

PROSTATE
PURIFY TO PREVENT
PROBLEMS

Sooner or later, just about every man will have a rendezvous with the prostate gland. This doesn't always mean cancer, although about 221,000 new cases of prostate cancer are diagnosed each year, and more than 29,000 men die from it. You're much more likely to get prostatitis, an infection or inflammation of the gland, or benign prostatic hypertrophy (BPH), a fancy name for age-related prostate enlargement.

The prostate is a small gland that en-circles the urethra, the tube that carries urine out of the body. When the gland is infected or enlarged, you may experience difficulty urinating, groin pain, or a burning sensation when you urinate.

Mainstream medicine is very good at treating severe problems, including cancer, but it isn't very helpful for men who have minor, day-to-day discomfort. In the last few years, the medical community has taken a hint from the world of alternative medicine and shifted the focus toward preventive strategies, including taking steps to cleanse the prostate of harmful molecules or hormones that fuel tumor growth, says Sheldon Marks, M.D., associate clinical professor of urology and clinical lecturer in radiation oncology at the University of Arizona College of Medicine, Tucson, and author of *Prostate and Cancer.*

Your Purification Plan

Strategy One: Take Steps to Prevent Cancer

The main treatments for prostate cancer—surgery, radiation, and drugs—can save lives, but they frequently cause impotence and other side effects. It makes a lot more sense for men to take the initiative and prevent cell changes that can eventually lead to cancer. Here's what Dr. Marks recommends.

Supplement with selenium. It's a trace mineral that improves the ability of your immune system to nail cancer cells at the earliest possible time, says Dr. Marks. Selenium is also an antioxidant that reduces the cell-damaging effects of high-energy, oxygen-based molecules (free radicals) that are naturally present in the prostate. One study showed that men at high risk of getting prostate cancer who took selenium cut their risk in half. A daily dose of 200 mcg is enough to significantly lower levels of prostate-damaging cells and molecules.

Load up on E. It's a very powerful antioxidant that works in the fatty portions of cells. Like selenium, it increases your immune system's ability to scour your prostate of cancer cells, and it has been shown to decrease the death rate from prostate cancer. You can get some vitamin E in nuts, seeds, egg yolks, and vegetable oils, but it's not enough to protect against cancer. Take a daily supplement that provides 150 IU.

Eat a lot of tomatoes. They contain lycopene, a plant pigment that mops up free radicals in the prostate and appears to slow the growth of cancer cells. A 5-year study of 48,000 men found that those who ate 10 or more weekly servings of tomatoes were two-thirds less likely to get prostate cancer than men who ate only two servings weekly.

The good news is, you don't have to fill your shopping cart with pallid, out-of-season (and tasteless) tomatoes. Ketchup, tomato sauce, and tomato paste contain even more lycopene than fresh tomatoes. So have yourself a big plate of spaghetti with tomato sauce, and know that that sauce is good for you!

Get used to tofu. It's still not a familiar food for most American men, but tofu, along with other soy foods, contains estrogen-like plant compounds, or phyto-estrogens, that reduce levels of dihydro-testosterone, a steroid hormone that stimulates the development of prostate cancer. Soy may also block angiogenesis, the growth of blood vessels that tumors need to thrive. Two or three weekly servings are enough.

Don't bother with soy supplements. They probably don't have the sought-after effects. Instead, try things like scrambled tofu in place of scrambled eggs, or "ice cream" made from tofu rather than cream. Soy milk and soy yogurt aren't bad, either. They come in delicious flavors.

Cut back on fat. Actually, it's fine to have olive oil or other kinds of mono- or polyunsaturated fats. The fat that you want to avoid is the saturated fat in milk, meat, and other animal products. It stimulates your body's production of testosterone-like hormones and increases your risk of prostate cancer.

"Be reasonable about fat," says Dr. Marks. "It's fine to have some, as long as you reduce the [overall] amounts and eat more fruits and vegetables."

Hang out in the sun. Worries about skin cancer have led many American men to avoid sunshine, but go ahead and work on your tan—in small increments—if you want to prevent prostate cancer. About 10 minutes of sun each day promotes your body's production of vitamin D, a nutrient that helps block the growth of cancer cells.

Strategy Two: Slow or Reverse Enlargement

If you're a man over age 50, you probably have some enlargement of the prostate gland. This enlargement isn't cancerous, and many men never experience problems. In some cases, however, the gland gets so big that it presses against the urethra and makes it difficult or painful to urinate. If you're having these or other symptoms, your doctor might decide to "trim" the gland and remove excess tissue. In many cases, though, you can slow or even reverse this uncomfortable

growth by purging the prostate of substances that cause the cells to multiply.

Take saw palmetto daily. Extracted from a small palm tree and available in supplement form, this herb contains a chemical compound that inhibits the action of an enzyme that converts testosterone into dihydrotestosterone, the "fuel" for prostate growth, says Dr. Marks. Several well-designed studies have shown that saw palmetto sometimes works as well as finasteride (Proscar), a prescription drug, and is less likely to cause side effects. The recommended dose is 160 mg twice daily.

Add pygeum to the mix. It's an herbal supplement that inhibits the body's production of prostaglandins, chemicals that can flood the prostate gland and cause swelling and inflammation. If you've tried saw palmetto for a few months without success, it's fine to combine it with pygeum. The recommended dose is 100 mg twice daily.

Get extra zinc. It's one of the key nutrients for prostate health, and low levels have been linked to prostate enlargement, says Dr. Marks. You can get plenty of zinc in shellfish, whole grains, and meats. Or take a daily supplement that provides 30 mg of zinc. If you do take zinc, be sure to include a daily supplement that provides 2 mg of copper because zinc has been shown to interfere with copper absorption. You might want to look for a multivitamin supplement that contains both minerals in the correct amounts; many do.

Strategy Three: Chase Away the Pain

A common source of male discomfort, and one that still has doctors scratching their heads, is prostatitis, a catch-all term for inflammation of the prostate gland.

A bacterial infection can certainly cause it, but many men who have symptoms, including painful urination or groin pain, don't have an infection or any other illness that doctors can pinpoint.

Prostatitis is rarely serious, but it can be extremely uncomfortable. Your best bet, after checking with your doctor, is to flush your prostate gland of inflammatory chemicals that cause discomfort. Here's the best approach.

The Crucifer Connection

IF YOU WANT TO GET SERIOUS about reducing your risk for prostate cancer, get in the habit of eating broccoli, cabbage, cauliflower, or other cruciferous vegetables at least a few times a week. They contain chemical compounds that appear to be among the most powerful cancer-fighters ever discovered. They also help the liver do one of its most important jobs: detoxifying the body.

One compound called sulforaphane, for example, boosts the body's production of cancer-blocking enzymes. The crucifers also contain compounds that appear to reduce tumor growth in hormone-sensitive cells. In a laboratory study done at Johns Hopkins, 68 percent of unprotected lab animals given a carcinogenic agent went on to develop cancer, compared to only 26 percent of those given sulforaphane first.

Outside of the laboratory, the evidence is clear that people who eat a lot of crucifers are protected against all kinds of cancer, especially those of the colon, breast, and prostate gland.

Harness the power of flowers. A flower-pollen extract called Prostat, available in health food stores, has been shown to lower levels of inflammatory chemicals in the prostate gland. Follow the directions on the package.

Drink water—a lot of water. It dilutes pain-causing substances and can help eliminate bacteria and other organisms before they have a chance to multiply, says Dr. Marks. The usual advice to drink eight full glasses is a good starting place.

Suck down cranberry juice. You can count it toward your water total, but it does more than provide extra fluids. Cranberry juice makes it harder for bacteria to cling to the walls of your bladder. If you drink several cups a day, you can prevent infections from spreading from your bladder to your prostate gland, and vice versa.

Soak away the pain. Relaxing in a hot bath once a day increases circulation in the prostate, which can help wash away pain-causing substances while bringing in healing blood and nutrients.

Eat fish at least twice a week. Fish oils, which contain omega-3 fatty acids, reduce levels of prostaglandins, says Dr. Marks. If you're not a fish lover, sprinkle a few tablespoonfuls of ground flaxseed on your breakfast cereal. It contains the same beneficial oils.

For a recipe featuring fish, see page 60.

SEXUAL DESIRE
PUT YOUR SEX DRIVE BACK IN GEAR

Ever since former senator Bob Dole found a second career touting the wonders of Viagra, advertisements for pharmaceutical sex enhancers have flooded the airwaves and magazines pages. The introduction of anti-impotence treatments for men, and new research into treatments for women, have improved the sex lives of millions of couples. But these approaches work only for the mechanics of sex; they don't increase desire. And without desire, none of the new drugs makes a bit of difference.

We all have peaks and valleys in our sexual desire. Everyday issues such as stress and fatigue can obviously act like a cold shower. Emotional issues can take the zip out of your sex drive. So can hormone imbalances or other physical problems.

Recent studies report that nearly one-third of women ages 18 to 59 suffer from a diminished interest in sex. Men are less likely than women to admit to sexual problems, but the numbers are probably about the same.

Scientists have only started to look at the effects of environmental toxins on sex drive, and what they've found is alarming. "There's been a huge increase in declines in libido," says Heidi Weinhold, N.D., a naturopathic physician at The Enhancement Center in McMurray, Pennsylvania. "We're living in a toxic world. We're exposed to chemicals from new carpeting, paints, dry cleaning, new office buildings, and thousands of other things—and the places these toxins affect first are the reproductive organs."

Your Purification Plan

Strategy One: Eat, Drink, and Be Sexy

Even if your sexual machinery hums right along, decades of exposure to environmental chemicals can leave you feeling tired, drained, and totally unsexy. "Cleansing is a big part of treating libido problems," says Dr. Weinhold. "Whatever you take in goes through the liver, and if the liver is overloaded, it throws you off mentally and emotionally."

Since medical problems are a common cause of libido loss, plan on seeing your doctor if you can't seem to get your sex drive out of park. In the meantime, here's a cleansing strategy using food, vitamins, and herbs that should get you back in the erotic swim.

Follow the three-quarter rule. Eat only organic foods that are free of chemical additives and preservatives, and make sure that 75 percent of the foods in your diet are eaten raw or lightly steamed. "This ensures that the natural nutrients aren't removed, which gives your body the tools it needs to remove chemicals and other toxins," says Janet Starr Hull, Ph.D., a nutritionist in the Dallas area and author of *10 Steps to Detoxification*.

Natural foods are also Nature's richest sources of antioxidants—plant chemicals that prevent artery damage that can interfere with bloodflow to the genitals. As a bonus, a plant-based diet means that you automatically get less fat. That's important because dietary fat can set the stage for circulatory problems, particularly for men with diabetes or vascular disease, says Dr. Weinhold.

Sip dandelion root tea. A cup or two daily, combined with schizandra berries, will clear contaminants from your liver. Other liver-protecting herbs include artichoke and milk thistle, but don't use them until you're several weeks into your cleansing plan, Dr. Weinhold says. "They're mainly involved in liver repair, and you don't want to add them until you've already cleaned out the contaminants." For all of these herbs, follow the directions on the package.

Clear your kidneys with cucumber. Your kidneys process a tremendous amount of waste each day. Along with your liver, they're responsible for purging your body of toxins that can drag your libido into the basement. To help them work more efficiently, add half a sliced cucumber to a quart of water, and drink the water daily. "Cucumber is great for detoxing because it's a very gentle diuretic," says Dr. Weinhold.

Count on cranberry. To give your kidneys an extra flush, add about 4 ounces of unsweetened cranberry juice to a pitcher of water, and drink several glasses daily, Dr. Weinhold suggests. It helps eliminate toxins from your kidneys, and it also promotes toxin drainage from your lymphatic system.

Knock out the caffeine. Even if you can drink a few cups of coffee without tossing and turning all night, caffeine is still a stimulant—one that can disturb normal sleep patterns even without your being aware of it. Since the liver cleanses itself at night, any interruption in your sleep can cause toxic buildups as well as fatigue, says Dr. Weinhold.

Strategy Two: Strip Away Toxic Thoughts

Sexual desire, like sex itself, involves a lot more than the physical components. It's not a coincidence that men and women with low libido invariably are coping with stress and fatigue as well. You can't have

good sex—or, indeed, any sex—when you can barely drag yourself through the day.

"People breathe shallowly when they're stressed, and shallow breathing increases levels of cortisol and other stress hormones," says Dr. Weinhold. These hormones, in turn, divert bloodflow away from the genitals. "Toxic, negative thoughts are among the main causes of low libido," she explains.

To get back in the mood, you first have to get out of the stress zone. Here's what Dr. Weinhold advises.

Get turned on. Start by turning off destructive self-talk, such as self-criticism about your appearance or mentally turning small problems into huge mental roadblocks. "All of that negative energy can make you feel very unattractive," says Dr. Weinhold.

"You have to turn the thoughts around," she explains. "When you find yourself in that negative state, catch it early and distract yourself. Pick up a book. Listen to an affirmation tape. Do something you enjoy. You'll be surprised by how easy and effective it is to turn negatives into positives."

Breathe life into your libido. Even if you do nothing else, breathing deeply for a few minutes a day will strip stress hormones out of your body, improve bloodflow, and help you relax and get into the mental place where you can start wanting sex again. "Once you get in the habit of breathing deeply into your abdomen, you'll notice that your head is clearer and you feel calmer," says Dr. Weinhold.

Focus on slowing down your breath. Get into a comfortable position, and breathe all the way to the bottom of your lungs. Breathe in for 2 seconds, hold it for a moment, then breathe out for 2 seconds. Keep breathing deeply in and out for 5 to 10 minutes.

Try breathing even slower. After a week or two, slow the rate of your breathing even more. Breathe in for a count of 4, or even 6 or 8, and then exhale at the same rate. "It gets easier with practice, and you'll find that your stress levels drop dramatically," says Dr. Weinhold.

SKIN CARE
PURIFY YOUR SKIN FROM THE INSIDE OUT

Your skin does more than protect your insides from the toxic external world. It also lets toxins out. When your body gets overloaded with toxins—everything from the natural by-products of metabolism to chemicals in air, food, or water—your skin does everything it can to sweat them out.

When you're young, it does a pretty good job both at blocking and releasing toxins. But as you get older, it starts to pay the price with wrinkles, age spots, and loss of tone. The only way to stop this downward spiral is to purify your body as well as your skin. Once you remove toxins, your skin cells will get firmer and healthier, and you'll look better all the way from your head to your toes.

The best way to regenerate tired-looking skin and take years off your looks is to start a program that includes toxin-blocking foods along with skin-healthy herbs and products. Here's a purification plan that will help.

Your Purification Plan

Strategy One: Improve Metabolism and Digestion

Purge with pungent spices. Drinking several cups of ginger tea daily or eating pungent spices such as basil increases metabolism and helps your liver and other organs remove toxins more efficiently, says Leanne Backer, an educator at The Chopra Center at La Costa Resort and Spa in Carlsbad, California. "Ginger also curbs food cravings, which means you're less likely to eat things that clog the system, like too much sweets," she adds.

Freshen your skin with popcorn. High-fiber foods like popcorn and brown rice improve digestion, which is essential for skin health because it speeds the passage of wastes through the intestine. The more quickly you move stools (and the toxins they contain) out of your body, the less likely they are to reenter your bloodstream and travel outward to your skin.

Strategy Two: Draw Out Toxins

Soothe with sesame. Once a day, rub every inch of your skin with sesame oil. It pulls out toxins and makes your skin feel soft and fresh, says Backer.

Soak and sweat. A hot bath does more than soothe away the day's cares. Hot water draws toxins in the body toward the skin's surface, and while the water cools, it pulls toxins all the way out. Adding Epsom or other salts to the bath will improve the detoxification process.

Pour water into your cells. The usual advice to drink eight glasses a day is about right, but more is usually better. "Water is almost a miracle cure," says Margaret Avery-Moon, a certified massage therapist at Desert Institute of the Healing Arts in Tucson. It helps the kidneys and liver process and remove metabolic wastes. It plumps the skin and makes wrinkles less visible. It can even help prevent those under-eye circles that can add years to your appearance.

Strategy Three: Clean Up the Damage

Keeping your skin beautiful and clear requires periodic cleansing of dead skin cells to make room for the healthier skin below to shine through. Here are two quick ways to make yourself glow.

Use a natural peel. Over-the-counter products that contain alpha-hydroxy acid, a natural substance found in fruits, sour milk, and sugar cane, help purge ugly, dead skin from your face. Clearing away the "trash" from the surface of your skin reveals the plump, living cells underneath and will help make your skin look younger.

Brush and stimulate. A process called dry brushing, in which you use a soft, natural bristle brush to rub every inch of your skin, moving from your extremities toward the center of your body, may improve your skin's ability to excrete toxins. It also removes dead cells and will make your skin look (and feel) fresher.

Strategy Four: Feed Your Skin

Happily, some of the best foods for your skin include delicious options like fish, nuts, and fresh vegetables. For mouthwatering recipes using many of the ingredients mentioned below, turn to chapter 4 on page 50.

Fight wrinkles with fish. Scientists have recently learned that "subclinical" inflammation (inflammation that slowly damages the skin even in the absence of immediate symptoms) is among the main causes of wrinkles.

Nicholas Perricone, M.D., assistant clinical professor of dermatology at Yale University School of Medicine and author of *The Wrinkle Cure,* advises everyone to eat at least a few servings of fish a week. Fish contains fatty acids that reduce or eliminate skin inflammation that increases the risk of wrinkles. A diet rich in fish can also reduce unsightly flare-ups from psoriasis or other skin conditions.

Firm up with vitamin C. This all-purpose nutrient is custom-made for healthy, toxin-free skin. It plays a key role in the production of collagen, the protein that keeps skin supple and tight. Just as important, it neutralizes harmful oxygen molecules (free radicals) that damage skin cells. You can get plenty of vitamin C from fruits, vegetables, and juices, along with a daily multivitamin, says Avery-Moon.

Get extra E. Vitamin C is very effective at quenching skin-damaging free radicals in the watery portions of the body, but you need vitamin E to protect the denser, fatty tissues, such as those in the underlying layers of skin. You can get some vitamin E from nuts, seeds, and vegetable oils, but to get the full amount you'll need, take a daily supplement of 150 IU as well.

Cleanse with carrots. That bright orange color comes from beta-carotene, an antioxidant that is converted to vitamin A in the body and is essential for skin health. The more polluted your environment (if you're a smoker, say, or you take prescription medications or live in a smog-filled city), the more carrots and other produce you should eat.

Strategy Five: Tighten Your Defenses

There's a good reason why pharmacy and beauty-store shelves almost collapse under the weight of skin creams, lotions, and masks. Many of these products provide a crucial barrier against environmental toxins, including skin-damaging UV rays from the sun. If you want to ensure that your skin stays taut and glowing throughout your life, here are a few things you should include in your daily plan.

Cool and tighten. Skin pores act as natural traps for oil and grit, which can lead to acne as well as less-than-fresh-looking skin. An easy way to seal out toxins is to splash your skin with cool water or witch hazel after washing. A bracing blast of cold water after a warm-water wash also increases the activity in your lymph glands and will help your body eliminate toxins more efficiently.

Smile big. While you're at it, open your

Detox Makeover

REMEMBER THE TOUGH YEARS OF PUBERTY? Most of us suffered from some combination of surging hormones, painful self-consciousness, and unpredictable outbreaks of acne. Just stepping in front of a mirror could feel like the ultimate torture.

Jane J., the timid teenager who walked through the doors of Betty's Bath and Day Spa in Albuquerque, New Mexico, had serious acne on her forehead and along her jaw. Not surprisingly, her self-esteem was almost in the basement.

"I knew right away that, like most teenagers, she probably had a terrible diet," recalls Sage Wise, head aesthetician at the spa. His first order of business was to explain the basics of good nutrition and exercise. After that, he went to work removing toxins from the surface of her skin.

He applied tea tree oil, which has been called Nature's antiseptic because of its antibacterial and anti-inflammatory effects. He applied a mineral mud mask to draw out toxins. He followed that with a toner to seal her pores, then an all-natural moisturizer to restore her skin's natural plumpness and shine.

"I saw her once a month initially, but she finally quit coming in," Wise recalls. "She did all of the things I told her, and now she has great skin."

eyes wide. Raise and lower your eye-brows. Make all the "big" faces that you can think of—and do it for a few minutes every day. "Moving your facial muscles helps keep the skin tight," says Avery-Moon. "Plus, moving the muscles helps remove accumulations of metabolic wastes."

Apply an antioxidant cream. These days, it's easy to find skin creams and lotions that contain green tea polyphenols, vitamin C, or other antioxidants. Studies have shown that daily applications of an antioxidant cream can help prevent cellular by-products from weakening skin tissues and causing wrinkles.

Get in the sunscreen habit. You probably don't think of sunshine as pollution, but exposure to UV rays triggers the production of skin-damaging free radicals. In fact, too much sun exposure is the main cause of tired-looking skin. Your best bet is to apply a sunscreen with an SPF (sun-protection factor) of at least 15 before going outdoors.

SMOKING
CURB NICOTINE CRAVINGS AND REDUCE THE DAMAGE

Smokers know by heart the reasons to quit: Smoking is the single greatest cause of preventable disease. In the United

States alone, more than 1,000 people die every day from smoking-related illnesses. Nearly every bodily organ you can name—the heart, lungs, and even the skin—is seriously damaged by the toxic chemicals in tobacco.

Cigarette smoke contains lethal combinations of carbon monoxide, hydrogen cyanide, and sulfur oxides. It contains tars, cadmium, nickel, and dioxin. It's one of the greatest sources of radiation. In fact, someone who smokes one to two packs a day might be exposed to radiation levels that are the equivalent of hundreds of annual chest x-rays.

More than 80 percent of smokers say that they want to stop, but they can't quite find the strength and willpower to make it happen. If you're ready to make the effort, you should certainly work with your doctor.

Studies have shown that the combination of medications and stop-smoking programs can double your chances of success, and people who are told by their doctors to quit smoking are twice as likely to try compared to those who try to quit on their own, says Jessica Nesseler-Cass, N.D., a naturopathic physician in private practice in Portland, Oregon.

In the meantime, you should detoxify your body to minimize the harmful effects of smoking, and also take advantage of proven strategies to reduce cravings and kick the habit for good.

Your Purification Plan

Strategy One: Cleanse Away Cravings

Withdrawing from cigarettes is never easy. The first 12 to 24 hours are generally the worst, and the first week can feel like years. If you've been smoking for a long time, your brain literally requires nicotine. It takes a powerful commitment to get through the withdrawal period. You can make it a little easier by reducing your body's demand for nicotine while at the same time practicing lifestyle habits that make it easier to get through those initial difficult days.

Eat organic foods. Smoking lowers your body's pH, which makes the cravings more intense. When you're trying to quit, eat a lot of organic fruits, vegetables, and whole grains, and minimize your consumption of meats and other high-fat foods. Your blood and tissues will get more alkaline and the cravings will be less intense, explains Elson M. Haas, M.D., director of the Preventive Medical Center at Marin in San Rafael, California, and author of *The Detox Diet.*

As a bonus, some of the components in produce bind to nicotine and help remove it from your body, adds Cynthia P. Buxton, N.D., L.Ac., a naturopathic physician and acupuncturist in private practice in Seattle.

Supplement with sulfur. A product called Sulfonil, available in health food stores, binds to nicotine receptors on your body's cells. "It makes the receptors less active and eventually causes cells to eliminate them," says Dr. Buxton. This process, called down-regulation, reduces your body's dependence on nicotine, she explains.

Curb cravings with bicarbonate. Available in pharmacies and health food stores, potassium or sodium bicarbonate tablets will make your body more alkaline and minimize your desire to smoke. Take five or six tablets daily until you've quit for good.

Optimize bowel function. The longer toxins from cigarettes remain in your body, the more intense your cravings are likely to be. The most efficient way to get them out is to have regular bowel movements, and the best way to achieve that is to get plenty of fiber in your diet, says Dr. Buxton. You'll almost automatically get enough if you make plant foods like fruits, vegetables, legumes, and whole grains the backbone of your diet. You can get even more fiber by taking several tablespoons of flaxseed daily. Flax is also high in omega-3 fatty acids, which reduce the inflammation that occurs when you're detoxing.

Snack smart. Keep plenty of raw foods in the house. Carrots, celery, and raw, unsalted sunflower seeds reduce the body's digestive burden and make it easier to eliminate toxins. At the same time, these easy-to-eat snacks replace the hand-to-mouth habit of smoking and can give you a psychological boost during the most difficult days.

Create a smoke-free lifestyle. Cigarettes are involved in nearly every part of your life if you're a smoker. The cravings will continue to be intense unless you replace your old habits with newer, healthier ones. Once you've made the commitment:

⚬ Banish reminders. Get rid of ashtrays and make your house a no-smoking zone.
⚬ Be squeaky clean. Brush your teeth often and get used to the fresh, minty feeling.
⚬ Divert your attention. Stay busy with hobbies, work, or anything else that keeps your mind busy. You're going to want to smoke for a long time. Staying active will make you feel good about making the change and less likely to dwell on your desire for cigarettes.

Strategy Two: Reduce Your Toxic Load

The chemicals in tobacco aren't the only things that make smoking so dangerous. Every time you light up, your body churns out free radicals, highly reactive oxygen molecules that damage cells in your airways, arteries, heart, and every other part of your body. The only truly effective way to reduce your risk of smoking-related diseases is to quit. But if you've only recently stopped smoking or you plan to do so at some point, it's worth taking steps to minimize the internal damage.

"Even if you can't bring yourself to quit, you'll be a healthier smoker if you eat well and get regular exercise," says Dr. Nesseler-Cass.

Load up on vitamin C. It's a potent antioxidant that reduces free-radical damage in the lungs and other tissues, says Dr. Nesseler-Cass. A study of more than 1,500 men found that those who got 138 mg of vitamin C daily—a little more than twice the recommended daily amount—were 37 percent less likely to die from cancer than those who got less.

Add vitamin E and selenium. These nutrients work together to quash the harmful effects of free radicals. Selenium is especially helpful because it improves your immune system's ability to recognize and destroy cancer cells caused by smoking. Since modern farming methods have depleted large amounts of selenium from the food supply, you might want to take a daily supplement that provides 200 mcg. Vitamin E is even harder to get from foods (the main sources are nuts and vegetable oils), so plan on taking 150 IU daily.

Eat a lot of produce. Experts aren't sure why, but smokers don't eat as many fruits and vegetables as nonsmokers do. So if you can't be a nonsmoker, at least try to act like one. Produce is loaded with chemical compounds that can help min-

imize the damage caused by smoking. Japanese researchers report that men who eat raw vegetables can lower their risk of lung cancer by an impressive 36 percent. Those who eat fruit daily do even better: They can reduce their risk of lung cancer by 55 percent.

Supplement with glutathione. Available in health food stores as well as pharmacies, it's an antioxidant that improves your liver's ability to break down and remove smoking-related toxins, says Dr. Nesseler-Cass. The recommended dose for smokers is 250 to 500 mg daily.

Take L-cysteine. It's an amino acid

Smoking with Fewer Risks

THERE'S NO SUCH THING as a safe cigarette, but natural-tobacco products such as American Spirit do appear to be less harmful than the big commercial brands because they don't contain chemicals that enhance burning, and they are cured without the use of chemical additives, says Elson M. Haas, M.D., director of the Preventive Medical Center at Marin in San Rafael, California, and author of *The Detox Diet.*

Another option, while you're working up the determination to quit, is to replace tobacco with a traditional "smoking herb," such as mullein leaf, rosemary, or sarsaparilla. Some herb shops carry lobelia leaf cigarettes. Also known as "Indian tobacco," lobelia is often used as a cigarette substitute because it has a similar taste.

that your body converts to glutathione—and glutathione is the most important antioxidant for the lungs as well as the liver, says Dr. Buxton. L-cysteine also protects your lungs from acetaldehyde, a chemical compound in cigarette smoke. Follow the directions on the label.

STRESS
DRAIN THE STRAIN FROM YOUR LIFE

Stress is a rational response to modern life. We're always in a hurry. Bills have to get paid. Family issues have to be dealt with. We get sick, fight, worry about our appearance, struggle through tough days at the office. Of course we're stressed.

The problem with stress is that it's an evolutionary response to physical danger. When we sense a threat, our bodies release adrenaline and other chemicals that make us more alert and increase our strength and reaction times.

But what happens when the stress is mental? The same chemical energizers course through our bodies, but they keep going all the time because modern stress never stops. We're not designed to withstand this nearly constant chemical rush, explains Dan L. Martin, N.D., O.M.D., a naturopathic physician and doctor of Oriental Medicine in Texarkana, Arkansas.

About 90 percent of doctors' visits are for stress-related disorders. Stress causes fatigue, insomnia, and low libido. It increases your risk of high blood pressure and heart disease. You're even more likely to get colds when you're stressed.

Since we can't eliminate stress from our lives, the only solution is to deal with its aftermath. This means purging your body and mind of stress-related toxins. And, as you might expect, there are a lot of them.

Your Purification Plan

Strategy One: Do Mental Detoxification

You don't need a degree in biochemistry to recognize that a negative, tension-filled mind saps strength and motivation and makes it harder to get through each day. It increases the activity of your sympathetic nervous system and unleashes floods of adrenaline, cortisol, and other stress-related hormones that have to be dispelled. The stress in your life may be a constant, but you can take control. Here's how.

Breathe! When you're stressed, it's normal to take short, uneven breaths. That's okay if it happens only for a minute or two each day, but when you're chronically stressed, as many of us are, your body is never able to fully dispel carbon dioxide from your blood. That means your tissues don't get enough oxygen. To turn things around:

◉ Breathe and hold. The next time you feel your stress level rising, take a deep breath, hold it in for about 5 seconds, then slowly empty your lungs. Repeat the cycle five or six times. It will permeate your cells with oxygen while at the same time removing toxic levels of carbon dioxide.

◉ Use alternate-nostril breathing. It's among the best ways to dispel stress chemicals and prevent them from accumulating throughout the day, says Peter Bennett, N.D., a naturopathic physician in Vancouver and coauthor of *7-Day Detox Miracle.* Exhale all the air from your lungs, then close your right nostril with your thumb and inhale deeply through your left nostril. Now, switch sides. Close your left nostril and exhale deeply through your right nostril. Repeat the same steps, only this time inhale through your right nostril and exhale through your left. Repeat the whole sequence 10 to 30 times.

Cleanse your mind of toxic thoughts. In fact, cleanse it of all extraneous thoughts for a few minutes every day. Because your mind is awash in thoughts, just as your body is awash in chemicals and wastes, clearing your mind with meditation gives it—and you—a chance to recover and rebuild.

Sit comfortably with your eyes focused on the floor. Pay attention to your breath as it enters your nostrils, fills your lungs, and then pours back out. Count each breath without allowing thoughts to interfere. Every time a thought does intrude (and this happens often), go back to number one. Try to count to 100 without letting a single thought, except for your counting, enter your mind.

Cleanse with yoga. Apart from its role in meditative stress-reduction, yoga improves your organs' ability to dispel stressful toxins. Nearly all health clubs offer yoga classes, sometimes for as little as $5 to $10 a session.

Strategy Two: Sweep Stress from Your Body

The conventional wisdom for managing stress is to maintain a positive attitude and to remind yourself that you can control how you react to the troubles life heaps up. To keep things in perspective, in other words, and to take the kinds of simple steps, such as breaking big jobs into smaller parts, keeping your expectations reasonable, and so on, that keep stress from overwhelming your life.

This is good advice, but you still have to take steps to cleanse your body of fatiguing wastes as well as the consequences of stress. Here's where to start.

Work it out. Exercise is one of the best ways to mop up adrenaline and other stress-related chemicals and to increase levels of endorphins, "feel good" brain chemicals that produce a sense of well-being. Recent studies suggest that getting as little as 20 to 30 minutes of easy to moderate daily exercise (walking, working in the yard, and so on) is enough to purge stress hormones as well as muscle and mental tension.

Double up on produce. "Nearly 100 percent of my patients are low in essential nutrients," says Dr. Martin. "Even if you eat an almost perfect diet, you're exposed to twice as much stress as humans were designed to handle." Your body works so hard dispelling stress and toxins that it depletes its nutritional reserves.

Supplement your diet. In addition to eating a lot more organic plant foods such as legumes, whole grains, fruits, and vegetables, Dr. Martin recommends taking a daily multivitamin supplement. It's especially important to get enough B vitamins because they appear to raise levels of dopamine, a brain chemical that's linked to feelings of confidence and well-being.

Rub it out. Researchers at the University of Miami report that massage helps mop cortisol from the blood while lowering blood pressure and tension-producing buildups of lactic acid. "Massage relaxes the endocrine system, especially the adrenal glands, which are responsible for producing stress hormones," says Dr. Martin. You can treat yourself to a professional massage. Or, better yet, you and your partner can alternate giving each other gentle, stress-relieving massages.

Purge your lymphatic system. Toxins that accumulate in your lymph nodes can overwhelm your liver and leave you feeling tired and stressed, says Dr. Martin. A Swedish massage will drain your lymphatic system to some extent, but you'll do better if you occasionally visit a massage therapist who specializes in lymphatic drainage.

Can the coffee. Duke University researchers report that four or five cups daily make the body act as though it's under constant stress. Coffee drinkers in a recent study showed a 32 percent increase in adrenaline, one of the main stress hormones. Caffeine is also a diuretic that accelerates the accumulation of toxins in the blood and causes low-level chronic fatigue, Dr. Bennett explains.

Refresh with ginseng. Commonly used for stress and anxiety, ginseng contains chemical compounds, ginsenosides, that protect the brain and nervous system from toxins and can improve emotional resilience. "It's like a reset button for the adrenal glands," says Dr. Martin. "It rebuilds the glands and helps the body adapt to stress." The recommended dose is 200 to 500 mg daily.

Feel better with St. John's wort. People who suffer from stress often experience mild depression, and treating the depression can lift the stress as well. The herb St. John's wort is as effective as prescription antidepressants for mild to moderate depression, and it has none of the side effects. The recommended dose is 300 mg three times daily.

Detox Makeover

FIVE OR SIX COLDS A YEAR. A persistent cough. One yeast infection after another. It took Liz Oates, a writer in the Philadelphia area, a long time to figure out that life wasn't supposed to be like that. It wasn't until a bout of pneumonia put her in bed for a week that the mental lightbulb went on.

On the advice of a friend, she went to see a naturopathic physician, who focused almost entirely on her emotional health. "She said I was stressed to the max, and that's where I needed the most work," Liz says.

On the advice of her doctor, she started an exercise program—a spinning class three days a week. She made an appointment with a massage therapist. She started doing breathing and meditation exercises before starting work in the morning. The most important change, she says, was in her thinking. "Whenever things used to go wrong, I always imagined the worst. Now, I ask myself, 'Is this really going to ruin my life?'

"I started really working on my stress about 2 years ago," Liz says. "I'm still pretty type-A, but I don't get sick as much, and I sleep better. My friends tell me I look happier. You know, I think I am."

Chapter 13

Quick Cleanups:
Fast and Easy Detox Tips
for Everyday Health Problems

SO YOU'VE MADE A FRESH START. Maybe you've gone through a 3-day fast, had hydration therapy, or even steam-cleaned yourself in a sweat lodge, and you feel absolutely wonderful. Your head is clear, your appetite for sweets is gone, and your body feels lighter. Then you drink a glass of water. Trouble.

The EPA lists 50 chemical and 10 microbial contaminants that may come out of your kitchen tap—even after your local water company has waved its purifying, clarifying, detoxifying magic wand over the reservoir. The air you breathe and the food you eat may be even worse. And all those nasty waste products your body produces in the normal course of metabolism constantly threaten to return you to the condition of a walking toxic dump. In other words, even if you've cleaned up your act, you will still accumulate toxins, and they can make you sick. What's a person to do?

Obviously, going on a juice fast or taking a high colonic every time you develop a headache or feel a little depressed isn't practical. It's easier, faster, smarter, and cheaper to target whatever particular toxin is causing symptoms or making a chronic condition worse. Often you can do that with a simple cleanup.

Below are some of the most common conditions caused by toxins, along with some quick strategies to help get them under control.

ARTERIOSCLEROSIS

"Arteriosclerosis" is a big word that simply means the hardening of the arteries. This condition is often caused by toxins, including fats, that inflame arterial walls. Here's how to keep your arteries clean and running smoothly.

Floss your teeth. "We have known for over a hundred years that there is a relationship between inflamed gums and circulatory health," says Decker Weiss, N.M.D., a naturopathic medical doctor at the Arizona Heart Hospital, a teacher at the Southwest College of Naturo-

---

Detox Makeover

DR. DECKER WEISS is perhaps the first naturopathic doctor ever to have completed a cardiac residency at a conventional medical hospital. Today he has staff privileges at the Arizona Heart Hospital in Phoenix, where he finds that detoxification is of tremendous help to his heart patients. He recalls one in particular: "I had one 89-year-old guy come to me and say, 'Dr. Weiss, I have one artery left, I've had stents three times, and I'm maxed on medication for chest pain. I want you to keep my artery open for 6 months until the next generation of stents comes out.' I told him, 'I'm not going to reverse your coronary artery disease just so you can go back on a stent.'"

Dr. Weiss put the patient on a detoxification program that, among other things, included a cleansing diet, ginger, cayenne, and magnesium supplements, as well as a health regime he calls The Weiss Method, which is described in his new book of the same name. A year and a half later, the patient's stress test was normal, he had normal blood pressure and heart rate, and he was nearly pain free. The foundation of his recovery was body purification. "Without detoxification," says Dr. Weiss, "nothing else works."

pathic Medicine in Tempe, and author of the book *The Weiss Method*. "That's because arteriosclerosis is an inflammatory process in the body," he says, "and some of the toxins that build up on your teeth and inflame your gums can also inflame your arteries. So get those teeth and gums taken care of." That means brushing, flossing, and regular visits to your dentist.

Reach for antioxidants. The antioxidant vitamins E and C neutralize free radicals—substances that cause inflammation. "I like any natural form of E," says Dr. Weiss. "If you have heart disease already, also take a separate mixed antioxidant supplement.

"The king of the antioxidants is alphalipoic acid. This is a spectacular medicine. Put me on a desert island with only a couple of supplements and this is one I want with me." Take 600 mg a day in capsule form.

BAD BREATH

Bad breath is more than just a social problem. It's a serious indication that your body is carrying a toxic burden that needs to be dealt with.

According to Decker Weiss, N.M.D., a naturopathic medical doctor at the Arizona Heart Hospital, a teacher at the

Southwest College of Naturopathic Medicine in Tempe, and author of the book *The Weiss Method,* "Bad breath is a cardinal warning sign that you have medical issues. It means you're at crisis level of not digesting and absorbing your food." Richard DeAndrea, M.D., N.D., a physician at the Akasha Center for Integrative Medicine in Santa Monica, California, agrees. Dr. DeAndrea is also medical advisor to the American Naturopathic Medical Association, the Physicians Committee of Responsible Medicine, and Earth Save International, as well as the co-creator of The 21 Day Detox program. "Bad breath is usually a sign that the plumbing in the body is backed up," he says. Here's how to clean up your act.

Go alkaline. "Reducing or eliminating sugars and animal proteins from your diet and eating lots of fiber can be very helpful over the course of a couple of weeks," says Dr. DeAndrea. This increases the overall alkalinity of your body and promotes better digestion.

Give your stomach a supplemental boost. "Supplement your diet with hydrochloric acid (HCL) and pancreatic enzymes," says Dr. Weiss. "If you have really, really bad breath and you're not digesting at all, try plant enzymes," he says. "They're super strong. But if you have an ulcer, they can increase pain, so it's best not to use them." Be careful as well with HCL; if it gives you any burning, stop taking it. Also, always take HCL in the middle of your meal, never before your food. Pancreatic enzymes, plant enzymes, and HCL are available at your local health food store.

BLADDER INFECTION

Infections of the urinary tract can be painful and annoying, and if not treated, they can lead to serious problems in the bladder or kidneys. Your kidneys play an important role in keeping your body free of toxins, so you need to do everything you can to keep these organs in good working order. If you're fighting an active infection, you need to be under a doctor's care, but you can also help yourself by flushing out some of the toxic microbes that are causing you misery.

Juice the germs. Cranberries can do more than simply add a crimson touch to your Thanksgiving dinner table. One study of 150 women showed that drinking cranberry juice on a regular basis can cut the risk for urinary tract infections in half. This detoxifier works by preventing bacteria from sticking to the lining of the urinary tract, and it's been shown to reduce urine odor, burning with urination, and calcium content in the urine. Studies show that drinking as little as 10 ounces a day can be effective, although it works better as a preventive measure than as a curative. Do not, however, drink juice with sugar in it. Sugar can make your condition worse.

Bear with it. Richard DeAndrea, M.D., N.D., a physician at the Akasha Center for Integrative Medicine in Santa Monica, California, recommends the herb uva ursi, also known as bearberry, to get rid of the microbes that cause bladder infections. Uva ursi contains a chemical called arbutin, which has an antiseptic effect on the mucous membrane of the urinary tract. Only the leaves are used medicinally, and it's easy to make an infusion from them. Just add 1 pint of boiling water to 1 ounce of leaves, let sit for 10 to 15 minutes, then strain and drink. Or you can take the herb in capsule form; just follow the dosage instructions on the package.

BREAST PAIN

When a woman develops breast pain, her first step should always be to see a doctor to make certain that it isn't the result of a serious medical condition. But if you suffer from tenderness and you're otherwise healthy, Decker Weiss, N.M.D., a naturopathic medical doctor at the Arizona Heart Hospital, a teacher at the Southwest College of Naturopathic Medicine in Tempe, and author of the book *The Weiss Method,* believes that the problem may be due to poor handling of hormones and toxins by your liver. Here's what to try.

Try liver herbs. "Milk thistle is wonderful," says Dr. Weiss. "It's a great antioxidant and it helps promote good liver function." Other effective herbs include dandelion root and artichoke, both of which increase your liver's ability to filter out toxins. Follow the dosage instructions on the package.

Add fiber. Dr. Weiss also recommends adding high-fiber foods to your diet. The liver uses bile as a way to eliminate toxins from the body. When bile, which helps digest fats, is released into the intestines, it takes a toxic load along with it. "When toxins get dumped into the bile," explains Dr. Weiss, "they've got to go 26 to 29 feet to get through the digestive system. Sometimes toxins can escape the bile and get back into the bloodstream." Fiber will help carry them out of the body more rapidly. Good sources of fiber include fruits, vegetables, legumes, and whole grains.

BUG BITES

Most bug bites and stings, which cause irritation and pain by way of toxic venom transferred to the victim, can be treated both topically and internally. However, if after a bee sting or spider bite you notice any significant swelling, redness, or difficulty breathing, you need to seek medical treatment immediately. For minor bites and stings, here's how to clean up the venom.

Get topical. There are a number of creams that work well to relieve the irritation of bites. "Calendula and burdock creams are wonderful," says Decker Weiss, N.M.D., a naturopathic medical doctor at the Arizona Heart Hospital, a teacher at the Southwest College of Naturopathic Medicine in Tempe, and author of the book *The Weiss Method.* There is also some evidence that calendula cream works well as a repellant. Echinacea is another excellent remedy, says Doug Schar, Dip.Phyt., M.C.P.P., M.N.I.M.H., a Washington, D.C.–based herbalist who was medically trained in Europe. It speeds the removal of insect toxins from the body and quickly reduces the pain and discomfort of the bite. Schar recommends putting a few drops of echinacea tincture on an adhesive bandage and strapping it right on the bite. Herbal tinctures are liquid drops, made by infusing herbs in alcohol, and are available at health food stores. (See page 113 for more information on tinctures.)

Try homeopathic treatments. "Homeopathics like urticarea apis and sulfur can bring relief," says Dr. Weiss. He recommends a low-potency dose every 15 minutes for 2 hours after you're bitten. Homeopathic medications are available at many natural food stores.

CELIAC DISEASE

Celiac disease is a condition that prevents your small bowel from absorbing food. The disease occurs due to damage caused by autoimmune reactions triggered by gluten, a substance in some grains such as wheat, barley, and rye. If you can digest gluten, there's no reason for you to avoid this substance. But if you're sensitive to it, gluten represents a serious toxic substance to your body.

Symptoms vary from person to person, but they may include pains in the gut, diarrhea, constipation, weight loss, fatigue, anemia, and joint pain. There is one good way to detoxify the gluten from your system.

Detoxify your diet. The way to relieve the symptoms of celiac disease is obvious: Keep gluten out of your system. Simply remove grass grains such as wheat, oats, barley, rye, and triticale from your meals. Even a teaspoon of the offending grains is enough to cause intestinal damage. Once gluten is removed from your diet, your body will begin repairing damage immediately.

Play detective. If you're not sure whether you have a sensitivity to gluten, you need to work with a health care professional who will likely put you on an elimination diet to determine whether you need to take the step of eliminating gluten from your diet. For more information on food sensitivities and elimination diets, see "Scoping Out Problem Foods" on page 38.

DANDRUFF

Spending a lot of time brushing the shoulders of your blazer with your hand? Your solution might not lie in a bottle of dandruff shampoo.

Check your oil. Body purification has two major effects: It purges the body of toxins, and it restores balance to the organ systems. If your scalp has been sloughing off a lot of snow lately, internal imbalance may be the problem, leaving your skin dry and flaky. "If you have dandruff, your internal oils are incorrect or off, or you're not getting enough good ones," says Decker Weiss, N.M.D., a naturopathic medical doctor at the Arizona Heart Hospital, a teacher at the Southwest College of Naturopathic Medicine in Tempe, and author of the book *The Weiss Method.* "Try using a good fish oil or a mixed plant oil." These oils are available at your local health food store. Follow the dosage instructions on the package.

DEPRESSION

Depression often indicates an overall toxic load, and studies show that getting those toxins out through aerobic exercise (walking, jogging, swimming, bicycling, and so on) can be as effective as any pill. If your depression is chronic, you need to be under a doctor's care. If your depression is mild to moderate, however, you may be able to deal with it on your own with these suggestions to help lift your mood.

Lift your spirits with aminos. "I'd do a large focus on amino acids, especially for depression," advises Priscilla Slagle, M.D., a holistic physician in Palm Springs, California, who specializes in the treatment of depression and is author of the e-book *The Way Up from Down.* "First get rid of sugar, red meat, and simple carbohydrates, which can cause mood swings. Then try a supplement of the amino acid l-tyrosine, which converts to neurotransmitters such as serotonin and dopamine." An imbalance of these chemicals in the brain is thought to be a major contributor to depression.

Get back to basics. When it comes to depression, "it's liver, liver, liver," says Decker Weiss, N.M.D., a naturopathic medical doctor at the Arizona Heart Hospital, a teacher at the Southwest College of Naturopathic Medicine in Tempe, and author of the book *The Weiss Method.* The liver is the body's most important detoxification organ, and it needs to be in good condition to deal with the general toxicity that causes low moods. So liver herbs such as milk thistle, dandelion, and artichoke may be helpful. It's also a good idea to adhere to a diet rich in high-fiber foods, such as beans, fresh fruits and vegetables, and whole grains.

Lighten up on sugar. "Sugar is a toxin," says Dr. Weiss. "It's an obstacle to health. It stresses your pancreas, it stresses your entire endocrine system, and it causes emotional ups and downs. Nicotine does the same thing. It causes emotional ups and downs. It's an addictive substance.

When you're trying to treat emotional issues, it's not the way to go."

DIABETES

When your blood sugar levels are regularly too high for good health, you have diabetes. Blood glucose is normally kept at acceptable levels by a hormone called insulin, which is released by the pancreas. People with Type 1 diabetes are born without the ability to produce insulin. People with Type 2 either don't make enough insulin, can't efficiently use the insulin they produce, or both. Type 2 diabetes often develops after age 40 and is associated with being inactive or overweight. If you have diabetes, you need to be under a doctor's care, but there are some cleanups you can do to help control your condition.

Take antioxidants. Decker Weiss, N.M.D., a naturopathic medical doctor at the Arizona Heart Hospital, a teacher at the Southwest College of Naturopathic Medicine in Tempe, and author of the book *The Weiss Method,* feels that Type 2 diabetes is a modern societal plague brought on by our culture of unhealthful habits. His first recommendation: "Take a lot of antioxidants because high glucose damages blood vessels." The damage is caused by inflammation, and where there is inflammation, there are toxic free radicals. Antioxidants include vitamin C and vitamin E. You can safely take 1,000 to 2,000 mg of vitamin C and 150 to 200 IUs of vitamin E daily.

Manage glucose levels with gymnema. "Botanicals such as dolberry, fenugreek, bitter melon, and gymnema can all help control glucose levels," says Dr. Weiss. "But you must continue to monitor your blood glucose levels to make sure they're working." His favorite is gymnema. It's often taken as a tea. Add ¾ teaspoon to an 8-ounce cup of boiling water. After several minutes, strain and drink. Two cups a day is optimal, taken an hour before breakfast and dinner. Gymnema works gradually, over a period of many months, so don't be surprised if you don't see immediate benefits. If your doctor has given you insulin, do not stop taking it. Gymnema is not a substitute.

EAR INFECTION

Otitis media, the medical term for an earache caused by an infection in the inner ear, is one of the most common conditions pediatricians see. But it doesn't have to be. There are some easy ways to drastically reduce the amount of suffering your kids go through.

Clear the air. A study in Canada of 650 first-graders demonstrated that young children who lived in homes with two smokers had up to an 85 percent increased risk for developing a middle ear infection. If only their mothers smoked, they had a 68 percent increased risk. So do yourself and your children a favor—detoxify your family by removing all tobacco products from your home. If you aren't yet ready to take the plunge and quit smoking, at least do your smoking outdoors.

Remove milk. Cows are not our friends when it comes to ear infections, so leave the milk products on the shelf at the grocery store. "Dairy products make you produce more phlegm, so reducing or eliminating milk, cream, and cheese consumption may help prevent earaches," says Richard DeAndrea, M.D., N.D., a physician at the Akasha Center for Integrative Medicine in Santa Monica, California.

You can find a tremendous number of substitutes for cow's milk in most grocery stores and in any natural food store. Try milk, cheese, and ice cream substitutes made from soy, rice, or almonds. For more information about cleansing your child's diet of problem foods, see "Scoping Out Problem Foods" on page 38.

FLATULENCE

The average person passes gas 14 times a day, but some people can run that number up a lot higher. When undigested food reaches the colon, harmless intestinal bacteria break it down in a process that releases nitrogen, hydrogen, and methane, as well as trace gases such as skatole, indole, and some sulfur-containing compounds, which give gas its characteristic smell. The challenge is to keep undigested food from reaching your large intestine. Here's how.

Cut the carbohydrates. Research suggests that, since most foods that reach your colon before breaking down are carbohydrates, you might want to cut sugars and starches from your diet as much as you can. The same goes for alcohol. This strategy, as many dieters will tell you, can also help you lose weight.

Fiber up. Any food that does happen to reach your colon should remain there, exposed to intestinal bacteria, as briefly as possible. Adding fiber to your diet, in the form of whole grain foods, fruits, and vegetables, can help move things along more quickly. Rye is a particularly good choice in that it contains more fiber—both heart-healthful soluble and bowel-healthful insoluble—than other grains do.

Some people who add fiber to their diets experience a temporary increase in the amount of gas they produce. The trick here is to add fiber in small increments, allowing your digestive system to become accustomed to it.

Combine foods properly. Many people find that certain combinations of foods produce more gas. "Eat proteins with vegetables and starches with vegetables, but never eat proteins and starches together," says Yvette Andrews, C.N., a nutritional consultant at Herbally Yours in Charlotte, North Carolina. "Don't eat acid fruits and sweet fruits together, and never eat melon with any other fruit. Drink water only after meals or about a half-hour before meals. And to make digestion easier, chew your food 20 to 30 times with each bite."

GALLSTONES

Toxic mineral deposits in your gallbladder can be painful and difficult to treat. If your body tries to excrete them, they can get stuck in the ductwork of your body and cause a medical emergency, so prevention is your best bet. Here's how.

Fatten up your food. Losing weight by eliminating fats from your diet may not be such a good idea. "Most people I've seen who have had gallstones have at one time or another been on a low-fat diet," says Decker Weiss, N.M.D., a naturopathic medical doctor at the Arizona Heart Hospital, a teacher at the Southwest College of Naturopathic Medicine in Tempe, and author of the book *The Weiss Method*. "When you eat fats, your body releases bile, which is full of salts. If you don't eat fats, the bile sits and forms stones." To get rid of the bile before it causes problems, add fats back into your diet in the form of quality fish (such as wild salmon or mackerel) and olive oil.

GOUT

"Gout was once known as the disease of kings and queens because they were the only people who could afford the expensive diet that leads to this painful condition," says Richard DeAndrea, M.D., N.D., a physician at the Akasha Center for Integrative Medicine in Santa Monica, California. "It's caused by an accumulation of toxins called purines, which form crystals in the joint of the large toe and damage the bone there." Here's how to keep those purines at bay.

Avoid meats. Animal flesh is taboo for people with gout, according to Dr. De-

Andrea. Why? "Purines come from concentrated sources of protein in the diet," he says. "So eliminating meats like steak, pork, and lamb can help reduce the amount of purines, which will break down into uric acid and be eliminated from the body." Anchovies, sardines, herring, mackerel, and scallops also have a high purine content.

Don't drink. Decker Weiss, N.M.D., a naturopathic medical doctor at the Arizona Heart Hospital, a teacher at the Southwest College of Naturopathic Medicine in Tempe, and author of the book *The Weiss Method*, says, "If you have gout, you can't drink alcohol or eat white sugar, either." Beer has especially high levels of purines.

Get milk. The *New England Journal of Medicine* published a study that shows that drinking a lot of milk can protect you against developing gout. No one knows why, but presumably, milk and other dairy products detoxify the body of purines.

Get more sulfur. "Eat more sulfur-containing foods, like eggs, asparagus, garlic, and onions," says Yvette Andrews, C.N., a nutritional consultant at Herbally Yours in Charlotte, North Carolina. Why? "Sulfur is excellent for helping the body repair bone and connective tissue."

HEADACHES

That pain in your head, whether it's dull, throbbing, or sharp, can signal anything from emotional stress to serious disorders in the brain, so if it lasts more than a day, see your doctor. Below are some ways you can use detoxification to ease the pain.

Watch what you eat. Richard DeAndrea, M.D., N.D., a physician at the Akasha Center for Integrative Medicine in Santa Monica, California, points out that what you put into your stomach can create problems for your head. "I would look for certain allergens in the diet that can be triggers, especially coffee, chocolate, burnt foods, and wine," he says. "These things can often exacerbate headaches or lead to migraine conditions."

De-hormonize. "If you get migraines and you're on hormone replacement therapy or birth control pills, you're going to have to do something else," says Decker Weiss, N.M.D., a naturopathic medical doctor at the Arizona Heart Hospital, a teacher at the Southwest College of Naturopathic Medicine in Tempe, and author of the book *The Weiss Method*. "Synthetic hormones cause headaches." You might try replacing your HRT with phytoestrogens made from plants, but talk to your doctor before changing any medications.

Double your relief with willow. "White willow bark is good for stopping pain, and it's also a diuretic," says Yvette Andrews, C.N., a nutritional consultant at Herbally Yours in Charlotte, North Carolina. Diuretics help the body lose excess water, and the urine is one pathway through which your body detoxifies. And studies have shown willow to be nearly as effective as aspirin at relieving pain. You can take this herb in the form of a tea or in capsules. Follow the dosage instructions on the package.

HEARTBURN

The sick, burning sensation you sometimes feel behind your breastbone is actually caused by a digestive chemical, hydrochloric acid, getting into the wrong place: your esophagus. Although heartburn has many causes, eating foods that are hard for your digestive system to handle is high on the list. Sticking to a diet that helps your body cleanse and purify itself on an ongoing basis (see chapter 3 on page 30) will go a long way toward helping to eliminate this problem. Here are some other ways to get that acid back down where it belongs.

Get aid from enzymes. "The sphincter muscle in your esophagus is like a cork in a bottle in that it keeps hydrochloric acid from escaping upward, out of your stomach," Decker Weiss, N.M.D., a naturopathic medical doctor at the Arizona Heart Hospital, a teacher at the Southwest College of Naturopathic Medicine in Tempe, and author of the book *The Weiss Method,* explains. "Sometimes it can become damaged by too much mechanical digestion, that is, when the digestive system does too much muscular grinding, rather than using chemicals, to break down food. To allow it to heal, you need to shift the emphasis back to chemical digestion. Plant enzymes would be my first choice for a digestive aid. They work extremely well and aren't likely to cause discomfort. Do not use hydrochloric acid (HCL) to fix this problem. It will only make things worse."

Drink lemon water. Limonene is a liquid terpene with a lemon odor found in lemons and oranges and other essential oils. "This helps fix the cork," says Dr. Weiss. "It works as well as Prilosec and other medications." Follow the dosage instructions on the package.

Limonene may be difficult for you to find in your health food store, so try drinking lemon water for the same effect, says Peter Bennett, N.D., a naturopathic physician in Vancouver and coauthor of *7-Day Detox Miracle*. "Squeeze the juice from half of an organic lemon into a quart of water. Drop in the remains of the lemon and the peel and leave them in the water," says Dr. Bennett. He suggests drinking the water throughout the day in place of, or in addition to, your regular water consumption. "You can even add half a cup of organic concord grape juice to the mixture if you find it too tart," he says.

High Cholesterol

Cholesterol is a waxy lipid that your body needs to make hormones, vitamin D, and bile acids. It also supports healthy brain function. Although you get some cholesterol from your diet, most is manufactured by your liver and travels to various organs in your body by way of your bloodstream.

Cholesterol types fall into two main categories: high-density lipoprotein (HDL), which protects your arteries, and low-density lipoprotein (LDL), which can damage them. In general, when you have a blood test, you want your blood level of HDL to be high (over 40 milligrams per deciliter, though over 50 mg/dL is optimal), and your LDL to be low (under 130 mg/dL, though under 100 mg/dL is optimal), to maintain good health. LDL can damage your blood vessels and cause heart disease, so it's considered a toxin. Fortunately, there are some very good ways to lower LDL levels.

Eat live foods. "To lower your cholesterol, first I would suggest a nutritional cleansing," suggests Yvette Andrews, C.N., a nutritional consultant at Herbally Yours in Charlotte, North Carolina. "Drink vegetable juice, add more live foods like fresh fruits and vegetables to your diet, and drink lots of water. This will bring the body back into balance and the body will begin to heal itself."

Beat it with beets. Adding beets to your diet can pay off with real benefits to your health. In laboratory animal studies, sugar beet root has been shown to lower LDL cholesterol levels by nearly one-third and triglycerols, another class of harmful lipids, by 40 percent. Researchers think beet root may work by improving the liver's ability to remove LDL from the bloodstream. It also raises HDL, and as an additional benefit, it seems to help protect you from colon cancer.

Fight fats with fenugreek. Fenugreek, an herb cultivated in both Europe and Asia, contains substances called steroid saponins, which lower the level of various harmful fatlike chemicals (lipids) in your blood. One study in France showed that people who consumed fenugreek seeds several times a day had lower blood levels of all types of harmful cholesterol (LDL and VLDL) as well as other lipids called triglycerides. Beneficial cholesterol (HDL), however, was not affected. By the way, fenugreek also helps keep blood sugar levels normal in people with diabetes.

Since fenugreek is a culinary herb, you can enjoy this herb in a variety of tasty dishes. You can also take the herb as a tea or in capsules. Simply follow the dosage instructions on the package.

IMPOTENCE

If the symptom is difficulty achieving or maintaining an erection during sexual intercourse, the problem may be erectile dysfunction, or, as it's more commonly known, impotence. Its causes are many and complex, not the least of which are accumulated toxins in the body. Here's how to detoxify your way to a better love life.

Reduce free radicals. Vegetables and fruits with red pulp, such as tomatoes, guava, and watermelon, all contain an antioxidant called lycopene, which can dramatically reduce free radicals that at-

tack the prostate. That's important, because prostate health is essential to good erectile function. An easy way for a man to get more lycopene is by simply eating a good tomato sauce twice a week.

Focus on heart health. Two major risk factors for heart disease—high cholesterol and smoking—also greatly increase your chances of developing erectile dysfunction. How many men would continue smoking if they knew that it could eventually cost them in the sexual performance department? Your quick action tip here is obvious: Take steps to quit.

IRRITABLE BOWEL

Irritable bowel syndrome (IBS), also known as leaky gut syndrome, can give you a whole palette of symptoms, including alternating constipation and diarrhea, gassiness, cramping, mucus-covered stool, and stool mixed with undigested food. No one knows what causes it. When examined, the bowels look perfectly healthy, so the toxin would seem to be in the stool itself.

Maintaining regularity and gut health are the goals, because as Richard DeAndrea, M.D., N.D., a physician at the Akasha Center for Integrative Medicine in Santa Monica, California, notes, "In alternative medicine, we say good health begins in the bowels. You should be having at least two bowel movements per day, or ideally, have one 35 to 40 minutes after every meal."

Bulk up. Any program to improve bowel function should begin with an internal cleansing, and one way to do that is with bulking agents. "Bulking agents will give you the same result as a colonic hydration, but not quite as quickly," says Priscilla Slagle, M.D., a holistic physician in Palm Springs, California. Bulking agents often contain psyllium along with other plant fibers that bulk the stool to lengths of over 4 feet. You can purchase these at any natural foods store.

Eat a diet high in fiber. Fiber-rich foods include beans, whole grains, fruits, and vegetables. You should be doing this anyway to support your body's ongoing detoxification efforts.

For stubborn symptoms, try flax. One study showed less constipation, abdominal pain, and bloating among people with IBS who took flax over the course of 3 months than among others who took psyllium, during the same time period. Take 1 tablespoon of whole or "bruised" seed with 8 ounces of liquid three times a day.

Bring back the bacteria. Try adding yogurt containing live cultures and acidophilus milk to your diet. Some research shows that you can relieve IBS by replenishing the level of friendly bacteria in your colon. Half of the acidophilus drinkers who participated in one study significantly relieved pain and other symptoms of IBS.

KIDNEY STONES

These stones form from minerals such as calcium, phosphate, oxalate, or uric acid, which accumulate around debris left by kidney infections. Don't try to remove them with home remedies. This is important, because you'll find many such remedies in popular books about how to detoxify your body.

Kidney stones can get stuck in your urinary tract and cause serious complications that can put you in the hospital. Instead, try to keep stones from forming by preventing minerals from getting out of balance and reaching toxic levels.

Pile on the vegetables. "Alkalinizing the diet by increasing raw fruits and vegetables is very helpful," says Richard DeAndrea, M.D., N.D., a physician at the Akasha Center for Integrative Medicine in Santa Monica, California.

Researchers agree. Studies show that the people least likely to form kidney stones eat lots of vegetables, especially those of the green, leafy variety, which are high in magnesium. Just by adding more of these veggies to your plate, you can halve your risk of developing stones. Switching to a vegetarian diet cuts your risk even more.

Demineralize with herbs and fruits. Stones form when urine stays in the bladder too long, says Doug Schar, Dip.Phyt., M.C.P.P., M.N.I.M.H., a Washington, D.C.–based herbalist who was medically trained in Europe. A simple solution is to keep the urine flowing. An easy way to make sure that happens is to use diuretic herbal teas. Regular cups of corn silk, elder, or buchu tea will do the job, and all are available in health food stores. Follow the dosage instructions on the package.

Make your body taboo to toxins. Taking foods high in oxalic acid out of your diet can significantly reduce your risk for kidney stones. Among the foods to avoid are meat, chocolate, cocoa, sugar, sodium, spinach, baked beans, blackberries, beet greens, rhubarb, peanuts, sweet potato, Swiss chard, coffee, regular beverage tea, and colas. If you often use herbal remedies, avoid sorrel and yellow dock leaves, as well. Many of the foods mentioned here are perfectly healthy for most people. You wouldn't want to eliminate these foods unless you'd been plagued by kidney stones in the past.

Use gravel to stop stones. According to Dr. DeAndrea, "Gravelroot seems to be very effective at reducing the incidence of stone formation in the kidneys by adding protective phytonutrients to the bloodstream." Gravelroot, also known as Joe Pye, is a native North American herb that is available in tincture and capsule form. Follow the dosage instructions on the package.

OSTEOARTHRITIS

The aches, pains, and stiffness you feel in your joints are caused by inflammation, and like smoke and fire, where there is inflammation, there are free radicals causing the mischief. Here's what you can do to mop them up and get them under control.

Seek sympathy from the devil. Devil's claw, an herb originally found in Africa, is a powerful antioxidant that can calm down red, hot, swollen joints; reduce pain; and even bring about some improvement in the condition of your

When Detoxing Is Dangerous

RICHARD DEANDREA, M.D., N.D., a physician at the Akasha Center for Integrative Medicine in Santa Monica, California, has been practicing integrative medicine for more than 10 years and is a strong supporter of body detoxification. However, he warns that detoxification may not be a good idea if you:

- Have cardiac arrhythmia, because changing potassium levels in your body can be dangerous
- Have anorexia or bulimia, because fasting and bowel cleansing may aggravate the problem
- Are pregnant, because changes in your blood chemicals may affect your baby
- Are breastfeeding, because toxins can be carried out of the body through breast milk
- Have had surgery in the past 2 weeks, because detoxification may affect healing
- Are on chemotherapy, because your body is already working overtime to clear out these toxic chemicals

joints. One study found that people who took 335 mg in capsule form three times a day for 3 weeks experienced significant relief from their symptoms. People who raised the dose to 400 mg actually felt improvement in the way they moved after 2 months.

Dump the dairy. Studies have shown that removing half the cholesterol from your diet can immediately help relieve the pain of osteoarthritis, according to Richard DeAndrea, M.D., N.D., a physician at the Akasha Center for Integrative Medicine in Santa Monica, California. "Any animal fat produces an inflammatory reaction in small blood vessels, which makes them contract. This in turn leads to congestion in the joint spaces, which then causes pain."

Add some fizz. One way to relieve any

type of chronic pain is to alkalinize the body, since changing a toxic acid pH to a base pH reduces irritation, says Priscilla Slagle, M.D., a holistic physician in Palm Springs, California. She has a simple method for doing that: "I tell my patients to take Alka-Seltzer Gold with 1,000 milligrams buffered vitamin C, or half a teaspoon of baking soda with 1,000 milligrams buffered vitamin C, three times a day." The buffering should reduce the risk of diarrhea, which can occur with high doses of vitamin C. If you experience this side effect, reduce your dosage until it subsides.

Premenstrual Syndrome

Moodiness, irritability, anxiety, depression, anger, fatigue, aches and pains, sore breasts, bloating—if a woman experiences these symptoms prior to the onset of menstruation every month, she suffers from premenstrual syndrome (PMS). The toxins causing all the problems are excess hormones, including estrogens and prolactin, produced by the pituitary gland. Fortunately, there are remedies that keep hormone levels under control.

Take the hormones out of your diet. "PMS is a condition that didn't exist up until 100 years ago," says Richard DeAndrea, M.D., N.D., a physician at the Akasha Center for Integrative Medicine in Santa Monica, California. "And it's very possible that it has been instigated by the use of hormones in animal products, such as bovine growth hormone. These hormones have been clearly demonstrated to affect the human glandular system, even when taken in through animal products such as milk, butter, eggs, cheese, and meat." Reducing or eliminating animal products from your diet is your first step toward reducing or eliminating your symptoms of PMS, he says. For more information on Dr. DeAndrea's approach to diet and detoxification, go to www.21daydetox.com.

Meanwhile, while working on reducing your total meat and dairy intake, switch to organic farm products, which are produced from animals fed only organic feed (grain or grass) and with no antibiotics, hormones, or animal by-products.

Chase away symptoms with chasteberry. In one trial, 1,600 women took chasteberry daily throughout their menstrual cycles. More than 9 out of 10 reported a significant improvement in symptoms. Chasteberry comes in both dry extract and fluid forms. Follow the dosage instructions on the package, but stop using chasteberry if you develop a rash. Pregnant women and nursing mothers shouldn't use it at all.

Soothe symptoms with SAMe. SAMe (methionine), a supplement well known for its ability to relieve depression, can also inactivate estrogens, the female hormones that, in excess, may cause symptoms of PMS. Take 200 to 400 mg daily. Don't use SAMe if you are pregnant or nursing, are using prescription antidepressants, have bipolar disease, or have liver disease. It's important to take a good vitamin B supplement (which should contain B_6, B_{12}, and folic acid) with SAMe. Without vitamin B supplementation, SAMe can raise levels of homocysteine in the body, a substance that can increase your risk for heart attack or stroke.

Get up and move. Exercise improves circulation, makes you breathe harder, and encourages sweating—all ways the body rids itself of waste. "Walking, swimming, and biking are all good for encouraging the body to get rid of the toxins that may be causing PMS," says Yvette Andrews, C.N., a nutritional consultant at Herbally Yours in Charlotte, North Carolina.

PSORIASIS

If your skin forms raised areas that become covered with silvery, dry scales, you may have psoriasis. Normal skin usually replaces itself in about 28 days. Psoriasis speeds up the cycle to 3 or 4 days, so you can't shed your dead skin fast enough to make way for the new. No one knows what causes it, but we do know that various enzymes in the liver and skin contribute to the process. Detoxifying your body and neutralizing those excess enzymes can help you keep your psoriasis under control.

Control it with Oregon grape. This Native American plant has been used to quell psoriasis for at least 200 years and is still working today, says Doug Schar, Dip.Phyt., M.C.P.P., M.N.I.M.H., a Washington, D.C.–based herbalist who was medically trained in Europe. "Beyond clearing up the uncomfortable condition, Oregon grape contains berberine, which stimulates the liver to enhanced activity and helps the body to rid itself of toxins at the root of the psoriasis, and toxins caused by the psoriasis." The herb works slowly so wait at least 2 months before you decide if it's working for you, according to Schar. Follow the dosage instructions on the package.

Try milk thistle. A psoriasis attack produces toxins, which the liver then neutralizes, so keeping the liver in peak form is essential to minimizing the effects or even preventing attacks. You can find milk thistle at your local health food store in tincture and capsule form. Follow the dosage instructions on the package.

Senior Moments

Have you noticed that as you've gotten older, the facts you once had at your beck and call now tend to stay on the tip of your tongue? Your brain is more vulnerable to oxidative stress—that is, free radical damage—than any other organ in your body, and as you get older, that damage sometimes shows itself as memory problems. Luckily for us all, some recent research has shown that getting rid of free radicals in the brain can be quick and easy.

Curry up! The American Physiological Society recently published a study suggesting that adding curry to your diet may protect your brain against free radicals, which can contribute to many kinds of dementia, including Alzheimer's disease. Although human studies are still to come (the study was done with lab animals), adding some curries to your diet may be a tasty and easy way to help get your memory back on track.

Grow younger with L-glutamine. L-glutamine is an amino acid that's essential to the functioning of the body, especially in recovering from stress. "One way it works," says Priscilla Slagle, M.D., a holistic physician in Palm Springs, California, who specializes in the treatment of depression and is author of the e-book

The Way Up from Down, "is by helping to remove ammonia from the body, and many people who are toxic have increased ammonia production. As a result, they may have fatigue, mental fog, and even depression. Overgrowth of candida, a yeast that lives in the gut, and low glutamine levels are also often seen together." You can find L-glutamine supplements at your local health food store. Follow the dosage instructions on the package.

Sinus Conditions

Your sinuses are bony cavities around and behind your nose. They're lined with membranes that create sticky mucus when you have a cold, allergy, or infection. That's not a bad thing. The mucus traps bacteria and incapacitates them. When you manufacture too much mucus, however, your sinuses become blocked and can cause you miserable pain. So for relief, you'll need to clear out your sinuses.

Steam clean the toxins out. A steam inhalant is a quick and effective method for draining your sinuses of excess mucus. Just add 2 ounces of dried thyme or eucalyptus leaves to a quart of boiling water. Remove the pot from the stove top and place it on a nonslip surface. Cover your head with a large towel, lean over the pot, and inhale. Be careful not to get your face too close to the steaming water, because there is a danger of scalding. Instead of using the leaves, you can substitute 10 drops of eucalyptus or thyme oil.

Get the mucus flowing. Certain plant foods help get mucus flowing out of blocked sinus passages, says Doug Schar, Dip.Phyt., M.C.P.P., M.N.I.M.H., a Washington, D.C.–based herbalist who was medically trained in Europe. Vegetables that relieve the pressure and prevent infections from building up include onions, garlic, leeks, and scallions. Hot, fiery foods also have the same effect. Use lots of hot pepper, wasabi, and ginger in your cooking when your sinuses are acting up. This will relieve blockages and work to prevent headaches and infections.

Use a neti pot. This is a nasal wash cup that helps keep your nasal passages and sinuses clear of pollutants and excess mucus. For directions on how to purchase and use a neti pot, see "Say Hello to Neti" on page 157.

STROKE

Stroke is the result of a blood clot moving and blocking circulation to the brain. "It's the cardiologist's nightmare," says Decker Weiss, N.M.D., a naturo-

pathic medical doctor at the Arizona Heart Hospital, a teacher at the Southwest College of Naturopathic Medicine in Tempe, and author of the book *The Weiss Method.* "Even if someone doesn't die from stroke, they can end up debilitated in terrible ways." While a blood clot may not exactly fit the definition of a toxin, it is certainly something you want to keep your body clear of. And a diet that supports the detoxifying efforts of your body (see chapter 3 on page 30) will also help prevent strokes.

Enlist some enzymes. Taking pancreatic enzymes can help prevent a stroke, says Dr. Weiss. This supplement is available at health food stores. Follow the dosage directions on the package.

Take some herbs. "Gingko, ginger, and cayenne can also be useful," says Dr. Weiss. "They help stop clot formation by keeping the blood cells too slippery to stick together. They're also anti-inflammatory." These herbal supplements are all available in capsule form at health food stores. Follow the dosage instructions on the package.

SUGAR CRAVINGS

The Atkins Diet, The South Beach Diet, and other popular weight-loss plans have prompted millions of Americans to ride the low-carb train. There's no question that these diets work, at least in the short run, but where do you find the willpower to overcome those sugar cravings?

Forget willpower. Just eat more complex carbohydrates, says Diane Spindler, Ph.D., N.D., a board certified naturopath and owner of Mountain Holistic Health in Indian Hills, Colorado. "When you eat simple carbohydrates such as sugar, you get a spike in energy that's followed by a hypoglycemic reaction." In other words, the initial energetic surge is followed by a crash. Your body then craves more sugar to get stimulated again. "Complex carbohydrates have a lot of fiber, so there's a slow, steady introduction of sugar into your system," says Dr. Spindler. "The pancreas is happy, the liver is happy, and your mental functions are happy, so you don't crave the sugar."

ULCERS

Ulcers in the stomach and the upper part of the small intestine, called the duodenum, can be extremely dangerous. "Any ulcer can be life threatening," warns Decker Weiss, N.M.D., a naturopathic medical doctor at the Arizona Heart Hospital, a teacher at the Southwest College of Naturopathic Medicine in Tempe, and author of the book *The Weiss Method*. "So if you have one, you should be under a doctor's care." You can, however, supplement medical care with some extremely effective detoxification techniques. The culprit behind your ulcer may be a microorganism, a bacterium called *Helicobacter pylori*, which embeds itself in the lining of your stomach or duodenum and makes you vulnerable to your own digestive acids and enzymes.

Eat more broccoli. This vegetable contains a chemical called glucoraphanin, which the body turns into sulforaphane, a very effective *H. pylori* killer. But not all broccoli is created equal. The younger the plant, the more potent it is. Broccoli sprouts contain 20 times more glucoraphanin than mature broccoli does, so adding them to your diet can be a real blessing to your upper digestive tract. Don't stop eating the mature variety, however. It contains more fiber, which is important for your lower digestive tract.

Do the licorice chew. "I get spectacular results with licorice," says Dr. Weiss, "but it should be the chewable kind." He means, of course, the kind of licorice actually made from licorice root, which you buy at your health food store, not the rubbery sugar sticks you give out at Halloween. The licorice should be deglyc-erolized (DGL), which will help prevent the elevations of blood pressure some-times seen with the use of this herb. Licorice works by providing a protective coating of a substance called mucilage to the walls of your stomach. Follow the dosage instructions on the package.

URINARY TRACT INFECTIONS

Urinary tract infections (UTIs) can be painful and persistent, and if left un-treated, they can lead to more serious problems. The urinary tract should be sterile; it's not a place for germs. Here are some ways to clean it out.

Flush your system. The first thing to do is to increase the amount of water you're drinking to at least 2 quarts a day, says Richard DeAndrea, M.D., N.D., a physi-cian at the Akasha Center for Integrative Medicine in Santa Monica, California. The more you urinate, the less time you'll give germs to hang around and cause trouble.

Go for the green. "Add parsley to your diet to prevent problems from devel-oping," advises Yvette Andrews, C.N., a nutritional consultant at Herbally Yours in Charlotte, North Carolina. "Celery also helps. Dandelion leaf tea is also a good diuretic. Just take some dandelion greens and boil them in water."

You can also buy the dried herb at any health food store. If you're picking fresh dandelion, find your plants well away from public highways or any other source of ground pollution. And don't just snip them from your own backyard unless you maintain an organic lawn.

YEAST INFECTIONS

"A yeast infection in a woman is a sign that the blood pH has shifted into the acid zone," says Richard DeAndrea, M.D., N.D., a physician at the Akasha Center for Integrative Medicine in Santa Monica, California. Here are some quick cleanups that can help you get rid of this irritating problem.

Shift your pH. "If you have an over-growth of yeast, especially vaginally, it's important to increase the alkalinizing potential of your body," advises Dr. De-Andrea. "A rapid way to alkalinize is to take 2 ounces of wheat grass juice every day, which you can find at any health food store. You can also make a douche by adding 1 to 2 ounces of wheat grass to 4 ounces of water." Wheat grass works because of its extremely high mineral content.

Get acidophilus on your side. Decker Weiss, N.M.D., a naturopathic medical doctor at the Arizona Heart Hospital, a teacher at the Southwest College of Naturopathic Medicine in Tempe, and author of the book *The Weiss Method*, agrees that yeast infections are a pH issue. Acidophilus can help. "Vaginal acidophilus douches can work wonders," he says. "If you want to take acidophilus by mouth, use the pearls. They work the best by far."

Juice it away. Priscilla Slagle, M.D., a holistic physician in Palm Springs, California, often sees overgrowths of candida, a type of yeast that can thrive in the intestines. Sometimes a general detox will help. One way to do that is with a 72-hour juice fast. "You'll go off of solid food for 3 days and replace it with vegetable juice, diluting it 50/50 with water. Drink 8 ounces every 3 hours. The juices should be freshly prepared, not stored.

Ginger root, red peppers, yellow peppers, parsley, carrots, celery, beets, greens, and tomatoes are all healthful ingredients you may want to use." She does offer one caveat: Fasting is not a great idea for people with low blood sugar.

For more information on fasting safely, see chapter 7 on page 143.

End the cycle. Rather than treating the condition every time you get its painful symptoms, you can get at the root of the problem, says Doug Schar, Dip.Phyt., M.C.P.P., M.N.I.M.H., a Washington, D.C.–based herbalist who was medically trained in Europe. Most yeast infections are caused by the antibiotics prescribed to treat bacterial infections. "You can prevent these bacterial infections by raising your immune system with herbal remedies such as echinacea, maitake, and calendula," he says. Buy them as tablets at the health food store and use them per the packaging instructions.

Chapter 14

Staying Clean: 45 Steps
to Toxin-Free Living

REMEMBER THE OLD ADAGE, "An ounce of prevention is worth a pound of cure?" It's absolutely true, especially when it comes to protecting yourself from the vast sea of toxins in which you swim each day. After all, it's a lot easier to prevent poisons from accumulating in your body than it is to eliminate them once they're there.

The first step is to reduce your exposure by as much as you can—and prevention starts at home, says Bruce Fife, N.D., a nutritionist and naturopath in Colorado Springs and author of *The Detox Book*. "That means being conscious of the food you eat, the quality of the air inside your house, and the products you use in your home and on your body," he says. "The fewer toxins you take into your body, the less stress you place on the organs that eliminate them."

It's not difficult to minimize your exposure to chemicals and pollutants. If you eat a plant-based diet, get regular exercise, replace toxic household cleansers with safer alternatives or all-natural products, and minimize or eliminate your intake of "optional toxins" such as those in cigarettes and alcohol, you're halfway there. And even one lifestyle change can make a significant difference in your body's toxic load.

What follows are 45 steps you can take that will reduce your body's toxic load on into the future. Feel free to pick and choose which steps you'll take—just keep in mind that the more steps you're able to implement, the cleaner your future will be and the better your health and well-being.

STEP 1: SMOKE OUT

Quit smoking, then start forking up loads of cruciferous vegetables such as broccoli, cabbage, cauliflower, brussels sprouts, and watercress. Research has shown that plant chemicals in these vegetables help counteract cancer in test animals.

Here's why: The smoke from cigarettes and other forms of tobacco contains more than 4,000 poisonous chemicals and gases. Many of these poisons cause cancer, and all of them alter the detoxifying enzymes that help break poisons down and eliminate them from your body. Common cancer-causing chemicals in cigarette smoke include polycylic aromatic hydrocarbons (PAHs), heterocylic amines, benzene, and nitrosamines. Cigarette smoke even contains radioactive materials such as polonium.

Smoking is toxic to everyone, including nonsmokers who inhale second-hand smoke. Women are particularly at risk, however. Between 1974 and 1994, lung-cancer deaths among women in-creased by 150 percent, compared with only 20 percent among men. Researchers believe that women may carry a genetic mutation that spurs tumor growth in response to some of the body's own hormones, particularly estrogen.

The good news is, detoxification procedures can help speed these poisons out of your body.

STEP 2: IF YOU DRINK, DRINK IN MODERATION

Indulge if you must, but when you do drink, make sure you drink at least one glass of pure water for every drink containing alcohol.

A special caveat to women: If you have a history of breast cancer in your family, you may want to consider not drinking alcohol at all. Some research suggests that even moderate drinking may increase a woman's risk of breast cancer.

Here's why: There's nothing wrong with an occasional beer or glass of wine. In fact, studies show that moderate alcohol consumption—one drink a day for women, two a day for men—lowers the risk of heart attack by 30 to 50 percent and may even protect against Alzheimer's disease. But chronic, heavy drinking can poison the body's main purification organ: the liver.

About 5 percent of the alcohol you drink is eliminated through sweat, urine, and breath. The liver handles the rest. The process of converting alcohol to energy or storing it as fat produces by-products, some of which are more toxic than the alcohol itself. These by-products include acetaldehyde, a close cousin to formaldehyde that is known to be toxic to the brain. Acetaldehyde is on the list of air toxicants regulated by the Environmental Protection Agency (EPA) and is thought to cause cancer.

Heavy drinking can also prolong your body's inflammatory process. Chronic inflammation leads to an overproduction of free radicals—unstable molecules believed to contribute to the aging process and degenerative diseases such as cancer. Alcohol abuse also depletes the body's store of glutathione and can cause changes in the digestive system that hinder its ability to absorb vitamins, minerals, and other nutrients in food.

STEP 3: CONTROL HOUSEHOLD PESTS NATURALLY

Every time you spray your kitchen for ants or roaches or you give Fido a flea dip, you're exposing yourself and your family to a chemical soup of poisons.

The solution? For starters, prevent pests from taking up residence in the first place. For mice, eliminate their entry points, such as cracks and crevices; for ants and roaches, keep all surfaces free of food crumbs, keep the lid to your kitchen garbage pail tightly closed at all times, and remove your pet's dish from the floor at night. In addition, explore the many ways to deter ants, roaches, fleas, and other indoor pests without man-made chemicals.

Scott Meyer, executive editor of *Organic Gardening* magazine, recommends sticky traps rather than pesticide sprays. These traps use an appealing scent or color to lure unwanted bugs onto a strip coated with a sticky substance from which they can't escape. When the strip is full of bugs, you can simply discard and replace it. These are available for flies, roaches, moths, and other household pests.

For ants in his home, Meyer uses the scientifically tested all-natural ant control formula described in "Pure Pest Power" on page 394. "It works like a charm," he says. You can find an assortment of resources for safe, natural pest control at *Organic Gardening*'s Web site, www.organicgardening.com.

Here's why: Pesticides are toxic products designed to kill living things. They include herbicides, disinfectants, rodenticides, fungicides, insecticides, and molluscicides. All pesticides must be registered with the Environmental Protection Agency (EPA). It is important to understand that EPA registration does not denote that a product is safe, just that it works!

In fact, pesticides must be treated with the utmost respect regarding their potential acute and chronic effects on human health. Pesticides can be absorbed through the skin, lungs, and eyes, and by ingestion. Absorbing these poisons can cause everything from neurotoxic effects (depression, headaches, rage, lack of concentration) to burning, itching, rashes, eye problems, and pulmonary difficulties.

Children are particularly vulnerable because of their small bodies and hand-to-mouth habits. Add to that the fact that their organs and central nervous systems are still developing, and it's easy to see why they are more at risk.

The EPA estimates that 75 percent of U.S. homeowners use store-bought pesticides every year. Pesticides contain both active and inert ingredients. Sometimes the inert ingredients are very toxic in their own right, and the synergistic relationship between the active and inert ingredients can make the overall pesticide more toxic than the active ingredient is by itself.

STEP 4: USE INTEGRATED PEST MANAGEMENT

Stop using garden pesticides and practice integrated pest management, or IPM. With IPM, you don't eliminate pests entirely, you just keep them at a tolerable level and aim for a healthy lawn rather than a perfect one. Often, man-made chemicals are replaced by microbial and botanical insecticides, such as Bt (*Bacillus thuringiensis*), which are derived from plants and break down more easily in air, sunlight, and moisture. For more information on IPM, visit the Environmental Protection Agency's Web page at www.epa.gov/pesticides/factsheets/ipm.htm.

One natural remedy that helps when practicing IPM is horticultural oil. You can use it to protect roses and other shrubs, trees, and even tomatoes. The oil smothers or repels pests like aphids, caterpillars, and beetles. But it won't harm your plants or bugs you're not targeting, according to Scott Meyer, executive editor of *Organic Gardening* magazine.

There are two reasons why today's light horticultural oils are an improvement over what was known as dormant oil:

First, you can use the light oil during the growing (not just the dormant) season—right when the pests are chewing on your garden. Second, the light oils are made from vegetable oil, rather than a petroleum by-product, which, no coincidence, is why they are not too overpowering to use during the growing season.

One more tip: If you or your children are walking on neighboring lawns that are treated with chemicals, keep the pesticides outside of your own home by leaving your shoes on your porch or outside your door, says Thomas J. Slaga, Ph.D., scientific director of the AMC Cancer Research Center in Denver and author of *The Detox Revolution*.

Here's why: Whenever you come in contact with a garden, orchard, or lawn that has been treated with chemical fertilizers or sprayed to keep pests or weeds away, you're exposing yourself and your family to poisonous substances that can be absorbed into your body and remain toxic to your system.

STEP 5: MAKE YOUR OWN BUG BEATERS AND WEED EATERS

In addition to shopping for less-toxic pest and weed killers for your lawn and garden, you can easily make your own natural formulas that can be your first line of defense against insect intruders and invasive plants. You can find resources for safe, natural pest control at *Organic Gardening*'s Web site, www.organicgardening.com. To get started today, look at the nontoxic garden savers in "Pure Pest Power" on page 394. As with any garden remedy, try the sprays on a few leaves first, then come back in 24 hours and check to be sure that the plants you're trying to protect do not have a bad reaction.

Here's why: It makes sense to use homemade natural pesticides, not only because they save you money, but because every effort you make to keep poisons away from yourself and your family can lessen the disease-causing toxic load that each of you must carry on into the future.

STEP 6: TOSS THE TOXIC CLEANING PRODUCTS

Take a careful look at all the cleaning products in your house with the goal of eliminating the ones that are potentially harmful. Conveniently enough, there's a sort of secret code on the product labels that can help you make intelligent choices.

These designations are placed on

products by order of the federal government, with the primary purpose of protecting you, and sometimes to tell you about the products' potential impact on the environment. Here's what to watch for.

⚅ POISON/DANGER means something very toxic; only a few drops could kill you.

⚅ WARNING means moderately toxic; as little as a teaspoonful can kill.

⚅ CAUTION denotes a product that is less toxic; 2 tablespoons to 1 cup could kill you.

⚅ STRONG SENSITIZER means the product can cause multiple allergies.

The most healthful home is one where no product is used that has a stronger signal word than "Caution." Detergents are labeled with a "caution" label. Furniture polish, with its petroleum distillates, would be labeled "Warning" and also probably "Flammable." Contact your local city government or hazardous household waste recycling organization to find the best means of disposal for these products.

Here's why: Each year, the average American uses about 25 gallons of household products that contain toxic chemicals, from air fresheners to oven and toilet-bowl cleaners to spot removers and carpet cleaners. You inhale them and absorb them through your skin, and they find their way into your body fat and tissues.

To give just a few examples: The phenol and cresol in many disinfectants can cause fainting, dizziness, and kidney and liver damage, while the nitrobenzene in furniture and floor polishes is linked to cancer and birth defects. More frightening, of the approximately 17,000 chemicals found in common household products, only 3 in 10 have been tested for their impact on human health.

Discarding just two or three chemical-laden cleaning products could significantly reduce your body's toxic load.

STEP 7: SWITCH TO PURE CLEANING POWER

The four best basic ingredients for less toxic cleaning are:

1. Baking Soda. This mineral, sodium bicarbonate, is slightly alkaline with a pH of 8.1, and it neutralizes many acid-based odors. It is also mildly abrasive.

2. Vinegar. Vinegar kills bacteria, mold, and germs. Numerous studies suggest that a 5 percent solution of vinegar kills up to 99 percent of bacteria, 82 percent of mold, and 80 percent of viruses.

3. Washing Soda. More alkaline than baking soda with a pH of around 11, washing soda is the mineral sodium carbonate. It is an excellent heavy-duty cleaner that will remove grease and even peel wax off a floor. It releases no harmful fumes, but it is caustic and you need to wear gloves when using it. Washing soda is available in the laundry section of most supermarkets. If you can't find it where you live, substitute borax.

4. Soap or Detergent. Soap and detergents cut grease and remove stains. Soap is alkaline, and detergent is usually close to a neutral pH of around 7. If you have hard water, choose a detergent, as it has been designed to not react with hard-water minerals and won't cause soap scum.

From the ingredients listed above you can make the following all-natural, all-purpose cleaning formulas that will leave your home squeaky clean—without the risk of toxic exposure. All of these can be applied with a sponge and should be rinsed well after using.

All-Purpose Cleaner: Combine ½ teaspoon washing soda, ½ teaspoon liquid soap or detergent, and 2 cups of hot water in a spray bottle. Shake to blend.

Soft Scrubber: Put ½ cup of baking soda in a bowl and add enough liquid soap or detergent to make a frostinglike consistency. Scoop the frosting onto a sponge and scrub the surface to be cleaned. This formula rinses easily.

Germ and Mold Killer: Put pure, straight, white household vinegar in a spray bottle. Make sure to avoid your eyes while spraying. Leave on for 10 to 15 minutes before rinsing.

Here's why: Having a clean house simply doesn't require loading up on the toxic chemicals that are so common in manufactured cleaning supplies.

STEP 8: GIVE YOUR TAP WATER AN EXTREME MAKEOVER

Make your own clean water by investing in a home water treatment device, says Dr. Slaga.

There are several kinds of treatment systems, including solid block carbon filters, reverse osmosis, and distillation. Some systems offer a combination of methods. You can choose from a point-of-entry system, which treats the water coming into the house, or a point-of-use system, which

(continued on page 396)

Pure Pest Power

TRY THESE NONTOXIC PEST CONTROLS you can make at home for just pennies.

Ant Control Formula. Scott Meyer, executive editor of *Organic Gardening* magazine (www.organicgardening.com), shares this recipe that's proven invaluable in his own home.

1. Start by making a 1 percent boric acid (available at any drugstore) and 20 percent sugar solution by thoroughly dissolving 1 teaspoon of boric acid and 6 tablespoons of sugar in 2 cups of water. Do this in a clear jar so you can see when all the boric acid crystals have dissolved. This is your bait solution; soak some cotton balls in it.
2. Make bait dispensers out of some old plastic cartons with lids (the kind you might take leftovers home in). Punch holes in them so the ants can get inside, then put the soaked cotton balls into the containers, and cover them with lids so the bait won't dry out.
3. Place the bait containers wherever you see ant trails, inside or outside your house.
4. Clean the containers and replace with fresh bait solution at least once a week.
5. Be patient! The key to effective control is to get worker ants to continually carry low doses of boric acid back to feed the ants in their nest. After a few weeks of using the 1 percent solution, reduce the boric acid content even further to ½ percent and use that for long-term control. Boric acid is mildly repellent to ants, and using a very low dose makes it more likely that surviving ants will continue eating the bait and taking it back to the nest.

Knockout Salsa

This favorite comes from the Santa Barbara, California, garden of Kathleen Yeomans, author of The Able Gardener. *This mixture yields about 3 cups of natural insecticide that quickly neutralizes aphids and other soft-bodied insects, as well as deters ants. And it's safe for use in the kitchen the next time you need to fend off an invasion of sugar ants!*

  2 pounds ripe, blemished tomatoes

  1 large onion

  1 pound fresh chile peppers

  2 cloves garlic

  1 cup vinegar

  ½ teaspoon pepper

  Disposable coffee filter or cheesecloth

Roughly chop the tomatoes, onion, chile peppers (wear plastic gloves when handling), and garlic. Blend in a blender or food processor until liquefied. Add the vinegar and pepper. Strain the mixture through the coffee filter or several layers of cheesecloth and pour it into a spray bottle. Spray the liquid directly on pests that you spot in your garden. But be careful: This spray can be highly irritating if it gets in your eyes or mouth, so spray it only on windless days.

The Gin Zapper

One application of this weed cocktail kills dandelions or just about any weed, but it's intended for spot use only. Apply it carefully and accurately to individual weeds because it can harm other plants as well—even grass blades. Thanks to Marion Hess of Northville, Michigan, for the recipe.

  1 ounce gin

  1 ounce apple cider vinegar

  1 tablespoon baby shampoo

  1 quart water

Combine the gin, vinegar, shampoo, and water in a spray bottle and set to the stream setting. Spray on a hot, sunny day, wetting all leaves and dousing the plant. Repeat the dose if the weed is not dead the following day (or simply pull out the weed, root and all).

delivers filtered water to a specific tap—say, your kitchen or bathroom.

How do you know which filtration system is best for you? Start by learning what's in your water. If your water comes from a municipal water system, call your water utility and ask for a copy of their Annual Water Quality Report (also called a Consumer Confidence Report). If you are on a private well, contact your local health department and ask for a list of the typical well-water contaminants in your area.

Choosing a water-filtration system can be confusing. For help, consult the National Sanitation Foundation (NSF) at www.nsf.org. This independent organization regularly evaluates most of the commercial filters on the market, rating their ability to remove pesticides, asbestos, lead, and various types of bacteria. The site has an entire section devoted to home water treatment devices. For more information on selecting a water-filtration system, see "Find the Right Treatment" on page 47.

The bottom line on water-treatment devices: "Decide what you can afford, do your research, and purchase one from a reputable dealer," says Peter Bennett, N.D., a naturopathic physician in Vancouver and coauthor of *7-Day Detox Miracle.*

Here's why: Pure, unadulterated water is perhaps the ultimate body-cleansing tool, both internally and externally. Alas, it's not that easy to find. Some of the more common contaminants that come out of the typical household tap include microorganisms, pesticides, heavy metals, and even asbestos.

STEP 9: DETOXIFY YOUR COSMETICS AND BODY-CARE PRODUCTS

Scrutinize the ingredients labels of the products in your medicine cabinet or shower caddy, and discard those that contain the potentially toxic chemicals below. And when you're shopping, don't buy any products that contain these ingredients.

Parabens (methyl-, propyl-, and butyl-) are preservatives, and they prevent the breakdown or spoilage of body-care products and cosmetics. However, some people are allergic to them and can develop skin rashes if they use them.

Dibutylphthalate (DBP), dimethylphthalate (DMP), and diethylphthalate (DEP) are chemicals known as phthalates. These are environmental estrogens (substances that mimic the function of the female sex hormone estrogen in both men and women) and are linked in animal studies to birth defects of the male reproductive system, including undescended or missing testicles and hypospadias, a defect of the penis. Phthalates are used in nail polish to keep it from cracking and in hair sprays to keep sprayed hair soft, rather than stiff. They're also in soaps, deodorants, lotions, and shampoos. The Environmental Working Group has a list of phthalate-free products on its Web site. Go to www.ewg.org/issues/cosmetics/phthalatefree.php.

Diethanolamine (DEA) and DEA-related ingredients, including cocamide DEA or MEA, lauramide DEA, and myristamide DEA. In 1998, a study conducted by the National Toxicology Program linked the topical application of DEA and certain DEA-related ingredients to cancer in test animals.

Here's why: The body-care and cosmetics industries use more than 5,000 chemicals to make body washes, hair dyes, cosmetics, and other personal-care products. However, the Food and Drug Administration (FDA) neither reviews nor approves cosmetics or their ingredients before they're put on the market. Because many substances applied to the skin end up in the bloodstream, it's up to you to make sure the products you use are safe.

STEP 10: USE CAUTION EVEN WITH "NATURAL" PRODUCTS

The best way to steer clear of body-care products and cosmetics that contain potentially toxic or allergenic ingredients? Become a savvy consumer. The FDA Web site has a whole area devoted to cosmetics ingredients, as well as labeling and label claims. You'll find it at www.cfsan.fda.gov/~dms/cos-prd.html.

Watch for reactions to any new products that you try. If you experience itching, rash, or skin irritations, discontinue use. If you know you're allergic to many substances, test any new product on a small patch of skin on your arm before slathering it over your whole body.

Here's why: While "natural" or "organic" cosmetics are usually an excellent choice, they contain ingredients extracted from plants or animal products that some people are allergic to. For instance, lanolin, extracted from sheep wool, is an ingredient in many moisturizers and is a common cause of allergies.

STEP 11: HUMIDIFY, BUT DO CLEAN YOUR HUMIDIFIERS

One simple way to minimize organic toxins—viruses and bacteria, molds and mildew, animal dander and dust mites—is to keep your home's humidity level at 30 to 50 percent. And if you use humidifiers in your home, keep them spotlessly clean and refill them with fresh water daily. A dirty humidifier is a breeding ground for biological toxins.

Here's why: Your home is under siege by organic toxins that can lead to infectious diseases like colds and flu, allergies, and some types of asthma. In addition, molds and mildews can cause allergies and release disease-causing toxins. Children; the elderly; and people with allergies, breathing problems, lung diseases, or weakened immune systems are particularly susceptible to these natural contaminants in indoor air.

STEP 12: LIMIT YOUR EXPOSURE TO PERFLOUROCHEMICALS

Minimize your exposure to Teflon, Stainmaster, Silverstone, Scotchgard, and Gore-Tex—chemicals known as perflourochemicals (PFCs), which are proving to be very persistent in the environment. Also, do what you can to avoid PFOA, another PFC. Start removing products that you have the most contact with first, such as Teflon frying pans, or clothes that you wear frequently that have stain protection. When it comes to personal-care products, choose those made with natural ingredients as often as possible, since it may be difficult to determine from the label whether or not a product contains PFOA. PFOA is found in so many consumer products that it's hard to list them all—from products designed to repel liquids, to shampoos, to brand-name products we are all familiar with, such as Stainmaster fabric protection.

Here's why: Any reduction in exposure to these potentially harmful substances is a good idea. In some cases these substances are so persistent in the environment that they won't *ever* degrade! The EPA took Scotchgard off the market in 2000, and it stopped the manufacture of an ingredient in Teflon soon after, according to the Washington, D.C.–based organization The Environmental Working Group (EWG).

The EPA classifies PFOA as a carcinogen in animals. It causes testicular, mammary, and liver tumors in rats. Five animal studies have shown that PFOA alters reproductive hormones in exposed rats, according to EWG. And 11 such studies show that PFOA damages the thyroid. "Three of the four tumors caused by PFOA are on the rise in people, including testicular, breast, liver, and prostate," notes EWG.

STEP 13: PAY SPECIAL ATTENTION TO LEAD REMOVAL

It's important for you to know whether your children are being exposed to lead. Children's blood lead levels can increase rapidly between 6 and 12 months of age, and they tend to peak between 18 and 24 months of age. Many states require lead testing for all children. If this is not the case in your state, ask your child's pediatrician to recommend and provide the best lead test.

If you suspect that you have lead paint in your home, consult your state health or housing department to find out how best to remove it and by whom the removal should be done. Do not try to remove lead paint yourself. You could be exposed to dangerously high lead levels. Here are some other actions you can take.

๑ Water usually does not contain lead unless the home has lead in its piping. If you're not sure whether this is a problem in your house, consult with a plumber. If you find lead, it's worth the expense to either have the lead removed or to buy a filtering system that will remove the lead. For more information on cleaning up your water supply, see "Water Fit to Drink" on page 45.

๑ The EPA recommends that you dust and vacuum frequently as an added precaution, since lead paint is powdery as it degrades and because lead is carried into homes on shoes. Lead and other heavy metals like cadmium and aluminum are by-products of vehicle operation and are found in high levels in "street dust." One study showed Seattle children who played and crawled on the floor were exposed to dangerous levels of these contaminants, which were tracked into the house.

๑ Use a solution of powdered automatic dishwasher detergent in warm water to mop floors and wipe window ledges, according to information from the EPA. Dishwasher detergent has a high phosphate content, and most all-purpose cleaners without phosphates won't remove lead. (This is one good use for phosphates.)

๑ If the exterior of your house was painted with lead-based paint, the soil near your house might be contaminated—even if that paint has been removed. Use doormats, and insist that people wipe their feet before entering your home.

⚘ In the year 2000, many vinyl window miniblinds were recalled due to lead contamination. If you have older blinds, check their labels. If the labels on the blinds read "Manufactured in Thailand for Ace Hardware Corp.," you'll need to replace the blinds.

⚘ For information on lead in dishes, see Step 27 on page 409.

Here's why: Lead is a highly toxic heavy metal that can cause serious damage to your brain, kidneys, reproductive system, nervous system, and red blood cells. In the United States, the most common source of lead in the home is dust from paint that was applied before lead paint was removed from the market in 1978. Other sources include dust from outside the home; tap water; dishes; and glazed pottery.

Children are particularly susceptible to lead poisoning, and it can cause delays in their mental development, lower IQ levels, and behavioral problems. Blood lead levels in children should not exceed 10 micrograms per deciliter, but this figure may be lowered even more in the near future. A screening lead test is ap-propriate for all children, but few medical doctors will think to do this. Consult a naturopathic doctor and ask for a stool or hair analysis to screen for lead in your child.

STEP 14: LIMIT EXPOSURE TO VOLATILE ORGANIC CHEMICALS

Volatile organic chemicals (VOCs) are gases that are emitted from liquids and solids. Common examples of VOCs include wet paint and paint strippers, fuels, glues, adhesives, permanent markers, and even the formaldehyde outgasing from pressed wood furniture.

Choose the least-toxic, most inert products you can so that your health isn't jeopardized by VOCs. You can substitute water-based paints, stains, sealants, and markers for those with solvents. Hint: The stronger and more persistent the chemical smell, the more likely the product contains VOCs. Choose non-toxic cleaning products and avoid all petroleum-based furniture-care products.

There are some rare exceptions when this isn't possible because there aren't viable, less-toxic, low-VOC alternatives. These include products such as strong glues or shoe polish, both of which can often be handled outdoors. Make sure that there is adequate ventilation anytime VOCs are present. If you do crafts in your home, pay special attention to this one. No matter how much you enjoy your beautiful creations, you don't want to undermine your health by regularly inhaling toxic fumes from glue or decorative paints.

Another way to reduce your VOC exposure is to remove the plastic bags from dry-cleaned clothes and let the clothes air outdoors before you bring them inside. This gives time for the chemicals to be released before you introduce them to your home.

Here's why: Many VOCs are carcinogenic; that means they can cause cancer. And many are also highly neurotoxic.

STEP 15: RECYCLE HAZARDOUS CHEMICALS

Take a good look under the sink, in your garage, in the garden tool storage shed. See any old chemicals that you've stashed away? Are you seriously thinking you might ever use them again?

Be rigorous in your decisions. If you're pretty sure you might use the products again, at least make sure the cans and bottles are fully sealed. (Wear gloves when you check!)

Now get rid of all the old cans of chemicals safely by contacting your local hazardous household waste recycling organization to find out where to take whatever you want to dispose of. Some places may recommend that you use up old paint and other materials before disposal. Be aware that with many products, especially pesticides, it is safer for you if they are removed and not used.

Here's why: Many of these can outgas toxic fumes as the containers deteriorate.

STEP 16: PROTECT YOURSELF FROM ELECTROMAGNETIC FIELDS

Buy or rent a gaussmeter to determine the overall electromagnetic field (EMF) readings in your home and appliances. There are a number of brands on the market costing $150 and up. The less-expensive meters are designed for consumer use. Make sure the meter is designed for use in America, where the power distribution network is 60 hertz.

EMFs from appliances can cause localized fields well in excess of 1 to 2 milligauss (mG), which is the level at which studies in Sweden determined that health effects occur.

It is important to note that these electromagnetic fields drop off almost completely within a few feet of the appliance.

Here are some basic rules of thumb to follow, to give you a general idea of how to reduce your EMF exposure from appliances.

⚭ Stay at least an arm's length away from any computer, whether you're using it or not.

⚭ Make sure not to put a bed on the other side of a wall that shares a big appliance, such as a refrigerator or an electric oven.

⚭ Sit 6 feet or more from a television set.

⚭ Don't sleep under an electric blanket that is on. Use the blanket to heat the bed before you get in, then turn it off.

⚭ If you have an electric clock on the nightstand next to your bed, move the clock across the room.

⚭ Don't keep a halogen lamp next to your bed. (They have a transformer that emits EMFs.)

Here's why: Controversy surrounds possible health effects of EMFs. Some research indicates that EMFs contribute to an increase in brain tumors and leukemia in children.

The concern about EMFs centers on low-frequency fields caused by our use of electric power. The sources of these fields are as common in our everyday lives as the beds we sleep on. Alarm clocks, dishwashers, electric lines, and television sets all give off quite predictable fields. High-tension power lines, electrical line transformers, and electrical power stations are other possible neighborhood EMF sources whose fields are very site-specific. The most unpredictable source of high EMFs is found in "askew" buildings. The buildings are called askew because they have unusually high EMFs, a result of faulty grounding and wiring. The Electric Power Research Institute estimates that up to a quarter of homes exceed the Swedish standard of 1 to 2 milligauss (mG) of overall background electromagnetic radiation.

STEP 17: CHECK YOUR HOME FOR ODORS

Pay careful attention to whatever it is that you smell when you first enter your home. If possible, do this after you've been away for a few days. Make sure that nobody in the home has been cooking anything within a few hours of your reentry, as the smell of food can overpower the sometimes-subtle house smells. Spend a few moments outside clearing your lungs by breathing deeply, and focus on paying attention to what you smell.

Once you have entered your home and your sense of smell has told you what the dominant smell or combination of smells is, you will need to identify the odor. This isn't always as simple as you might think it would be; however, most people will be able to easily identify the source of a smell.

Some ideas to consider when you're trying to identify the odor include heating and cooking fuel, new carpets, mold, perfumes, scented candles, and animals. Try to isolate the smells in your mind.

Once you have isolated the most dominant odor, determine its toxicity. An oil burner in need of cleaning and venting is not healthy, and if you smell strong oil burner fumes, the situation needs to be remedied immediately. The cause of mold needs to be addressed, if that is the smell dominating your home. (See Step 19 on page 404 for information on how to do this.) Most importantly, use your intuition. Tend to the smells that bother you.

Here's why: Not all smells need attending to, of course, but keep in mind that the healthiest home is the one that has the most inert ingredients. Those generally don't have any smell at all.

Interestingly enough, the first thing you smell upon entering your home is most likely something that is problematic for your health—something that is not necessarily the most toxic smell, as some toxic fumes have no odor, but something that could be causing problems nonetheless. Different people can smell different dominant odors in the same home. If one family member is allergic to pine terpenes, for example, then the smell of pine paneling might be very strong to them. Another family member may not smell pine, but might be strongly aware of the "new" carpet smell, because they are sensitive to it.

Many homes have characteristic odors, such as cork tiles, oil burner fumes, or pine wall panels. What to you is the characteristic smell of your home? Do you remember what you smelled the first time you entered it?

STEP 18: DECLARE WAR ON MOLD

The key to mold control is moisture control. Clean any mold you find with a weak bleach solution, 10 parts water to 1 part bleach. (Do not mix bleach with ammonia.)

Once you've cleaned the mold, get rid of excess water or moisture. Fix leaky plumbing and get rid of any standing water in your basement. If the basement or any other room has been flooded, use the bleach-and-water solution to clean walls and other water-damaged items immediately. You'll probably have to replace carpeting, ceiling tiles, insulation, and wallboard.

Here's why: Mold: It's alive, it's unpleasant, and sometimes, it's toxic.

There are more than 100,000 species of mold. The spores can waft into your house through open windows and heating, ventilation, and air conditioning systems. They can even attach to people and animals, turning your shoes or pets into mold-delivery systems.

Mold loves moisture, and it thrives in areas where leakage or flooding has occurred. Many building materials (including ceiling tiles, wood and wood products, insulation materials, and drywall) provide nutrients that encourage its growth.

Common molds such as cladosporium, penicillium, aspergillus, and alternaria don't pose a danger to healthy people. However, a few dozen molds are toxic and are associated with health problems. One of these is *Stachybotrys chartarum*. This greenish-black mold produces chemicals (mycotoxins) that can cause allergic reactions, asthma, rashes, respi-

ratory complaints, seizures, memory loss, and severe fatigue. According to the CDC, it's not necessary to clean *Stachybotrys chartarum* any differently than you would other molds.

In the past 15 years, toxic mold has become a significant health problem. "Sick building syndrome," the result of indoor air contamination from the stachybotrys and penicillium molds, has forced office buildings and schools to close because workers and students got sick. In 2002, Johnny Carson's former sidekick, Ed McMahon, sued his insurance company for $20 million, claiming that toxic mold in his Los Angeles home killed his dog. Some mold experts have linked stachybotrys to the deaths of some infants from a fatal lung condition, pulmonary hemosiderosis, but the CDC says the link hasn't been proven.

STEP 19: BANISH MILDEW ALONG WITH MOLD

Three natural ingredients work very well for killing mildew and will also work well on mold. The most successful is Australian tea tree oil, a broad-spectrum fungicide. Some people find the smell too strong for their liking, but the smell from the formula on page 406 does dissipate after a few days. Another killer, and a material that doesn't smell, is grapefruit seed extract. The third material that works well is borax, but it isn't as successful as the first two. None of these materials are practical for big jobs, and the mold and mildew will just return unless the source of moisture feeding the mold is removed. Make sure to spot test when using any of these formulas, especially on material that isn't inert, such as fabric. Make sure you have adequate ventilation in enclosed places such as a shower stall. For the formulas and instructions on using these cleaning solutions, see "Mold and Mildew Busters" on page 406.

Here's why: If you have mildew in your home, you probably also have mold. The same damp conditions provide ideal living conditions for both. While mildew just smells bad, many different mold species are toxic. And many people are allergic to mold spores.

STEP 20: HAVE YOUR HOME TESTED FOR RADON

If radon is a problem in your area, contact your state to have your home tested and to find a contractor certified in radon remediation.

Here's why: It is critical to your health to have your home tested. Radon is an odorless gas that seeps up from the soil and can cause lung cancer.

STEP 21: PAY ATTENTION TO CARBON MONOXIDE

Don't forget to install carbon monoxide detectors along with fire detectors. If you heat your house with gas, oil, or some other fuel, make sure you have a detector installed.

Here's why: Carbon monoxide is a poisonous, completely odorless gas given off by faulty heating systems. If you have a carbon monoxide problem in your house, it could cause headaches and fatigue. Having an alarm that detects carbon monoxide can even save your life if your furnace malfunctions and this gas seeps into your living quarters. Without an alarm, you could be dead before the problem is discovered.

STEP 22: PROTECT YOURSELF FROM FORMALDEHYDE

Many modern kitchen cabinets are made of a plastic laminate applied over pressed wood, particleboard, or plywood that could be outgasing formaldehyde. What do you need to do about it? The answer

Mold and Mildew Busters

KEEPING YOUR HOME FREE OF MOLD AND MILDEW IS CRUCIAL in the fight against toxins that compromise your health. Here are some effective, natural cleaning solutions.

Tea Tree Mold and Mildew Killer

> 2 teaspoons tea tree oil (available in
>   health food stores)
> 2 cups water

Combine the oil and water in a spray bottle and spray this formula on the object you need to clean. (Make sure to spot test first.) Don't rinse. The smell will dissipate in a few days, as will the smell of mold and mildew. After the smell of the tea tree oil is gone, clean off the mold stain, if present.

Grapefruit Seed Extract Mold Killer

> 2 teaspoons grapefruit seed extract
>   (available in health food stores)
> 1 cup water

Combine the extract and water in a spray bottle and spray this formula on the object you need to clean. (Make sure to spot test first.) Don't rinse.

Basic Borax Deodorizer

> 2 cups borax
> Enough water to make a thick paste

Note: This formula takes a lot of rinsing and should be used only on materials that can handle water.

Scoop the paste onto a sponge and scrub onto the mold or mildew. The key is to let the dry mineral set on the object (be it a wall or tile grout) until it is fully dry. Then vacuum up as much of the residue as is possible, and rinse to remove what remains.

to that question depends on how old your cabinets are. The amount of formaldehyde outgased from cabinets diminishes over time, and after 10 years or so the amount may be minimal. If the cabinets are older than 10 years, you can simply leave them be.

Another factor to consider is where the

cabinets are located. Formaldehyde out-gases more when it is heated up, such as when the sun shines on the cabinets, or if a cabinet is next to a stove and warms when the stove is on. You need to be more concerned about cabinets that are regularly exposed to heat.

Cabinets that may be outgasing formaldehyde can be sealed thoroughly with a specially designed sealer that blocks formaldehyde. The American Formulating and Manufacturing Association (AFMA) manufactures sealants for toxic materials such as formaldehyde and carpets. (They also make safe paints, stains, and cleaning products designed for those sensitive to chemicals.) They can be contacted at:

AFMA, 350 West Ash Street, Suite 700, San Diego, CA 92101; (619) 239-0321 or (800) 239-0321; www.afmsafecoat.com.

Here's why: Formaldehyde is not only a suspected carcinogen, but it's also a substance that can sensitize you to a number of potential allergens.

Step 23: Throw Away Disinfectant Sponges

If your current sponges exude a distinctive disinfectant smell, throw them out and search for a source of sponges made of pure cellulose. Buy only pure cellulose sponges and avoid sponges in packages that use language such as "kills odors." Finding sponges without disinfectants in supermarkets has become increasingly more difficult, but hardware stores usually sell pure cellulose sponges.

You can sterilize sponges by boiling them in a pan of water for 3 to 5 minutes or by placing them in your automatic dishwasher whenever you do a load of dishes.

Concerned that you'll be losing all the disinfectant power in those chemical sponges? Don't be! It's simply impossible to sterilize your kitchen using a sponge impregnated with disinfectants.

Instead, follow good handling practices with meat (cut it on plates that can be washed with soap and hot water or in the dishwasher), and keep your kitchen clean using soap and water.

Here's why: Almost every sponge now sold in U.S. supermarkets is impregnated with a synthetic disinfectant—usually triclosan—that has been registered as a pesticide with the Environmental Protection Agency (EPA). Common disinfectants may contribute to drug-resistant bacteria, just as antibiotics do. Out of concern for the environment, Scotland has banned triclosan from their stores!

But that's not the only reason to avoid

triclosan. This chemical is possibly toxic to both the skin and the immune system. It is more hazardous than most chemicals in an EPA ranking system of chemicals that are hazardous to aquatic systems. The jury may still be out on just how serious it is to come in daily contact with triclosan, but why chance it when you don't have to?

STEP 24: USE CAUTION WITH GAS STOVES

If it's possible for you to switch to an electric range, consider doing so. If you must cook with gas, make sure that your kitchen is vented and that your stove has an automatic pilot. Automatic pilots have an automatic shutoff valve that turns the system off if the pilot light goes out. Those without automatic pilots allow gas to leak when the pilot light goes out.

Here's why: Studies have shown that being in a kitchen with a gas stove provided the highest concentrations of nitrogen dioxide (NO_2) that a person who worked outside the home was exposed to all day, including during their commute.

NO_2 is a cardiovascular, developmental, reproductive, respiratory, and endocrine toxicant. It is also a suspected immunotoxicant and neurotoxicant. It is more hazardous than most chemicals listed in five government and academic ratings.

As if that wasn't bad enough, some mostly rural gas companies in the United States add a toxic additive to gas, usually mercaptan or a similar sulfur-based compound. Its strong odor is meant to serve as a means of letting people know when there is a gas leak. Breathing this additive is dangerous to your health.

STEP 25: DON'T HEAT COOKING OILS TO THEIR SMOKE POINT

The ideal way to reduce smoke from burning cooking oils is to choose your oils carefully, cooking with oils that can handle high heat without smoking. For example, refined avocado oil can be heated to just under 500°F before smoking, while unrefined safflower oil will smoke when heated to just under 225°F. The smoke point for unrefined olive oil is 325°F. Contact the manufacturer of the brand of oil you use to find out its smoke point.

Also, a kitchen stove hood or vent is a very good way to help reduce this form of indoor air pollution in your home.

Here's why: Heating cooking oils to their smoke point can cause serious indoor air pollution. There is simply no reason to expose yourself and your family to these toxic particles when there are such easy alternatives.

STEP 26: DON'T CONSUME ARTIFICIAL FOOD COLORING

Read product labels and avoid any product that contains artificial colors. And don't let up on your vigilance when you're doing creative baking, either. You can make your own food dyes easily using the natural dyes from foods. The rule of thumb is that any food that will stain your clothes should work really well as a food dye: blueberries, beets, cranberries, turmeric, or even tea!

When making colored cake or cookie frosting, or dough, for example, substitute a tablespoon or two of berry juice for the few drops of food dye, and reduce the liquid required by the same amount. You can use turmeric powder for yellow without changing the liquid amounts in the recipe.

Here's why: Doctors from the University of Southampton in the United Kingdom have found in their research that food additives such as artificial dyes have a significant impact on the behavior of ordinary children and boost levels of hyperactivity. The doctors urgently recommend that these additives be removed from children's diets.

STEP 27: GET THE LEAD OUT OF YOUR DISHES

Test any china that you use on a regular basis. Do-it-yourself lead tests are readily available; you can find one through a simple Internet search. Test results are available within minutes of swabbing the china.

When purchasing new dishes, look for white china, stoneware, china without any added decorations, or china labeled as lead-free. Also, avoid drinking anything stored in crystal decanters. (It is not uncommon for people to store brandy and other liquors in crystal decanters.) Glass crystal contains lead, and liquid, especially acidic liquid, leaches lead from the glass and into the fluid.

Three rules of thumb to follow to avoid lead exposure from suspect utensils and dishes:

1. Do not store food and beverages in them for longer than an hour or so.
2. Never store acidic foods in them, as the acid will help facilitate the lead leaching into the food. Acidic foods include wine, salad dressings, tea, dairy products, and tomato sauces.
3. Never heat food in questionable china.

Here's why: Lead is so toxic that you should protect yourself and your family from unnecessary exposure in any way possible. Lead is highly neurotoxic, a suspected carcinogen, and it is toxic to the blood system and kidneys. Any amount of lead is unsafe for children, pregnant women, and nursing mothers.

STEP 28: DON'T STORE OR HEAT FOOD IN PLASTIC

Never use plastic containers to heat food in a microwave. Never use boil-in-a-bag foods. Avoid storing wet food in plastic.

We all know the flavor of bottled water that has been left in a hot car; it tastes like plastic. If the water tastes like plastic, don't drink it! And particularly avoid storing acidic liquids, such as tea, juice, and wine, in plastic.

Look to plastic recycling classifications to protect yourself. The safest plastics are:

#2—high-density polyethylene (HDPE)
#4—low-density polyethylene (LDPE)
#5—polystyrene (PS)

Note that #7, polycarbonate, should be avoided even though commercial sports water bottles are commonly made of it. To find out whether your containers are made of one of the safer plastics, check the bottom of the water bottle or container and look for the number inside the recycling symbol.

The best choices for storing food and drink? Stainless steel thermoses (for bottled water to go) and glass.

Here's why: Many plastics leach the hormone-disrupting chemicals phthalates and Bisphenol-A, which in turn migrate into food that comes into contact with it. Plastic especially migrates into hot, fatty foods, such as packaged cheese that has been left in the sun. Ingesting these chemicals can cause disruption of the hormonal systems of your body and affect the thyroid and reproductive systems.

STEP 29: PROTECT YOUR HANDS WHEN DOING DISHES

Switch to a "green" brand of dish detergent that doesn't have synthetic fragrances and other added chemicals. Or you can simply wear gloves whenever you wash dishes.

Here's why: Your skin is a major organ of protection. It many cases, it's all that stands between you and exposure to toxic chemicals. Many chemicals can be absorbed right through your skin. That's something to think about whenever you plunge your hands into a chemical on a regular basis, as you do whenever you clean up just a few dishes.

STEP 30: TOSS THE AIR FRESHENERS IN THE TRASH

You can easily sweeten the smell of a bathroom by making or buying a natural potpourri or by placing a few drops of your favorite essential oil in a bowl of water to evaporate.

Here's a great recipe for a natural potpourri.

Rose Potpourri

5 cups rose petals*

1 cup lavender stems

¼ cup orrisroot, powdered

4 bay leaves, broken

1 cup sea salt

⅛ to ¼ cup allspice, crushed

¼ cup broken cinnamon sticks

¼ cup broken cloves

Combine the rose petals and lavender stems with the orrisroot powder. Add the bay leaves, salt, allspice, cinnamon, and cloves and stir. Place the potpourri in an open bowl or a bowl with a top that you can remove whenever you want to scent the room.

Some people sprinkle the potpourri with brandy every few months to refresh the scent. If you choose to do this,

*A store that sells supplies for herbalists can provide bulk rose petals, lavender, and orrisroot. The other ingredients can be found at health food stores.

simply stir a few drops of brandy into the mixture.

Here's why: Commercial air fresheners might smell good, but they are notoriously toxic. It isn't uncommon to read on the label that the product is banned in California because it is thought to cause cancer. Researchers at the EPA note that plug-in air fresheners can react with ozone on smoggy days to synergistically generate formaldehyde and other VOCs.

STEP 31: PUT THE LID ON ARTIFICIAL FRAGRANCES AND PERFUMES

Naturally scented personal care products are readily available in health food stores, but not all such products use natural scents, so you need to read labels. Look for products that state that the source of the fragrance is an essential oil, or product labels that name the specific oil, such as "honeysuckle oil." If you are sensitive to essential oils, look for fragrance-free brands.

And whenever possible, buy scent-free products, such as detergents. Let's face it, there is simply no good reason to add scent to your clothes when they're drying or to have scented toilet paper hanging in your bathroom.

Here's why: Synthetic fragrances are complex mixtures of solvents, aroma chemicals, possibly natural essential oils, and alcohol. They are found in every type of personal care product available and also in tissues, toilet paper, and even garbage bags. Up to 600 ingredients may be used for any one fragrance. Toluene, which the EPA detected in every fragrance sample collected in 1991, may be a toxic VOC. The Food and Drug Administration (FDA) reports that fragrances are responsible for 30 percent of all reactions to cosmetics.

STEP 32: COLOR YOUR HAIR WITH CARE

Switch to demi-permanent or semi-permanent dyes. And consider using pure vegetable products. Their colors are very natural looking. The added bonus is that the products condition your hair while coloring it.

Here's why: If you use permanent hair dyes at least once a month, you have twice the risk of bladder cancer, according to a 2001 study from researchers at the University of Southern California. You have three times the risk if you have used permanent hair dyes for 15 years at least once a month. The concern is a family of chemicals known as arylamines, which are found in many hair dyes. Darker hair dyes come with a higher risk because of the increased number of chemicals.

STEP 33: DON'T USE LINDANE FOR HEAD LICE

If you have kids, the likelihood is that at least once in their lives they'll bring home a crop of head lice. And if you have close contact with the public as part of your work, you might even catch them yourself. The usual product recommended for banishing lice is lindane.

Safer alternatives to lindane include combing the hair carefully with a nit comb and then washing the hair with an olive oil castile soap. Add a few drops of tea tree or lavender essential oils to the rinse water. (Make sure the individual isn't allergic to the oils, and pregnant women should always consult with their doctors before using essential oils.)

For scabies infections, which are also commonly treated with lindane, apply pure lavender oil to the site that is affected by the scabies every 30 minutes for 4 hours. Repeat for 4 consecutive nights.

Here's why: Don't even think about using lindane. It is a chlorinated hydrocarbon, a xenoestrogenic pesticide that is stored in body fat and is very long-lasting in the environment. This chemical should be avoided, and in the opinion of many doctors of environmental medicine, it should never be used on children.

STEP 34: SEAL YOUR WALL-TO-WALL

The best wall-to-wall carpet to have is either 100 percent pure wool or 100 percent cotton. Even better, replace your wall-to-wall with hardwood floors and cotton or wool throw rugs. Not too many people have the luxury of these options. If you can't replace carpets that are causing health problems (really the best option), then apply a sealant. The American Formulating and Manufacturing Association offers a carpet sealant that works remarkably well. (See contact information on page 407.)

Here's why: Regarding wall-to-wall synthetic carpets, the prevailing wisdom is that the highest potential for carpets to be unhealthy is because of synthetic chemicals from two sources. The first comes from carpets that have been glued down. The glues give off neurotoxic VOCs. The second major problem comes from those that have a backing

made of styrene-butadiene-rubber latex, which gives off VOCs.

Unfortunately, the potential health risks don't end there. Other problems associated with carpeting come from stain repellents and biocides. Carpets also serve as a home for dirt, dust mites, molds, and pesticide residues.

STEP 35: REPLACE POLYURETHANE FOAM CUSHIONS

Ideally, cushions should be stuffed with cotton or wool batting. Polyester fill is your next best option. Have the stuffing in your cushions replaced.

Here's why: Polyurethane foam outgases a wide range of neurotoxic chemicals, as do toxic fire retardants.

STEP 36: COVER YOUR MATTRESS

Replace your mattress with organic cotton, wool, or natural latex, or cover the mattress with a cotton barrier cloth. Wool is naturally fire-resistant and is not chemically treated, although most sheep are regularly dipped with pesticides to control parasites, so you must specify organic wool if you want a truly pure mattress.

Encasing your mattress will help reduce your exposure to mattress emissions and protect against small allergen particles, including dust mites and animal allergens. The cloth won't completely eliminate exposure, but it will reduce it. Don't use plastic, however. Plastic will outgas chemicals. A natural cotton barrier cloth is much preferable. Do a search on the Internet to find a mail-order provider for a cotton barrier cloth.

Here's why: Standard mattresses can contain fire retardants, pesticides, stain protectors, and other toxic chemicals. Polyurethane foam mattresses are even worse. Those outgas neurotoxic chemicals, usually including the fire retardants polybrominated diphenyl ethers (PBDEs). PBDEs are, like their cousins PCBs, long-lasting in the environment, and they accumulate in people's fat. Nationwide tests by The Environmental Working Group (EWG) found "record levels" of PBDEs in the breast milk of American mothers in 2003.

STEP 37: NEVER USE MOTHBALLS

Use herbal sachets to repel moths. Look for sachets made with the traditional weaver's herbs rosemary, mint, thyme, and cloves.

Clean all your woolens thoroughly be-fore storing them. If you do discover moths, place the clothes in the freezer for 2 days.

Here's why: The Environmental Protection Agency requires that mothballs, made from paradichlorobenzene, carry a label warning users to "avoid breathing the fumes." Have you ever had mothballs around that you *couldn't* smell? Their odor is insidious and so pervasive that after a while you can't smell them any more. They're also seriously toxic.

STEP 38: DON'T USE OIL-BASED PAINTS

Low-VOC latex paint is a much better choice, or better yet, a low-VOC paint without biocides. These are hard to find, but worth an Internet search. All exterior paints have fungicides, and stains have even greater amounts of fungicides. The best choice for an exterior paint is a water-based paint that has zinc oxide as the fungicide.

Sources of safer paints include NEEDS (www.needs.com) and The Environmental Home Center (www.environmentalhomecenter.com). Both companies are experienced in the field of nontoxic building supplies and offer the best products available.

Here's why: Believe it or not, most

paints contain pesticides to prevent mildew growth. These pesticides can be detected up to 5 years after the paint has been applied. Oil-based paints are very high in VOCs, and the petroleum solvents are neurotoxic.

STEP 39: CHASE FLEAS WITH ORANGE

Citrus peel extract is an excellent weapon to use against fleas on dogs, because its components—d-limonene and linalool—kill all stages of the flea's life cycle.

D-limonene, although natural, is a VOC, so don't use it if someone in your family has asthma. It shouldn't be used around cats, either. However, assuming you don't own a cat and you keep your windows open when applying the d-limonene, you can rid your house of fleas by:

- Washing the floors a couple of times a week with a solution of ¼ cup citrus peel extract (available in health food stores) in 1 to 2 gallons of water.
- Spraying bedding with a mixture of 2 teaspoons citrus peel extract and 2 cups of water. (Use a spray bottle.)
- Washing your dog with an orange-based shampoo.

You can also try mixing a little garlic and brewer's yeast into your pet's food;

the ingredients make your pet's flavor unappetizing to pests.

A good herbal repellent for fleas on cats is a tea made from rosemary or sage. Just put 1 teaspoon of the spice, taken right out of your spice rack, in a cup. Pour a cup of boiling water over it and let it steep until cool. Strain, then rub the liquid into your cat's fur. (Start by doing just a small patch of fur to make sure Kitty can tolerate the herb.)

Here's why: Your pets come in contact with almost everything in your house, including you and your family. Keeping them free of both pests and potent chemicals should be a priority.

STEP 40: CLEAN UP YOUR HEAT SOURCE

If you heat with wood, make sure to use the most modern, efficient woodstove you can find. Avoid gas and kerosene space heaters at all costs, and make sure gas heating systems are running efficiently.

If you have forced hot air heating, make sure that you have the ducts professionally cleaned on a regular basis. If you have an oil burner, make certain that it is well ventilated. And for any of these heating sources, consider having high-performance air filters installed in your home. These include electrostatic air cleaners, pleated media filters, and electronic air cleaners.

Here's why: An EPA study concluded that breathing wood smoke particles outdoors on days of high pollution is equivalent to smoking 4 to 16 cigarettes a day. Imagine how much worse the problem can be indoors if your fireplace or woodstove is not properly vented.

STEP 41: PROTECT YOUR FAMILY FROM ARSENIC-TREATED LUMBER

Do you have treated lumber in your yard or garden, or on your deck? For that matter, has treated lumber been used in your local playground? Then you should be aware that wood that has been pressure-treated with chromated copper arsenate (CCA) results in wood impregnated with 22 percent pure arsenic.

The Consumer Product Safety Commission is working on a sealant for CCA. At the time of this printing, the sealant hasn't yet been developed. Until the sealant and details about how to handle existing CCA are available, you need to use common sense. Don't grow vegetables in flowerbeds made of CCA-treated wood. Be aware that CCA can leach into the soil near treated wood. If you have arsenic-treated wood anywhere near your vegetable garden, it is especially important to have your soil tested. Call your county's agricultural extension service for suggestions. Growing flowers in this soil is fine, as long as you don't intend to ingest any part of them.

If you have a well and have pressure-treated lumber, test your water for arsenic, since it may have leached into it from the yard.

If you can remove the CCA-treated wood, do so if it is possible without causing wood dust. Instead, use recycled plastic lumber or sustainably grown, naturally rot-resistant wood.

Here's why: Arsenic is a known carcinogen of the lung and bladder. Children are very vulnerable, particularly because backyard play sets were almost exclusively made with CCA for years. Children touch the wood and absorb the arsenic when they put their hands in their mouths. Arsenic can also leach from outdoor structures into wells, contaminating drinking water.

STEP 42: REPEL INSECTS WITH ESSENTIAL OILS

Here's a recipe for repelling a wide variety of insect pests without chemical pesticides. (Pregnant women should consult with their doctors before trying essential oil repellents.)

Insect Repellent Base

10 to 25 drops essential oil (see recommended oils, below)

2 tablespoons vegetable oil or olive oil

1 tablespoon aloe vera gel (optional)

Combine the essential oil, vegetable or olive oil, and aloe vera gel (if using) in a glass jar. Shake to blend. Dab a few drops on your skin or clothing. This easy-to-make repellent has a shelf life of around 6 months. If you make multiple varieties, label the jars "mosquito," "tick," and so on, for quick identification.

Mosquitoes: Try citronella, thyme, or lavender oils, alone or in any combination. (Since mosquitoes breed in stagnant water, make sure you empty all containers, such as bird baths and old tires.)

Blackflies: Try lavender, eucalyptus, pennyroyal, cedar, citronella, or peppermint oils, alone or in any combination.

Ticks: Rose geranium is the essential oil of choice. (To protect your dog, put just one drop of oil on her collar; avoid using on cats.)

Here's why: There is no need to expose your skin to the neurotoxic chemicals in commercial-grade insect repellents when these natural alternatives work just as well.

STEP 43: DON'T SWEAT THE SMALL STUFF (OR THE BIG STUFF)

You can't escape stress any more than you can escape your own shadow. But how do you handle those traffic jams, your demanding boss, the spats with your partner or kids? Do you let them roll off your back, or do you let them poison your heart with frustration, anxiety, anger, and depression?

Practice some form of stress control every day, says Phoebe Yin, N.D., a naturopathic physician at the Bastyr Center for Natural Health in Seattle. You'll find many relaxation techniques in chapter 8 (see page 161), including positive thinking, affirmations, prayer, meditation, and even ancient purification rituals that you can use to battle 21st-century stresses.

Or try "moving meditation," such as yoga or tai chi. Both incorporate breathing, movement, and posture to achieve a union of mind, body, and spirit. People who practice these ancient forms of movement say that they achieve a deep feeling of tranquility.

You could also try walking meditation,

which is just what it sounds like—combining a walk with quiet reflection. While you can practice it anywhere, even a city sidewalk, it's best in a peaceful setting, such as a quiet path in your local park. Don't focus on a destination; with walking meditation, it's the journey that counts. The key is to focus on the mini-movements that make up the act of walking. For example, as you lift each foot, silently say, "lifting." As you move your leg forward, say, "moving." Then, as you place your foot on the ground, say, "placing." Repeat these words silently as you walk (or use other words, if you like).

Here's why: Learning to let go of these negative emotions can help clear your mind, which will in turn have a positive effect on your physical health, says Dr. Yin. Think of your capacity to deal with stress in terms of a bucket. There's only so much a bucket can hold, right? While you can't empty your bucket completely—there's no such thing as no stress—you can learn to keep it from overflowing.

STEP 44: BECOME AN ACTIVIST

Visit the Web site www.scorecard.org, put in your zip code, and you will be given a list of all the industrial polluters in your vicinity. Armed with this information, you can then work locally with other citizens to protect yourselves.

Another important step is to establish your neighborhood as a pesticide-free zone. Try formally contacting everybody in your neighborhood and asking for compliance. There are sometimes one or two families that are holdouts for chemical lawn care, but the majority are generally delighted to unite to protect their kids, pets, and wells.

Here's why: It is amazing what even one person's complaints can do to change the course of events.

STEP 45: FOLLOW THE PURIFICATION PLAN

We've introduced you to a number of the best detoxification and purification methods that medical science and the healing arts have to offer. Following the advice of the leading doctors and healing practitioners in this book will not only make a measurable impact on the current levels of toxins in your body, but will also keep you on the path of purification. While some of the methods, such as herbs, spa treatments, and fasting and cleansing may have been new to you, others such as diet, exercise, and stress reduction have long been recognized as the mainstays of healthy lifestyles. But now you can practice them with an eye toward their detoxifying effect.

For example, if you want your body to stay healthy, start by eating clean, says Peter Bennett, N.D., a naturopathic physician in Vancouver and coauthor of *7-Day Detox Miracle.* "Diet has a strong effect on the liver's detoxification enzymes," he says. "Eating foods that support the liver can reduce your susceptibility to damage from toxins." That means loading your plate with vegetables, fruits, beans, nuts and seeds, and whole grains.

You also need to keep moving. "Regular exercise helps the body's purification organs to do their work," says Phoebe Yin, N.D., a naturopathic physician at the Bastyr Center for Natural Health in Seattle.

Most health experts advise that we engage in moderate exercise at least 30 minutes a day, most or all days of the week. Brisk walking, cycling, jogging, and swimming all fit the bill. You might also consider rebounding—jumping on a mini-trampoline, says Dr. Bennett. Rebounding delivers a great cardiovascular workout and also improves circulation of the lymphatic system, a part of the immune system. Yoga may be particularly effective in eliminating the effect of toxic emotions. In one study, people who took a 60-minute yoga class once a week scored lower on anger tests than those who didn't.

Here's why: In today's world, practicing a healthy lifestyle must include a healthy diet, adequate exercise, and choosing from the full array of detoxification methods offered to you in the techniques described in this book.

Index

Underscored page references indicate boxed text. **Boldface** references indicate photographs.

F

T

U

V

W

X

Y

Z